# Wheeling and Dealing

# Wheeling and Dealing

## Living with Spinal Cord Injury

Esther Isabelle Wilder

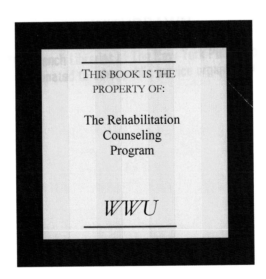

Vanderbilt University Press
NASHVILLE

This book is the recipient of the 2004 Norman L. and Roselea J. Goldberg Prize
from Vanderbilt University Press for the best project in the area of medicine.

Designed by Wendy McAnally

Library of Congress Cataloging-in-Publication Data

Wilder, Esther I.
Wheeling and dealing : living with spinal cord injury / Esther Isabelle Wilder.
p. ; cm.
Includes bibliographical references.
ISBN-13: 978-0-8265-1534-6 (cloth : alk. paper)
ISBN-10: 0-8265-1534-7 (cloth : alk. paper)
ISBN-13: 978-0-8265-1535-3 (pbk. : alk. paper)
ISBN-10: 0-8265-1535-5 (pbk. : alk. paper)
1. Spinal cord—Wounds and injuries—Case studies.
2. Spinal cord—Wounds and injuries—Psychological aspects—Case studies.
3. Spinal cord—Wounds and injuries—Social aspects—Case studies.
4. Paralytics—Rehabilitation—Case studies.
[DNLM: 1. Spinal Cord Injuries—psychology—Case Reports.
2. Disabled Persons—psychology—Case Reports.
3. Disabled Persons—rehabilitation—Case Reports.
4. Models, Psychological—Case Reports.
5. Socioeconomic Factors—Case Reports.
6. Spinal Cord Injuries—rehabilitation—Case Reports.
WL 400 W564w 2006] I. Title.
RD594.3.W532 2006
617.4'82044—dc22
2005035363

To William H. Walters

# Contents

# Acknowledgments

There are many people whose kindness and support have made this book possible. I am especially grateful to the study participants, who welcomed me into their homes and shared their life stories with me. Their warmth and willingness to discuss a wide range of issues gave me a compelling mission to tell their stories. I am also grateful to Jeffrey Henderson, who inspired me to investigate the lives of individuals living with spinal cord injury.

I have received strong institutional support for this project from a variety of sources. In particular, funding for this research has been provided by the People's Staff Congress of the City University of New York and by the George N. Shuster Foundation at Lehman College. The Lehman College administration and the staff in the Office of Grants and Contracts have provided strong support for the preparation of the manuscript.

I feel indebted to my students at Lehman College, whose passion for knowledge and interest in my scholarship continually remind me of how fortunate I am to teach at the City University of New York. My colleagues in the Department of Sociology and Social Work at Lehman College and in the Sociology Program of the CUNY Graduate Center have also enthusiastically supported this project. The library staff at Lehman College, especially Gene Laper, have gone well beyond the call of duty in helping me track down information.

I thank Michael Ames, my editor at Vanderbilt University Press, and the other editorial and production staff for their commitment and expertise. William H. Walters has provided advice and loving encouragement throughout this project, and his editorial skills have been invaluable. I am also grateful to Dick and Annie Bower for their meticulous preparation of the index.

This book would not have been possible without the loving support of my family. In particular, I thank Teresa Wilder, Martin Wilder, Elizabeth Wilder, Kenneth Wilder, Edythe Erdman, Robert Erdman, and Elizabeth McGhee. I am especially grateful to Saam Trivedi for his unwavering love and affection. As always, my colleagues and friends have provided kind encouragement and support.

# 1
# Introduction

Travis is a 29-year-old history student at Flagship University. He is 6′3″ and has fair skin, a shaved head, and a blondish-brown goatee. He has a broad build and is somewhat overweight. Travis has something to say about almost every issue, ranging from national politics to the Israeli-Palestinian conflict. When he isn't busy with school, Travis spends time at the mall with his fiancée, Mary, and plays with his black poodle, Sadie. According to Travis, Sadie is "extremely hyper and requires a great deal of attention—at least she thinks she does."

As I spoke with Travis, Sadie ran around the room and jumped on both of us. Travis is paralyzed from the nipple down and has limited mobility. He sustained a spinal cord injury 15 years ago in a motorcycle accident at the age of 14. Travis described his life before the injury:

> My whole concept in life was I was going to play pro ball. That was my thing. I wanted to be famous. I was so arrogant I used to sit and practice my signature because I knew that all the great players had footballs with their names on them and I wanted my signature to look really cool.

Travis feels that the injury changed his outlook on life. "I think it's probably made me a little bit more intelligent because I've relied on my intelligence more than I probably would have otherwise." He plans to go to law school, and he views his situation in both negative and positive terms:

> At times it's a pain in the ass—literally and figuratively. But at times it has allowed me to be a better person. It allows me to look at things

differently and not be as threatening to some people where I can have interaction with them that I maybe wouldn't if I was still an athlete. Because a lot of times male interaction is done on the basis of pissing contests: "I'm bigger, I'm tougher, I'm stronger, I'm smarter." When you're in a chair they don't look at you like that.

At the same time, Travis feels that many people don't know how to interact with him. "People are so uncomfortable they don't know how to deal with me, and I would rather you make a mistake and deal with me than not deal with me at all."

## Biomedical and Social Models of Disability

Although spinal cord injury (SCI) can lead to personal, intellectual, and spiritual growth, it also brings major physical and social challenges. This book describes the experiences of 32 individuals with spinal cord damage—men and women who became paralyzed as a result of car accidents, gunshot wounds, sports injuries, or underlying physiological conditions. It explores how the physical and social changes associated with spinal cord injury influence economic well-being, employment patterns, family and friendship networks, intimate relationships, religious beliefs, and ideological perspectives. For those who have been recently injured, this book provides a roadmap for what lies ahead. That is, it tells the stories of those who have already taken the journey. While each individual is unique, the common physical and social responses to spinal cord injury represent shared concerns, challenges, struggles, triumphs, and hopes.

Historically, the study of disability has been grounded in the biomedical model—the view that disability is chiefly or solely a medical problem. This approach, dominant since the early twentieth century, focuses on pathology, diagnosis, impairment or functional limitation, and remedial action (Barnes, Mercer, and Shakespeare 1999; Hahn 1994). It treats human variation as deviance from the norm and regards disability in individual terms as a deficit, a personal burden, and a tragedy (Linton 1998). Both the causes and manifestations of disability are thought to be primarily internal. Thus, the remedies for illness are those procedures designed to restore normal function with regard to the individual's physical, mental, or emotional health (Hahn 1994). The definition of disability as a medical problem also "presumes a corresponding solution and so encourages the domination of disabled people's lives by a vast army of allied professionals" (Barnes, Mercer, and Shakespeare 1999: 25).

By the 1970s and 1980s, disability activists were increasingly critical of the biomedical model. Linton (1998: 11) summarizes the limitations of the biomedical approach:

> Society, in agreeing to assign medical meaning to disability, colludes to keep the issue within the purview of the medical establishment, to keep it a personal matter and "treat" the condition rather than "treating" the social processes and policies that constrict disabled people's lives.

Consequently, many disability activists have tried to dispel the stigma associated with disability by viewing deviations from the norm in nonmedical terms (Albrecht 1992; Anspach 1979). While the social approach to disability gained prominence in the post-civil rights era, evidence of this perspective can be seen as early as 1948, when Myerson (1948: 111) wrote that the "psychologically disabling effects of physical disability rest upon the highly negative values assigned to certain atypical physiques in our culture. It is predominantly a social phenomenon and can be remedied by social action."

Recent perspectives on disability have therefore emphasized disabling environments and hostile social attitudes, and scholars and activists have increasingly argued in favor of policies that locate the causes of disability within society itself rather than within individual impairments.[1] Many British authors have examined disability within the context of political power, social relations, and material factors, and some have suggested that disability and dependence are an outgrowth of industrial capitalism (Abberley 1987; Barnes 1996; Finkelstein 1980; Oliver 1990, 1993a, 1993c, 1996c).[2] The predominant view in the United States has focused more broadly on the cultural and historical factors that influence the definition and experience of disability (Marks 1999; Shakespeare 1998). Most of the relevant theoretical work has been rooted in structural functionalism and deviance theory, and the social construction of disability has been characterized as an inevitable outcome of the evolution of contemporary societies (Barnes 1998). For example, Stone (1984) contends that capitalist development is linked to rationalization and bureaucratization—that "disability" has been used as a distributive category that relegates people to either work-based or needs-based systems of commodity distribution. In a related line of research, Hahn (1988b) shows that two critical values of twentieth-century Western society—personal appearance and individual autonomy—have a major impact on the treatment of disabled individuals. Specifically, those who fail to meet prescribed standards of physical attractiveness and functional independence are stigmatized as biologically inferior. Our definitions of disability, and our responses to it, are therefore based on "a vocabulary of acknowledgement and modification" that implies "what should be" (Kroll-Smith 1994: 5).

Criticism of the medical model has also led to an increased emphasis on community-based services and social welfare programs (Finkelstein 1993). The independent living movement has attempted to demedicalize disability by arguing that the problems of those with severe disabilities are embedded in a physical and cultural environment that incorporates the social control mechanisms of society at large (DeJong 1979, 1983). The disability rights movement in the United States has emphasized the minority status of individuals with disabilities as well as their consumer rights and cultural differences (Fine and Asch 1988a, 1998b; Gliedman and Roth 1980; Hahn 1986, 1988a, 1988b, 1994; Marks 1999; Nagler 1993b; Safilios-Rothschild 1976; Stubbins 1988; Wright 1960). To some extent, the discrimination and social exclusion faced by individuals with disabilities mirror the experiences of other minority groups.[3] While people with disabilities have much in common with other minority-group members (identifiability, differential power, pejorative treatment, etc.), they may be less likely to adopt a minority-group consciousness because environmental and social barriers make transportation and group participation difficult (Fine and Asch 1988a).

In spite of the dominance of the biomedical model, disability has been increasingly viewed through a social lens (Finkelstein 1993).[4] Writing from the United Kingdom, Leach (1996: 88) argues that "the 'social model' and the policies of the disabled people's movement have seemingly replaced the discredited 'medical model' of disability." Even the health care professionals whose autonomy has been challenged by this new approach (physicians, medical technologists, etc.) have adopted certain aspects of the social model of disability (Leach 1996). For example, "the social work task is no longer one of adjusting individuals to personal disasters but rather helping them to locate the personal, social, economic and community resources to enable them to live life to the full" (Oliver 1983: 31). In spite of these efforts, however, "sociologists have never been able to dislodge the primary position of the health professions in efforts to identity and ameliorate disability, and the medical model has remained the core element of traditional approaches to the study of this subject in the social sciences" (Hahn 1994: 11). As a consequence, "powerful metaphors of disease and health dominate our perceptions of disability" (Gliedman and Roth 1980: 301).

Just as the biomedical approach to understanding disability has come under attack, so too has the social model of disability. Several authors have argued that the social model does not fully recognize the physical difficulties associated with impairment (Crow 1996; French 1993a; Morris 1991; Williams 1998). As Wendell (1996: 154) notes, "Many people with disabilities . . . admit that there are often heavy personal burdens associated with the physical and mental consequences of disabling physical conditions . . . that no amount of accessibility and social justice could eliminate." The pain associated with chronic illness and disability can be oppressive (Williams 1998), and an exclusive focus on social factors denies "the personal experience of physical or intellectual restrictions, of illness, of the fear of dying" (Morris 1991: 10).

The social approach has also been criticized for its failure to fully consider the extent of variation in the experience of impairment and disability (Barnes and Mercer 2003).[5] Some disabled individuals—those with learning impairments, for example—may be marginalized within the social model of disability. The experience of disability is often exacerbated by the interaction of disability status with other forms of minority status (Vernon 1998), and some authors contend that other forms of oppression (racism, sexism, and homophobia, for example) have not been fully incorporated into the social model (Oliver 1996a, 1996c). Abberley (1987: 16) argues that while oppressive theories of disability have a tendency to "stereotype the identities of their putative subjects by constituting them only in their 'problem' aspects, the most fashionable but equally unacceptable liberal reaction . . . is to deny all difference," thereby devaluing the authenticity of each person's experience. As a result of these criticisms, a new generation of scholars operating from feminist and postmodern perspectives has begun to focus on the everyday experiences of disabled people (Barnes 1998).

## Research Methods and Sampling

The research described here was undertaken from April 2000 to January 2002. Questionnaires were first administered to 32 individuals with spinal cord injury living in a particular state of the American Heartland. (The Heartland generally refers to the midwestern states, or to those between the Mississippi and the Rockies. The name of the state has been suppressed to protect respondents' anonymity.) Afterward, 31 in-depth interviews of approximately two hours each were conducted in the individuals' homes. Each interview was taped, and I personally transcribed the recordings to protect the participants' confidentiality. Because I was especially interested in social adjustment during the prime reproductive years, I restricted the sample to individuals aged 18 to 55. This restriction also minimized the confounding effects of age.

Study participants were identified through (1) meetings of the local SCI association, (2) an advertisement that ran for several days in the student newspaper of a large public university, and (3) referrals from other partici-pants. Of the thirty-two individuals who completed the survey, sixteen were present at one or more meetings of the SCI association, six responded to the newspaper ad, and ten were contacted through referrals. At the time of the study, all participants lived within a 100-mile radius of a city of half a million people. Twenty-five were originally from the American Heartland, one had been born in India, and the remainder were from non-Heartland states such as New York, Pennsylvania, and Texas (Appendix provides basic information about each participant). Pseudonyms are used for the individu-als I interviewed, and I have occasionally changed physical descriptions, identifying occupational characteristics, and names of places and schools in order to protect the study participants' anonymity.[6]

Much has been written about interviewer effects, and it is important to acknowledge that the interviewer's appearance, presentation, and com-munication style influence the data-gathering process. While I have tried to remain a neutral observer, my own personal characteristics may have influenced the results presented in this book. I am able-bodied, Jewish, and single. At the time of the study, I was from 32 to 34 years old and had long, frizzy hair. (Many people tell me that I look distinctively Jewish.) During the interviews, I usually wore casual clothing, and several of my hosts told me I looked too young to be a professor. In the course of the interviews, some of them asked me personal questions about my age, marital status, and religion. When asked, I provided honest answers to these questions or jokingly asked "who's interviewing whom?" in order to return the focus back to the interviewee. I did sometimes volunteer anecdotal information of a personal nature, however, and I felt that I had befriended many of the participants by the time the interviews were over. The overwhelming majority of study participants had not yet met me when they completed the twelve-page questionnaire that solicited basic demographic information (age, race, religion, living arrangements, etc.) and posed questions about their attitudes on a wide range of topics.[7]

Because the sample was restricted to residents of the American Heartland, the findings presented here do not necessarily apply to the population of all individuals with SCI in the United States. Since it included many students and members of the local SCI association, my sample is also likely to be biased in favor of individuals who have adjusted well to SCI and are more actively engaged in the community. I did not, for instance, interview people residing in nursing homes or independent living centers. (I did learn, however, that at least two of the study participants had moved to nursing homes after their interviews.) Previous research suggests that individuals with the greatest difficulty adjusting to their disabilities tend to remain disengaged and are unlikely to volunteer to participate in these kinds of studies (Chubon, Clayton, and Vandergriff 1995).

The narratives presented here paint a picture of what it means to have a spinal cord injury while living in the American Heartland. Although the central states of the U. S. play a major role in defining the nation's social and political landscape, this region is conspicuously absent in the literature on disability studies. Heartland residents tend to be politically conservative, with strongly held moral values and a tendency toward religious fundamentalism. In some parts of the study—the discussion of religion and spirituality, in particular—this cultural context is readily apparent. In other sections it is less evident. Overall, however, the study participants were a diverse group whose personal narratives are likely to resonate with many individuals in the Heartland and elsewhere.

## The Language of Disability

In response to considerable debate regarding the language of disability (see, for example, Bury 1979; Haber and Smith 1971; Hamilton 1950; and Wright 1960), the World Health Organization (WHO) developed a typology that distinguishes among the concepts of *impairment, disability,* and *handicap.* According to the WHO's *International Classification of Impairments, Disabilities and Handicaps* (1980: 47), *impairment* can be defined as "any loss or abnormality of psychological, physiological, or anatomical structure of function." Some examples include the loss of a limb, paralysis, loss of vision, or brain damage. In contrast, the WHO initially defined *disability* as "any restriction or lack (resulting from impairment) of ability to perform an activity in the manner or within the range considered normal for a human being" (WHO 1980: 143). *Handicap,* in turn, has been defined as "a disadvantage for a given individual, resulting from an impairment or a disability, that limits or prevents the fulfillment of a role that is normal (depending on the age, sex, and social and cultural factors) for that individual" (WHO 1980: 183).

Although the typology put forward by the World Health Organization in 1980 was favorably received by most social scientists, many disability activists found the term *handicap* objectionable because it implies that the difficulty lies within the individual rather than the physical or social environment (Albrecht 1992) and because of its connections to the potentially degrading role of charities in the lives of disabled people (Oliver 1996c).[8] Critics have also argued that while the 1980 WHO classification was a major advance over previous biomedical approaches to understanding disability, it remained heavily grounded in medical assumptions (Barnes and Mercer 2003; Ingstad and Whyte 1995; Marks 1999). Although the distinction between *disability* and *impairment* is central to the disability rights movement (Hevey 1993; Oliver 1996c), many disability scholars have criticized the 1980 WHO typology for taking the environment for granted and presenting disability as a static state (Barnes and Mercer 2003; Hahn 1994; Oliver 1990). According to the 1980 WHO definition, *impairment* is identified as the cause of both *disability* and *handicap*—a situation that "privileges medical and allied rehabilitation and educational interventions in the treatment of social and economic disadvantages" (Barnes and Mercer 2003: 14).

As a result of extensive criticism from disabled people, disability rights organizations, and medical researchers, the WHO has since revised its classification scheme. As presented in the *International Classification of Functioning, Disability and Health*, the new scheme retains the concept of *impairment* but replaces *disability* and *handicap* with a series of new terms designed to "extend the scope of the classification to allow positive experiences to be described" (WHO 2001: 3). Alternative definitions have also been put forth over the years. In keeping with the idea that disability can be viewed as an oppressive relationship between the social/physical environment and an individual with an impairment (Finkelstein 1980; Oliver 1983, 1990; Stubbins 1998), the Union of the Physically Impaired Against

Segregation (UPIAS) defined *disability* as "something imposed on top of our impairments, by the way we are unnecessarily isolated and excluded from full participation in society" (UPIAS 1976: 3). The definition put forward by Disabled People's International (DPI) contends that disablement has nothing to do with the body—that it results solely from the physical and social barriers that prevent participation in community life (Oliver 1996c). The acceptability and usefulness of these definitions have not yet been established, however.

Throughout this book, I use the term *impairment* to refer to the biomedical condition of spinal cord injury. *Disability* was interpreted by the participants in the study in different ways, but most seemed to view it as encompassing the physiological, psychological, and social manifestations of physical impairment, as well as the consequences of that impairment. I have avoided the terms *handicap* and *handicapping* except in direct quotations and in reference to specialized parking or housing.

Along with definitional concerns, there has been much controversy about the appropriate language to use when discussing individuals with disabilities (see, for example, Linton 1998). Many people in the disabled community, particularly those in the therapeutic professions, have called for *people-first language* (e.g., *individuals with disabilities* rather than *disabled people*) on the grounds that it treats each person first and foremost as an individual and only secondarily as a person with a disability (Blaska 1993; Hadley and Brodwin 1988; Kailes 1985; La Forge 1991; Vash 1981). As Zola (1993: 19) writes, "a 'disabled car' is one which has totally broken down. Could a 'disabled person' be perceived as anything less?" Becker (1978: xv), who herself has a spinal cord injury, writes that she shares in the "collective anger of many spinal cord injured women who labor under the destructive impact of negative labels such as *crippled, handicapped*, and *disabled*." At the same time, the call for people-first language has not been adopted consistently by scholars of disability studies, and references to *disabled individuals, disabled persons*, and simply *the disabled* abound in the literature (La Forge 1991).[9]

More recently, a number of activists and scholars have claimed that people-first language may have the unintended effect of further stigmatizing individuals with disabilities. Vaughn (1997), for example, describes people-first language as an "unholy crusade." While positive pronouns such as "intelligent" generally precede the word *person,* putting disability-related adjectives after *person* emphasizes disability in an "ungainly new way" (Vaughn 1997). Indeed, an overemphasis on putting the person first and the disability second may appear to reinforce the notion that it is bad to have a disability (La Forge 1991). Oliver, who himself has a spinal cord injury, writes,

> It is sometimes argued, often by nondisabled professionals and some disabled people, that *people with disabilities* is the preferred term, for it asserts the value of the person first and the disability then becomes merely an appendage. This liberal and humanist view flies in the face of reality as it is experienced by disabled people themselves who argue that far from being an appendage, disability is an essential part of the self. . . . Consequently, disabled people are demanding acceptance as they are, as disabled people (Oliver 1990: xiii).

Indeed, some individuals with SCI are unhappy with the use of "politically correct" disability terminology (Cole 2004).

To the extent that nondisabled persons maintain distance from individuals with disabilities because they fear offending them or saying the wrong thing (Lenney and Sercombe 2002), the controversy over language may generate further uncertainty and contribute to avoidance. Moreover, the divisive struggle over language may threaten the essential unity of the disability rights movement and detract from the need to address more pressing problems (Wendell 1996; Zola 1993). While it is self-evident that some of the less subtle and more idiomatic terms for disabled person are clearly offensive and hurtful (e.g., *cripple, vegetable, dumb, deformed, retard,* and *gimp*) (Linton 1998), none of the people I interviewed emphasized the importance of people-first language, and all stressed that they had far more pressing concerns. "You can't see the forest through the trees," said Stan, a 50-year-old quadriplegic man. While some of the study participants—most notably the students—were familiar with people-first language, several had never heard of it. At least a few were mildly amused when I attempted to explain it to them. Several stated that language was a nonissue for them. For example, Todd, a 34-year-old quadriplegic man, said, "I don't care what you call me. . . . I call myself all sorts of things: *gimp,* whatever."

In this study I use a variety of terms to refer to individuals with spinal cord injury: *paraplegics, quadriplegics, disabled individuals,* and, of course, *individuals with spinal cord injury.* These expressions were commonly used by my study participants to identify themselves (and others) and were not perceived negatively. Like Waxman (1996), I take the position that disability is a social identity, much like being African American or Latino.

To the extent that expressions such as *disabled individuals* are perceived to be offensive, I believe the problem lies in one's perception of *disabled* as a negative condition.

As Shapiro (1993: 32–33) notes, "disabled people resent words that suggest they are sick, pitiful, childlike, dependent, or objects of admiration—words that . . . convey the imagery of poster children and supercrips." For example, the language of victimization (e.g., "Mr. Smith *suffered* a spinal cord injury") is problematic (Lynch and Thomas 1994). Consequently, I have tried to avoid language that contributes to the victimization or glorification of individuals with physical disabilities. At the same time, I have not consistently avoided the phrase *in a chair* because I feel that *wheelchair user* (the preferred term in the rehabilitation literature) misrepresents the language most often used by my study participants.

Several of the people I interviewed used slang and derogatory terms such as *para*, *quad*, *gimp*, and *crip* to refer to themselves and others. Indeed, the term *cripple* has been revived by some in the disability community—including both disability activists and performers—who refer to each other as *crips* or *cripples* (Linton 1998; Shakespeare 1993). While such terminology is unlikely to become widespread in general usage, the increasing popularity of the term *cripple* "shows that the stigma of disability is being rejected and replaced with pride in being identified as disabled" (Shapiro 1993: 34). Meanwhile, slang terms such as *crip* and *gimp* are generally reserved for exclusive, internal use by the people with particular disabilities (Shapiro 1993). As a consequence, I have avoided using these terms (except in direct quotes) because they are not mine to adopt.

# 2
# Physical Trauma, Social Consequences

I spoke with Kevin the day before his 34th birthday. Kevin lives at home with his parents in a two-story house that has been made wheelchair accessible on the ground level. At the time of the interview, his young niece and nephew were visiting. They climbed up on top of him as he moved around in his wheelchair. We conducted the interview in Kevin's bedroom to avoid being disturbed by the children. His bedroom is a small room with a twin bed, a desk with a computer, and a few Christian posters.

Kevin was injured when he was 18 years old. He'd been at college for just two days and was taking the Labor Day weekend off. He was on his way to go camping with his brother and several friends when he stopped to put gas in his car. "All of a sudden my back started hurting real bad," he said. He stayed at the gas station for five more minutes, but the pain just intensified, so he drove himself to the hospital. Thirty minutes after arriving at the hospital, Kevin was no longer able to move. An aneurysm had ruptured in his neck, causing damage to his spinal cord. As a result, he is a quadriplegic and has no control or movement below his neck.

Kevin has a handsome face and light blond hair, a small potbelly, and very slender arms and legs that show evidence of muscle atrophy from lack of use. He looks somewhat frail and fatigued, and during the interview sweat permeated the back of his shirt. Kevin has a leg bag that collects urine on his left leg, and he uses a sip-and-puff wheelchair for mobility. When he reflected on the ways in which his disability had affected his life, he was especially preoccupied with the biomedical aspects of his impairment—in particular, the chronic back pain:

> Suicide runs through my brain about 40 times a day. . . . [But] I
> pretty much decided against it. I like my little nephews too much. I
> want to see what happens to them when they grow up.

Kevin's problems with chronic pain also limit his work and his social activities:

> I went to college and got my degree. . . . thought I was getting ready
> to start [work], and then I started having all these problems with
> my back and it just got worse ever since. . . . I don't even like going
> places in a van—the way it bumps and stuff; it hurts like hell.

He frequently clashes with his parents, especially his mother, because she "just doesn't understand back pain." Although he feels that going to a chiropractor has helped a little, he isn't optimistic that things will ever improve: "It keeps getting worse and worse." Kevin especially resents how his injury has interfered with his excretory functioning:

> The bowel problem—that really pisses me off and humiliates me. . . .
> Lay me down in the bed, put a suppository in, wait about an hour,
> and get back up. Sit on the shower chair and Mom does that digital
> stimulation, and it pisses me off anybody would have to do it.

In his view, bowel complications are one of the "top three major gripes about being paralyzed." When I asked what the other two were, he mentioned his inability to use his arms ("I used to love to drive like a bat out of hell") and the fact that he could no longer shoot his guns.

## The Demographics of Spinal Cord Injury

More than thirty Americans become paralyzed each day (National Spinal Cord Injury Association n.d.). While the National Spinal Cord Injury Association (2005) estimates that there are between 250,000 and 400,000 Americans with SCI, many scholars cite figures closer to the lower end of this spectrum (see, for example, Lasfargues et al. 1995). The incidence of spinal cord injury ranges from 30 to 50 cases annually per million population (the higher figures usually include deaths prior to arrival at the hospital).[1] As the population has aged, there has been an upward trend in the ages of individuals incurring SCI. From 2000–2003, 40% of spinal cord injuries occurred among persons ages 16 to 30 years old, and 27% were to individuals ages 31 to 45 (Jackson et al. 2004). During this same period, the average age at injury was 38 and the median was 34. By way of contrast, the average and median ages during 1973–1979 were 29 and 24, respectively (Jackson et al. 2004).

Along with mobility impairment, spinal cord injury is associated with a wide range of physical complications, including loss of bowel and bladder control, blood clots, edema, excessive sweating, low blood pressure, loss of muscle tone, inability to regulate body temperature, chronic pain, pressure sores, and recurrent urinary tract infections (Staas and Ditunno 1992; Stover, DeLisa, and Whiteneck 1995; Sullivan 1990a; Whiteneck et al. 1993). In fact, the overwhelming majority of individuals with SCI experience one or more secondary complications (Post, de Witte, et al. 1998).[2] The self-care regimens most often used to minimize these complications include medication compliance, routine pressure releases, good nutritional habits, daily skin inspections, and hygienic bladder and bowel management techniques (Herrick, Elliott, and Crow 1994b; Jubala and Brenes 1988). As Jonathan, a 49-year-old paraplegic, noted,

> There's just lots of things that you have to do on a daily basis to stay healthy. A lot of guys don't do it, don't live very long, don't stay very healthy. . . . [You need to] drink a lot of water. . . . You got to have certain seating requirements as far as where you're sitting, what you're sitting on—cushions, just pressure spots, things like [that]. You have to just really pay attention to those, and I have a lot friends that never do.

On average, individuals with SCI make 18 physician visits and 48 visits to nonphysician practitioners each year (Harvey et al. 1992). Their rate of physician visits is nearly four times that of nondisabled working persons (DeJong, Brannon, and Batavia 1993).

## The Physiology of Spinal Cord Injury

Spinal cord injury (SCI) occurs when trauma to the spinal cord produces a lesion or severs the cord. This can result in a loss of motor function, paralysis in certain parts of the body, and a corresponding loss of sensation. The

# Figure 2.1  *The Spinal Cord and Nerve Supply*

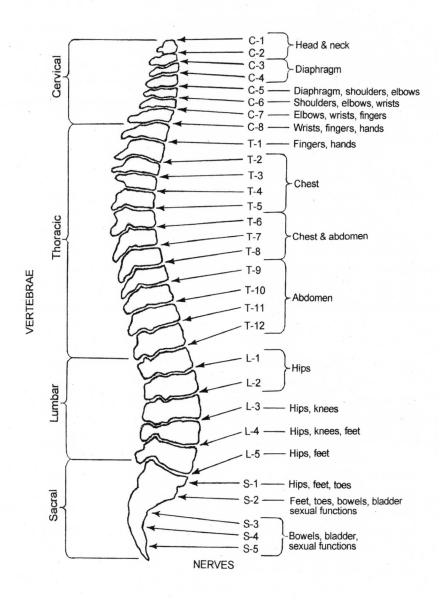

Figure courtesy of Teresa M. Wilder.

Sources: Cole 2004; Morris 1989; Trieschmann 1988; Williams 1997.

spinal cord is surrounded by rings of bones that are numbered according to location; there are seven cervical (C) vertebrae in the neck, twelve thoracic (T) vertebrae in the upper back, five lumbar (L) vertebrae in the lower back, and a fused group of vertebrae called the sacrum (S) at the base of the spine. Spinal cord injuries are described by their root level—the location at which the nerve has been damaged. The most commonly occurring spinal injury is at the C-5 level (16%), followed by C-4 (13%), C-6 (13%), T-12 (8%), C-7 (6%), and L-1 (5%) (Go, DeVivo, and Richards 1995). Figure 2.1 shows the functions associated with each spinal root level.

Cervical (neck) injuries result in quadriplegia (weakness or paralysis in all four limbs and the trunk) whereas injuries at the thoracic level and below result in paraplegia (weakness or paralysis in the legs, with full use of the arms and hands). The *Standards for Neurological Classification of Spinal Cord Injury* further classify spinal cord injuries as either *complete* or *incomplete* (Stover 1996). With complete injury, there is no motor function and no sensation (touch, temperature, position sense, or pain) below the level of the injury. With incomplete injury, there is at least partial preservation of motor or sensory functioning below the level of the injury. The combination of neurological level (C-5, T-12, etc.) and completeness of injury (complete or incomplete) provides a reasonably clear picture of each individual's condition.[3] Quadriplegia (54%) and complete injuries (56%) are more widespread than paraplegia and incomplete injuries (Jackson et al. 2004) and the most common neurological category is incomplete quadriplegia, followed by complete paraplegia, complete quadriplegia, and incomplete paraplegia (Go, DeVivo, and Richards 1995; National Spinal Cord Injury Association 2005). Slightly less than one percent of individuals with SCI experience complete recovery by the time they are discharged from the hospital (Go, DeVivo, and Richards 1995), possibly because their nerves are crushed rather than severed (Dreifus 2004). Women are more likely than men to recover, a finding that may be related to estrogen levels (Sipski et al. 2004).

In general, the higher the level of injury and the more severe the cord damage, the more extensive the paralysis and loss of sensation. For instance, individuals injured at cervical levels 1 and 2 (C-1 and C-2) can move only their facial muscles. They usually rely on sip-and-puff wheelchairs for mobility and on mouthsticks for activities such as computer use and environmental control (Trieschmann 1988). Individuals with complete injuries at these levels experience paralysis of the diaphragm and require mechanical assistance for ventilation (Kocan 1990).

Injuries at the C-3 level allow for mobility in the shoulders but result in paralysis below the neck. Individuals with C-3 injuries may rely on respirators, and extensive personal assistance is usually needed.

Individuals injured at the C-4 level may be able to breathe on their own, since this is the level at which the diaphragm is innervated (Jubala and Brenes 1988; Trieschmann 1988). The upper extremities are paralyzed, however, and independence of function is severely constrained.

Those injured at the C-5 level are able to use their shoulders and biceps, but most lack the power to straighten their elbows (Cole 2004). They may be able to feed themselves and to participate unassisted in some activities. For these individuals, an electric wheelchair is the usual means of locomotion (Trieschmann 1988).

Individuals with injuries at the C-6 level are considerably more likely to be independent. They generally lack hand functioning but are able to use their wrists, and many are able to transfer in and out of wheelchairs on their own. They may be able to use manual wheelchairs and to drive through the use of hand controls. Finger dexterity is usually quite limited, however, since the nerves that control the fingers are found at the C-8 and T-1 levels (Cole 2004).

Injuries below the T-1 level result in paraplegia rather than quadriplegia. Because the spinal nerves between T-2 and T-8 control the chest muscles, persons injured at lower levels are able to breathe more easily and to better control their balance and trunk stability. The abdominal muscles are controlled from T-6 to T-12, so individuals with lesions at or above this level often experience "a lax and large abdomen" (Cole 2004: 15).

Individuals with injuries at the T-12 level have good abdominal control, resulting in better trunk stability and good balance while sitting. Some many be able to walk with leg braces and crutches, although this may require considerable energy (Trieschmann 1988).

For those with injuries at L-4 and below, walking is possible. Short leg braces may be needed, along with crutches or canes (Trieschmann 1988). Among those with injuries at the sacral level, only short leg braces may be needed (Jubala and Brenes 1988). Unfortunately, bowel, bladder, and sexual functions are coordinated at the S-2 level and below, so these functions are often impaired even when the level of injury is low.

## The Epidemiology of Spinal Cord Injury

Spinal cord injury is far more common among men than among women. Although there has been a slight increase in the percentage of females over time, the four-to-one male/female ratio has changed little over the years (Jackson et al. 2004; National Spinal Cord Injury Statistical Center 2005). Among those who sustained spinal cord injuries from 2000 to 2003, the racial/ethnic distribution was approximately 67% white, 19% black, 10% Latino, and 3% other (Jackson et al. 2004). Blacks and American Indians are overrepresented among those with SCI (Go, DeVivo, and Richards 1995; Stover 1996).[4] My sample was 78% white, 9% African American, 6% Native American, 3% Latino, and 3% Asian Indian.

Data from 2000–2003 reveal that the causes of spinal cord injury are motor vehicle accidents (50%), falls (24%), acts of violence (11%), sports accidents (9%) and other (6%) (Jackson et al. 2004). Notably, two-thirds of sports-related SCI cases can be attributed to diving accidents (National Spinal Cord Injury Association 2005). While data from the 1970s through the 1990s showed that the percentage of people who had sustained injuries due to violence was rising dramatically (Jackson et al. 2004; Waters, Cressy, and Adkins 1996), more recent evidence from the 2000s points to a reversal of this trend, compensated for by an increase in motor vehicle accidents (Jackson et al. 2004). Injuries due to motor vehicle accidents, sports, and falls are considerably more likely to result in quadriplegia, whereas violence and other etiologies are more likely to result in paraplegia. With the exception of motor vehicle accidents, where the male to female ratio is 3:1, the ratio in all other etiology groups is approximately 4:1 (Jackson et al. 2004). Among the participants in my study, 50% had been injured in vehicular accidents (38% automobile, 9% motorcycle, and 3% pedestrian), 19% in swimming accidents, 16% due to physiological conditions (e.g., aneurysm, tumor, etc.), 9% as a result of gunshot wounds, 3% in sporting accidents, and 3% in falls.[5] Females were considerably more likely than males to have been injured as a result of automobile accidents.

## Fault and Blame

While about half the study participants had sustained injuries unrelated to their own actions—they had been passengers in car accidents or victims of violence, for instance—the other half had engaged in activities that were somehow related to their injuries. Some had been injured while driving recklessly, for example, or while diving in shallow water.

Some evidence suggests that individuals whose own behavior played a part in their injuries adjust more successfully than those who were "innocent victims" (Bulman and Wortman 1977; Decker and Schulz 1985). For example, Athelstan and Crewe (1979: 317) demonstrate that individuals who were at least partly responsible for their injuries tend to have personality traits that complicate rehabilitation in the short term but foster positive adjustments in the long term. In particular, they tend to be "energetic, adventuresome, and adaptable."[6] Similarly, Stewart and Rossier (1978) assert that chronic anger (which sometimes leads to depression and other adjustment problems) is more common among individuals whose own actions played no significant part in their injuries.

Other studies point to the opposite conclusion, however. Self-blame is generally regarded as a negative coping strategy, and several studies suggest that individuals who blame themselves cope less effectively—that they have higher levels of pessimism, depressed states, anxiety, and hostility (Nielson and MacDonald 1988; Sholomskas, Steil, and Plummer 1990). These difficulties seem to subside over time, however (Hanson et al. 1993; Nash 1988; Richards, Elliott, et al. 1997; Schulz and Decker 1985; Van den Bout et al. 1988).

A third body of research suggests that there is no significant link between an individual's perceived role in his injury (active or passive) and his subsequent adjustment to SCI. For example, Marini and associates (1995) found no association between self-esteem and attribution of blame. Likewise, several authors have found that the perceived avoidability of the disabling injury is only a minor or insignificant determinant of well-being among middle-aged and elderly individuals with SCI (Cecka 1981; Rodriguez 1991; Schulz and Decker 1985).

My findings support the assertion that those individuals who were in some way responsible for their injuries adjust better than those whose own actions played no part in their injuries. For example, 93% of those in the first group but only 73% of those in the second group reported that they were happy. The individuals who expressed the highest levels of unhappiness were two men who had been injured as a result of medical conditions (a spinal tumor and a neck aneurysm), a man who had been shot, and a man who had been a passenger in a car at the time of his injury. Kevin, introduced at the beginning of this chapter, wished he had someone to blame for his injury. When I asked him if he was angry, he replied,

> Yep, but I don't know at who. If you put one person down in front of me and said, "This is who made you be like who you are," I'd want to kill that person slowly. Or put them in a wheelchair.

Edward, a walking quadriplegic, had been shot in the neck by a volunteer at the library where his then-girlfriend worked. He remained intensely angry at the man who had shot him:

> Prison wasn't enough for him. 'Cause he was a computer nerd and now he's sitting in prison—probably got his own computer and all this stuff and I don't like that.
>
> EIW: You would prefer that he got the death penalty?
>
> Or ice pick in his spinal cord so he could get a spinal cord injury. [*laughter*] That would have been better than death.

## Spinal Cord Injury and Mortality

The earliest documented reference to spinal cord injury dates from the Edwin Smith Surgical Papyrus written about 5,000 years ago by an unidentified Egyptian physician. This reference includes an accurate diagnosis of spinal cord injury followed by an unfavorable prognosis:

> One having a dislocation in a vertebra of his neck while he is unconscious of his two legs and his two arms, and his urine dribbles. An ailment not to be treated (Breasted 1930: 327).

During the 19th century, neurosurgery began to flourish with the introduction of cerebral localization, antisepsis, and anesthesia (Goodrich 2004). Despite limited successes, however, approaches to treating SCI remained conservative. Most physicians considered SCI surgery to be dangerous and unjustifiable (Lifshutz and Colohan 2004). Prior to World War II, approximately 80% of people who sustained spinal cord injuries died within a few weeks as a result of infection, bed sores, or catheterization (Carroll 1970). In 1943, Donald Munro, a neurosurgeon at Boston City Hospital in Massachusetts, came forward with a new philosophical approach toward SCI, since referred to as the "Munro doctrine":

> Every patient with a spinal cord or cauda equina injury who has preserved the innervation of upper extremities and is intelligent and co-operative, can after proper treatment lead a social life and can gain his living according to his abilities (Beneš 1968: 6).

The first rehabilitation programs were established at about the same time, in Stoke Mandeville Hospital in the United Kingdom by Sir Ludwig Guttman, another neurosurgeon, and in West Roxbury, Massachusetts, by Munro (Kennedy 2001). In subsequent decades, a number of developments—including the advent of sulfa drugs in the 1940s; discoveries of antibiotics in the 1940s, 50s, and 60s; and the emergence of spinal injury treatment centers—have greatly enhanced survival rates among individuals with SCI (Gutierrez, Young, and Vulpe 1993; Trieschmann 1988; Whiteneck et al. 1992).[7]

Since the mid-1970s, the leading cause of death among individuals with SCI has been pneumonia. The other major causes of death are nonischemic heart disease, septicemia, pulmonary embolus, ischemic heart disease, suicide, unintentional injuries, and cancer (Stover 1996). While the likelihood of dying from renal disease has declined over time, the rates of death from suicide, liver disease, and alcohol abuse have all increased (Geisler et al. 1983). Although the life expectancy of individuals with SCI has improved dramatically over the years, it still remains significantly lower than that of the general population, in part due to elevated mortality from pneumonia, pulmonary emboli, and septicemia (DeVivo and Stover 1995). Respiratory and genitourinary mortality rates are also considerably higher for individuals with SCI than for the general population (Whiteneck et al. 1992).

Death rates and causes of death among individuals with SCI vary with age and severity of impairment. Quadriplegics have mortality rates 1.4 times higher than those of paraplegics (Whiteneck et al. 1992), and individuals who rely on respirators have especially high mortality rates (DeVivo and Stover 1995; Lanig and Lammertse 1992; Trieschmann 1988). Pneumonia is the leading cause of death among quadriplegics and individuals older than 55. Suicide and unintentional injuries are the leading causes of mortality among paraplegics and individuals younger than 55 (DeVivo et al. 1989).[8]

Sedentary lifestyles may contribute to premature death among individuals with SCI (DeVivo et al. 1989). Those who are socially and vocationally active have higher survival rates, as do those with better emotional adjustment (Kjorsvig 1994; Krause 1991; Krause and Crewe 1987; Krause, Saari, and Dykstra 1990). Survival rates are especially high among individuals with high levels of excitement, joy, and vigor, and low levels of caution and restraint (Krause, Saari, and Dykstra 1990). Health status, economic status, personal independence, and community integration also influence survival rates (Krause, DeVivo, and Jackson 2004; Trieschmann 1988).

## Physical Health and Psychosocial Well-Being

Physical health and psychosocial well-being are strongly related among individuals with spinal cord injury (Hampton 2004). In particular, those who experience secondary complications (e.g., severe pain and pressure sores) tend to be preoccupied with present needs (Martz and Livneh 2003) and to have lower levels of life satisfaction and psychological well-being (Coyle et al. 1993; Post, de Witte, et al. 1998; Ville et al. 2001). Likewise, chronic pain is often accompanied by a higher likelihood of psychological distress, depression, substance use, and suicide (Barrett et al. 2003; Boekamp, Overholser, and Schubert 1996; Craig, Hancock, and Dickson 1994; Nagumo 2000; Putzke, Richards, and Dowler 2000). Repeated hospitalizations are associated with elevated rates of depression, substance abuse, and other psychological problems (Weingardt, Hsu, and Dunn 2001). The converse is also true, however. Individuals with SCI who have relatively few health problems and perceive themselves to be better-adjusted to their impairments are more likely to feel integrated into their communities (Anson, Stanwyck, and Krause 1993; Boschen, Tonack, and Gargaro 2003; Hammell 2004b). In turn, those who are socially integrated tend to have a lower risk of depression (Fuhrer, Rintala, et al. 1993).

While poor adjustment to SCI seems to exacerbate preexisting medical conditions (Heinrich and Tate 1996), the resolution of psychosocial issues has been shown to reduce somatic complaints (Mathew et al. 2001). For example, depression and low levels of nurturance have been linked to a variety of health complications, including inadequate self-care, substance abuse, and lack of attention to nutrition and hygiene (Herrick, Elliott, and Crow 1994b; Krause, Saari, and Dykstra 1990; Malec and Neimeyer 1983). Self-destructive neglect and noncompliance with medical instructions increase the likelihood that individuals with SCI will develop secondary complications such as pressure sores, phantom pain sensations, urinary tract infections, autonomic dysreflexia, and severe spasticity (Stern and Slattery 1975).

Individuals with spinal cord injury exhibit lower levels of physical self-esteem than their able-bodied counterparts (Mayer and Eisenberg 1982). Many are especially dissatisfied in the areas of health, health care, finances, and community safety (Kemp and Krause 1999). Perhaps not surprisingly, subjective health and satisfaction with life are inversely correlated with depressive symptomatology (Bombardier, Richards, et al. 2004).

## Health Problems Associated with Spinal Cord Injury

### *Pressure Sores*

Pressure sores (decubitus ulcers or ischemic ulceration) are the single health problem that most often accompanies SCI (Whiteneck et al. 1992). These sores, which occur almost exclusively over bony prominences, are caused by sustained pressure on a small area of soft tissue—most often, from lying or sitting in one position for too long. They afflict between 42% and 85% of all individuals with spinal cord injury (Gordon et al. 1982), and approximately one-third of all community residents with SCI exhibit one or more pressure sores at any particular time (Fuhrer, Garber, et al. 1993). While skin care is seldom rated as an area of high need, severe pressure sores can be costly in both economic and social terms (Cox, Amsters, and Pershouse 2001).

Pressure sores frequently result from a failure to adhere to proper medical protocols. They can often be prevented by "releases," whereby individuals with SCI reposition their bodies to restore the blood flow to constricted areas. Repositioning can be difficult, however, especially when spasticity is present (Smith and Porter 1992).[9] Individuals with SCI are also encouraged to consume adequate amounts of water and to observe a healthy diet to ensure proper nutrition for the skin (Herrick, Elliott, and Crow 1994b; Smith and Porter 1992). A number of demographic characteristics place individuals with SCI at even greater risk of pressure sores; these include male gender, minority group membership, older age, complete injury, and a lesser degree of voluntary muscle control (see, for example, Anderson and

Andberg 1979; Fuhrer, Garber, et al. 1993; Gerhart et al. 1997; Yarkony and Heinemann 1995).[10]

Pressure sores have been linked to a variety of psychological and emotional variables, such as poor emotional adjustment, poor social adjustment, and low self-esteem (Gordon et al. 1982; Hundley 1985).[11] The association between pressure sores and psychosocial adjustment may be linked to a variety of factors. For example, the need to remain in bed during healing may impede social activity. Individuals prone to pressure sores may also have distinct psychological characteristics that make them less compliant about monitoring their health (Gordon et al. 1982). For example, depressed persons may stop doing pressure releases or turning in bed (Yarkony 1993).

Over half the study participants described experiences with pressure sores. Rosa, a 38-year-old single mother, summarized the sentiments of many others when she stated,

> We've all had those pressure sores. Those are a pain in the you know what. . . . You have to go right to the doctor with those. You can't heal those up yourself. . . . They always want to put you right into the hospital; they don't like sending you home unless they know you've got someone at home to help take care of it.

Indeed, the healing process demands patience and therapeutic vigilance—virtues that do not come easily to everyone. Brad, a 32-year-old quadriplegic who works as a PC technician, had to postpone getting his own apartment so that he could pay the surgical bills that had resulted from a pressure sore.

## Temperature Regulation

Spinal cord injury adversely affects two of the processes needed for temperature regulation: shivering (which heats the body) and sweating (which cools it). In particular, temperature regulation is a common problem for those with lesions above the T-6 level (Jubala and Brenes 1988). The larger the portion of the body that is paralyzed, the greater the impairment of the body's ability to shiver or sweat (DeLoach and Greer 1981). Thus, for example, many people with quadriplegia cannot regulate their internal body temperatures and are dependent on external temperature control—a condition known as *poikilothermia* (Palmer, Kriegsman, and Palmer 2000).

As a result, quadriplegics may experience hypothermia when temperatures drop below 70°F and run fevers in response to hot weather.

Concerns about hypersensitivity to temperature were voiced by numerous participants with quadriplegia, and several commented that this problem adversely affected their social lives. Stan, a slender 49-year-old quadriplegic man who works at a nonprofit organization, complained about difficulties withstanding the heat. He regularly attends a Wednesday night Bible study group, but not when "the hot weather sets in." Similarly, Adam, a 26-year-old quadriplegic, lamented the need to be careful participating in outdoor activities on hot days:

> I do still go to the lake. We've got some friends with a boat and I go tubing and stuff. . . . [I] still like being outside. I have more limitations now because being a quadriplegic I have temperature limitations. I guess the thermostat doesn't work anymore. I get really hot easily because I don't sweat so I have to be really careful with that during the summer. . . . I don't sweat at all unless I'm sick and then I sweat really bad. [*chuckle*]

Others complained about sensitivity to the cold. Todd, a very thin 34-year-old quadriplegic man, reported that his social activity was severely constrained during the cold months:

> The worst part about being paralyzed is my inability to handle weather. I don't even like going out in the winter time; I'd rather be home, it's warm in my house. . . . I live for summer. [*laughter*]

Derrick, a 39-year-old quadriplegic, complained that his "hands are cold, miserably cold all the time," and Jeremy, a 46-year-old quadriplegic, said, "I always feel like I'm standing in a vat of ice."

## Bladder and Bowel Dysfunction

Spinal cord injury generally results in urinary and bowel dysfunction. Bladder management—the routine maintenance and use of apparatus for emptying the bladder at predictable intervals—is therefore essential. The most common bladder-emptying techniques include stimulation, intermittent catheterization procedures (ICP), and the use of an indwelling or suprapubic catheter introduced through the abdominal wall.[12] As many as 95% of individuals with SCI also use some form of therapeutic method to initiate defecation. These techniques include manual evacuation, digital stimulation, and suppositories (Glickman and Kamm 1996).[13] Constipation, diarrhea, nausea, and fecal incontinence are also common complications of SCI (Glickman and Kamm 1996). The prevention of urinary tract infections (UTIs) and kidney stones is an ongoing challenge that requires the scrupulous cleaning of catheters and the careful use of ICP techniques (Herrick, Elliott, and Crow 1994b). All else equal, minority-group members are at especially high risk of UTIs (Waites, Canupp, and DeVivo 1993).

For many individuals with SCI, the inability to control excretory functions results in shame and embarrassment (Hayes, Potter, and Hardin 1995; Hendrick 1981; Stewart and Rossier 1978). Urinary incontinence and repeated infections also interfere with many activities of daily living (Lundqvist et al. 1991). Bowel management is often a source of emotional distress (Glickman and Kamm 1996), and the incidence of bowel accidents is a significant determinant of life satisfaction (McColl and Skinner 1996).

All of the participants mentioned that their spinal cord injuries had affected their bladder and/or bowel regimens,[14] and over half a dozen reported that their inability to effectively manage these routines prevented them from having the kind of active social lives they would have liked. Several complained that they had very limited warning before they had to use the bathroom. For instance, Edward, stated, "When I gotta go pee, I've got to go—even if I'm in a gas station at the gas pump." Travis felt that his bowel problems were probably worse than most because he suffered from irritable bowel syndrome:

> It turns into a vicious circle because if you're stressed and then you have a bowel accident, it's going to stress you even more. And so sometimes it just turns into this situation where it almost becomes like you're basically managing bowel accidents because your body's not regular enough that you can manage it the way you normally do.

Travis said that he'd sometimes go a week without having a bowel accident, but that other times he'd have three or four in a single day. At the worst times,

You can't even hardly leave the house. Every time you get cleaned up from one and get dressed and get ready to go, you have another. And so that's when it's really like detrimental as far as being able to attend class or things of that nature. There's no consistency in it.

Travis was considering getting a colostomy, since he felt this would allow him to better manage his bowel problems: "There are days when I would do it myself if I thought I had a sharp enough knife." He said he had reservations about the procedure, however, since he was uncomfortable with hospitals and felt that the operation would move him "further away from being normal." In general, however, colostomies do not reduce the quality of life of individuals with SCI (Randell et al. 2001), and they may actually enhance it. Several months after the interview, Travis reported that he had gotten a colostomy and was very upbeat about the procedure.

Andrew, a 36-year-old quadriplegic who worked as a computer programmer, recalled how he had once rushed home when he was having problems with loose stools at work. While he was wheeling to his car, he looked back and saw a trail of stool leaking behind him. Fortunately, it rained before he returned to work again. Likewise, Chris—a married 48-year-old quadriplegic—lamented that his bowel problems had kept him out of the labor force and interfered with his ability to participate in recreational activities.

On the other hand, Jonathan felt that bowel and bladder problems need not interfere with social and recreational activities. He described how he had reacted to one of his friends who was having problems:

Jerry would [say], "Well I can't go here, I can't control my bowels, I can't do this. I have a lap full of pee, blah blah." I was going, "Jerry, Jerry. Look." I just kinda tell him some of the things that I've worked through and what I try to do. I said, "You can do it."

### Sympathetic Nervous Dysfunction

Autonomic hypertension, also called "autonomic dysreflexia," is a pathological reflex in which the blood pressure suddenly rises to dangerously high levels (Trieschmann 1988). These crises often occur as the result of increased autonomic activity caused by a noxious stimulus below the level of injury (Hanak and Scott 1983; Palmer, Kriesgman, and Palmer 2000). Common triggers include overdistension of urine (accumulation of too much urine) or fecal impactions (stool retained in the lower bowel), but autonomic dysreflexia may also be caused by pressure on the skin, rectal stimulation, bladder stones, pressure sores, ingrown toenails, severe menstrual cramps, temperature changes, a blocked catheter, or spasticity of the pelvic floor (Palmer, Kriegsman, and Palmer 2000; Staas et al. 1988; Weiss 1968). The symptoms include excruciating headaches, flushing of the face, seeing spots in front of one's eyes, goose bumps, sweating, blurred vision, and nasal stuffiness (Hammond et al. 1992; Staas et al. 1988; Weiss 1968). Autonomic dysreflexia can constitute a medical emergency and has the potential to result in a stroke if the condition is not brought under control.

Autonomic dysreflexia is an underrecognized clinical entity that affects approximately 50% of those with injuries above the T-5 level (Freehafer 1997; Krassioukov, Furlan, and Fehlings 2003). Several individuals with high-level injuries described how they had faced this complication. For example, Harry, a 33-year-old quadriplegic student, reflected,

> I was on a lot of medication back then so what would happen is I would be so relaxed and sleep and my bladder would fill up so hard, so full that I'd wake up and be in the middle of dysreflexia with my blood pressure sky high and my brain about to blow and explode.

Al, a 28-year-old quadriplegic student, described how he experienced autonomic dysreflexia:

> Your body sends you these messages on what's going on. Like if you need to pee real bad, they'll get [a] bad headache. I know if my back's pinched off and I need to pee, I'll get goose bumps. My face will turn red, I'll start sweating.

A few mentioned how they suffered from dysreflexia during sexual intercourse (see Chapter 4). Despite its severity, however, autonomic dysreflexia did not interfere with the social lives of the people I interviewed in the same way that some other complications did.

## Chronic Pain

Chronic pain is one of the most serious complications associated with SCI (Benrud-Larson and Wegener 2000; Cole 2004; Siddall, Yezierski, and

Loeser 2002; Widerström-Noga 2002; Widerström-Noga and Turk 2003; Yezierski and Burchiel 2002), and many individuals with SCI have an unmet need for pain management (Cox, Amsters, and Pershouse 2001). Because different classification schemes have been used, estimates of the incidence of chronic pain among individuals with SCI have ranged from 11% to 94%.[15] However, most studies report prevalence rates between 60% and 70% (Benrud-Larson and Wegener 2000; Cohen et al. 1988; Conant 1998; Henwood and Ellis 2004; Mariano 1992; Maynard et al. 1995; Richards 1992; Summers et al. 1991) with severe pain in approximately one-third of all cases (Siddall, Yezierski, and Loeser 2002). Low-income individuals, members of ethnic minorities, and individuals who sustained gunshot wounds are especially likely to experience chronic pain (see, for example, Go, DeVivo, and Richards 1995; Richards, Stover, and Jaworski 1990).

Three kinds of chronic pain are common among individuals with SCI: central, dysesthetic pain (characterized by burning, tingling, or aching sensations below the level of the lesion); mechanical pain (sharp and localized at the site of injury); and radicular pain (associated with nerve damage and radiating in a dermatomal pattern—down the affected leg, for example) (Benrud-Larson and Wegener 2000). While the experience of chronic pain is quite variable, most studies indicate that it does not dissipate over time (Störmer et al. 1997; Widerström-Noga 2002) and is often unresponsive to pharmacological and surgical interventions. Nonetheless, the recommended treatments include the use of anticonvulsants, tricyclic antidepressants, Lidocaine, and opioids (Finnerup and Jensen 2004). Some nonmedicinal strategies for coping with chronic pain include massage, stretching, heat, exercise (especially swimming in warm water), vocational and social activity, and distraction (Henwood and Ellis 2004). Approximately half of those who experience chronic pain report that their symptoms are either eliminated or considerably reduced by physical therapies of one type or another (Widerström-Noga and Turk 2003).

The etiology and pathophysiology of SCI-related pain are only partly understood (Mariano 1992; Richards 1992). Most studies report that this pain cannot be adequately conceptualized as either a purely physiological or a purely psychological phenomenon (Mariano 1992; Widerström-Noga 2002). Some evidence suggests that SCI pain is more readily explained by psychosocial than physiological factors, however (Summers et al. 1991; Störmer et al. 1997). For example, the incidence or severity of chronic pain has been linked to poor quality of life, depression, anxiety, fatigue, anger, familial/social difficulties, and general psychosocial impairment (Barrett et al. 2003; Benrud-Larson and Wegener 2000; Conant 1995; Gerhart et al. 1997; Giardino et al. 2003; Henwood and Ellis 2004; Lundqvist et al. 1991; Widerström-Noga 2002). Acceptance of disability and an internal locus of control have both been associated with the absence of chronic pain (Conant 1995; Li and Moore 1998), although it is not clear whether psychosocial problems result in pain or vice versa—or if the two conditions simply reinforce one another.

The role of physiological factors in explaining SCI pain remains a topic of considerable debate. While most studies fail to find any systematic relationships between chronic pain and the characteristics of the injury itself (level, completeness/incompleteness, and operated/non-operated status) (Störmer et al. 1997; Wang et al. 2004), some evidence suggests that the area of the injury may be an important site for generating pain (Finnerup and Jensen 2004) and that those with thoracic and lumbar injuries have a greater incidence of pain (Wang et al. 2004). Recent research suggests that damage to the spinothalamic tract is a necessary but insufficient condition for the occurrence of chronic pain (Defrin et al. 2001), and clinical observations and autopsy evidence indicate that neuropathic pain is more common in those with incomplete lesions (Siddall, Yezierski, and Loeser 2002). Many physical and environmental factors appear to exacerbate pain, including urinary tract infections, constipation, prolonged sitting or lying down, cold or hot temperatures, humidity, and weather changes (Henwood and Ellis 2004).

Many individuals with chronic pain resulting from SCI report that this complication interferes with daily activities such as sleep, work, exercise, and household chores (Barrett et al. 2003; Loeser 2002; Widerström-Noga, Felipe-Cuervo, and Yezierski 2001). Indeed, several of the people I interviewed—especially the quadriplegics—volunteered complaints about problems with chronic pain. For example, Derrick reported "terrible pain in my left ischel" and Meghan said that her back pain was only getting worse over time. Interestingly, many of the individuals who complained about chronic pain also reported problems with hypersensitivity to the weather.

Phantom sensations (e.g., pain, burning, tingling, vibrating, or numbness) are another common problem among individuals with SCI. For example, Todd experienced phantom pains in his stomach:

> It's just a sensation you have of burning—an uncomfortable situation. I went to numerous doctors to figure out what was going on and they never could.

Unlike other kinds of SCI-related pain, phantom sensations have been found to decline in severity over time (Allden 1992).

## *Weight and Nutrition*

Weight and nutrition are important concerns for individuals with spinal cord injury, especially due to their impact on general mobility, ease of transferring, joint functioning, and risk of fracture (McColl and Skinner 1996). Individuals with SCI sometimes demonstrate nutritional deficits due to physiological changes (Formal 1992), and glucose intolerance and anemia are common sequelae of spinal cord injury (Blissitt 1990). Fortunately, the provision of nutritional care at the onset of SCI decreases the likelihood of secondary complications and enhances rehabilitation outcomes (Houda 1993).

Weight guidelines for individuals with SCI are ten to fifteen pounds lower for paraplegics and fifteen to twenty pounds lower for quadriplegics than the Metropolitan Life Insurance ideal body weights (Blissitt 1990). At the same time, individuals with SCI are especially likely to be either underweight or overweight (McColl and Skinner 1996). The former condition often represents loss of muscle tone and muscle atrophy due to paralysis, while the latter may be linked to a sedentary lifestyle. Both excess and insufficient weight may result in problems of skin breakdown among individuals with SCI, either because of too much weight over pressure points or insufficient muscle between bones and skin (Hammond et al. 1992).

While most of my study participants appeared to be average or slender, approximately 20% were visibly overweight. Several voiced weight-related concerns and mentioned the difficulty of losing weight while in a wheelchair. Shannon, a 43-year-old paraplegic woman who looked about 40 pounds overweight, reported,

I've put on a lot of weight since I've been in a wheelchair

EIW: Does it fluctuate?

No, it just keeps going up. It has never gone down. [*laughter*]

EIW: Do you do any kinds of exercises right now?

No, I have a desk job. I sit at a desk ten hours a day. It makes it more difficult. It's not that I couldn't, but I really don't enjoy arm exercises, never did. I used to like jogging and doing aerobics and all that stuff, and now you can't really do jogging, aerobics. I like the leg stuff a lot better than the arm stuff. And weights, I hate it.

Shannon has a desk job where she sits "ten hours a day," and this makes it difficult for her to schedule exercise. Rosa, a 52-year-old paraplegic woman, also struggles with her weight:

That's because you're sitting in your chair there. All my weight's from the waist down. I've asked RNs if they can tell me how to lose weight and they said they've never had anyone ask them that's in a wheelchair how to lose weight.

Several participants in the study described how hospitalizations and paralysis had made them too thin. A few of the men were especially upset that their injuries had affected them in this way. For example, Kevin described how his physique had changed following his injury:

I used to be built pretty good and all, but a few weeks of being in the hospital and the IV food, that will do it to you. . . . I got pretty skinny.

Similarly, Todd reported:

Now that my muscles atrophied away, what's left? Not much. My legs are skinny and everything. . . . But if I tried to gain weight, all the weight, it seems like on people, goes right to their guts. 'Cause you look at people and 90 percent of them have a gut on 'em, whereas I'm still pretty skinny and I want to keep it that way. I don't want one of those big old potbellies.

Meanwhile, Derrick complained about weight gain in his belly:

Hopefully one day I'll be able to do a sit-up again, and once I get to then I'll be able to get rid of my gut which just kills me, but everybody calls 'em "a quad gut."

A few of the people I spoke with, including Andrew and Harry, described how they had gained weight due to heavy drinking in the aftermath of their injuries. Both had subsequently lost weight, however.

## The Daily Dose

Approximately 80% of individuals with SCI use at least one type of prescription drug in any given year (Harvey et al. 1990). Many are given low-dose antibiotics for the prevention of urinary tract infections, low-dose anticoagulants for the prevention of deep vein thrombosis, and antispasticity drugs for the management of spasticity (DeJong, Brannon, and Batavia 1993). For the overwhelming majority of the individuals I interviewed, daily medication—prescribed, over-the counter, and/or illicit—had become a routine part of life. Virtually all the study participants had received pharmacological treatment for one or more health problems: muscle spasms, neurogenic bladder,[16] pain, recurrent urinary tract infections, anxiety, depression, etc.

My study participants seemed to resent their dependence on any kind of medication. This finding is consistent with the fact that the use of multiple medications is positively correlated with depression among individuals with SCI (Shnek 1995). Several described how they had gradually reduced their use of various medications or had simply quit taking them altogether. When Edward had problems with muscle spasms and stiffness in his lower back, aspirin was the only medication he took:

> I used to take Baclofen. I had to wean myself off of those. . . . I finally got off of 'em. I have muscle spasms but . . . I don't really care for taking drugs. I take Bayer just because my left leg bothers me all the time and it just eases that enough that I can get to sleep.

Ryan, a 20-year-old paraplegic student, had also weaned himself off antispasm medications. When I asked him if he ever took any medication related to his injury, he responded:

> I used to when I was ten or eleven. I used to take the pills for muscle spasms all the time; muscle relaxers. I was taking some sort of muscle relaxers and they would put me through such mood swings and I was always tired and they just put me out like that so my

mother gradually took me off of 'em and said, "We don't need that anymore."

Several participants reported having taken psychotropic medications, usually antidepressants. The use of psychotropic drugs for individuals with SCI is controversial. While some researchers advocate the use of medication to treat post-injury depression (Judd et al. 1989; Knorr and Bull 1970), others have advised against this treatment, noting that the use of antidepressants may interfere with the mourning process (Frank, Elliott, et al. 1987; Stern and Slattery 1975). Many individuals with SCI experience secondary (reactive) depression, a type that is less responsive to antidepressant medication (Jubala and Brenes 1988; Stern and Slattery 1975). While a combination of antidepressants and psychotherapy does appear to reduce depressive symptomatology (Kemp et al. 2004), additional research is needed (Elliott and Kennedy 2004). Of particular concern is the fact that many antidepressant medications have potentially serious side effects.[17]

Several individuals who had taken antidepressants reported favorable results, although most of them also seemed uncomfortable with this acknowledgment and emphasized that their use of such medication had been short-term. Stacy, a 20-year-old paraplegic student, described how her mood had been closely linked to her use of antidepressants:

> It's been about only six months since I stopped taking [Prozac]. . . . I would feel like I didn't need it anymore and I'd stop taking it and I'd get run down; I'd get tired and I'd stay home more so I'd start taking it again.

Stacy reported that since she stopped using Prozac, she no longer experienced depression. Interestingly, the majority of the women in the sample—but not the men—reported that they had taken antidepressants.

A few of the individuals I interviewed reported that they had been prescribed antidepressants, not for the treatment of depression but for various other physical problems they had encountered (phantom pains, sleep problems, etc.). For example, Todd had been prescribed the antidepressant amatriptiline for chronic pain, but he was not certain whether it had helped. He quit taking it after a while.

## Substance Abuse

Individuals with SCI are especially prone to substance abuse and related problems (Alston 1994; Asch 1970; Charlifue and Gerhart 1991; Glow 1989; Heinemann, Doll, and Schnoll 1989; Heinemann et al. 1987; Heinemann, Mamott, and Schnoll 1990; Kennedy et al. 2000; Kewman and Tate 1998; Kishi and Robinson 1996; Moore and Polsgrove 1991; O'Donnell et al. 1981–1982; Tate et al. 2004). In particular, the first post-injury year is associated with relatively high rates of exposure to tobacco, amphetamines, cocaine, and marijuana and other hallucinogens (Heinemann 1993; Heinemann, Doll, and Schnoll 1989).[18] Substance abuse remains problematic in later years as well. Cannabis and stimulant use are each about three times as high among individuals with SCI as among the general population (McColl and Skinner 1996), and estimates of marijuana use among individuals with SCI have ranged from 16% to 42% (Tate et al. 2004). Surprisingly, however, studies of veterans with SCI have revealed especially *low* rates of substance use within this group (Kirubakaran et al. 1986), and an incidence of smoking no different from that of nondisabled veterans (Spungen et al. 1995).

The nature of the link between SCI and alcohol abuse is not entirely clear. Although some studies suggest that alcohol use declines in the aftermath of spinal cord injury (Heinemann, Doll, and Schnoll 1989; McMillen and Cook 2003), others show a post-injury decline followed by an increase in alcohol use thereafter (Bombardier 2000). While Tate and associates (2004) report that individuals with SCI are more likely than the general population to meet the diagnostic criteria for alcohol abuse, McColl and Skinner (1996) find no such relationship. In an effort to characterize the various patterns of alcohol use among individuals with SCI, Glass (1980–1981) distinguishes between Type A drinkers (those whose drinking problems predate SCI) and Type B drinkers (those whose drinking problems began only after the onset of SCI). This distinction may be useful in determining the kind of treatment that is necessary. Type A problem drinkers require specific treatment for alcohol abuse, while Type B problem drinkers have a good likelihood of experiencing improvement when they are provided with broad-spectrum evaluation and skills training as well as cognitive therapeutic training (Glass 1980–1981). The diversity of alcohol-related problems among individuals with SCI suggests a need for multidimensional treatment efforts (Turner, Bombardier, and Rimmele 2003).

In some cases, substance abuse is associated not with SCI itself, but with the personal characteristics of the individuals most likely to incur spinal cord injuries. It is noteworthy, for instance, that between 17% and 68% of the individuals who have sustained spinal cord injuries were intoxicated at the time of their accidents (Heinemann 1993; Heinemann, Doll, and Schnoll 1989), and as many as three in five had been heavy drinkers prior to their injuries (Kolakowsky-Hayner et al. 1999). In fact, drug and alcohol use can be regarded as "sensation seeking" behaviors that fit the personality type most often associated with SCI (Alston 1994). These characteristics also predispose individuals with SCI to subsequent injuries (Krause 2004). Because intoxication at the onset of spinal cord injury is a marker of pre-injury substance use, it is important to screen for substance abuse in persons who incur traumatic injuries (Heinemann 1993; Heinemann et al. 1987; Heinemann, Mamott, and Schnoll 1990; Rohe and Basford 1989). Individuals with SCI who have a history of problem drinking tend to progress more slowly during rehabilitation and are at greater risk of developing post-rehabilitation complications (Bombardier, Stroud, et al. 2004).

Substance abuse may also represent an effort to medicate the secondary complications of spinal cord injury (Radnitz and Tirch 1995; Richards, Kewman, and Pierce 2000; Tate et al. 2004). For instance, the tendency to self-medicate spasticity with marijuana can sometimes lead to abuse (Malec, Harvey, and Cayner 1982; Radnitz and Tirch 1995). Individuals with SCI who drink report that it helps to reduce tension and to enhance social assertiveness, mood, and sleep (Heinemann, Schmidt, and Semik 1994). In addition, the impetus for drug use can sometimes be external; doctors may overmedicate or prescribe potentially addictive drugs because they feel unable to help in any other way (Greer 1986). Similarly, friends and family members may express attitudes that fail to discourage substance abuse (Radnitz and Tirch 1995).

Drug and alcohol abuse can have especially adverse health consequences among individuals with SCI, since the usual risks associated with substance abuse (diseases of the liver, pancreas, brain, cardiovascular system, respiratory system, endocrine system, and musculoskeletal system) are combined with the effects of drugs and alcohol on the ability to manage self-care and to perform activities of daily living (McColl and Skinner 1996; Radnitz and Tirch 1995).[19] Among other things, those who drink alcohol on a regular basis are less likely to spend time in productive activities such as rehabilitation therapy (Heinemann et al. 1989). Substance use has also been linked to secondary complications, including the development of pressure sores

(Hawkins and Heinemann 1998). Since substance abuse may be especially dangerous for individuals with SCI, abstinence seems to be the most appropriate treatment goal (Radnitz and Tirch 1995). Moreover, given that the best "cure" for drug abuse is a meaningful life, these programs should aim to help individuals find such lives (Sweeney and Foote 1982).

Approximately half a dozen people I spoke with volunteered that they had turned to either alcohol or illicit substances (primarily marijuana) to cope with their disabilities. Interestingly, there was very little overlap between those who had used antidepressants and those who had used illicit substances. Many reported that they had used drugs and alcohol in order to cope with the emotional pain and physical complications associated with their disabilities. For example, Harry described a period when he was abusing a wide range of substances:

> I used to get drunk quite a bit. I'd go to the doctor, take every medication he'd give me. Of course, I was having a lot of muscle spasms, too. . . . I was taking about 18 to 20 pills a day. I was taking stuff like Librium, Valium, Dantrium, Lioresal, Soma, which is really good.[20] [*laughter*] . . . And I was drinking about a twelve-pack of 5-percent beer from Missouri on top of that probably at least five times a week. So I was way overweight and I was having back problems.

When I asked him how he had overcome his substance abuse, he reflected,

> I was sitting on my porch one night and my face was like flashing— like I was gonna have a stroke or something. . . . And I was like, "Look, you probably hit bottom as far as you can hit right now. You've got a choice to make. You can either go set some goals for your life, you can get out of this crap and do something with your life, or you can just go ahead and go past this step and go ahead and die. . . . It's gonna go one way or the other." And I knew it.

Harry then made a conscious decision to get his life back on track:

> This was probably one of the most grueling things I ever went through. . . . I couldn't sleep at night so I would try to stay as active as possible during the day because I was weaning myself on the

medication and my body was freaking out. I was going through hell. So what I did was I had to stay active so as soon as it started getting dark at night I started pushing up and down the street. . . . And I did that like all summer.

Eventually, Harry was able to wean himself off the drugs. He now takes only Ditropan, vitamins, and herbs.

Like Harry, Rosa turned to substances to numb the pain of her disability. She describes the period immediately after her car accident as one of "doing nothing":

[I] sun-bathed and cleaned [my sister's] house and cooked and did house-keeping and stuff. . . . [I was] depressed. . . . I think my friend was alcohol. I'm a reformed alcoholic. I drank a little bit before the injury. After, the injury intensified it.

At the time of the interview, Rosa had been sober for at least two years. Not only had she quit drinking, she had stopped using marijuana—another of her coping mechanisms. When asked how she had achieved sobriety, she responded, "The good Lord above."

Unlike Rosa, Andrew continued to rely on marijuana for its antispasmodic effect:

I don't take any kind of medication for muscle spasms. And whenever I did, what was prescribed was Valium. Well, Valium would always kind of just bring me down and just kind of zap me, so I couldn't really take Valium. Plus I had a problem with incontinence when I would take Valium. . . . It seemed like I was peeing on myself all the time. So I had to stop taking the Valium and when I stopped taking the Valium I was smoking pot and when I quit smoking pot my muscle spasms just tripled.

Todd also felt strongly that marijuana had been helpful to him. He smoked pot several times a week and described it as "the best spasticity drug there is." He had tried a variety of drugs and treatments (including Valium) to deal with his muscle spasms, but none had been as effective as marijuana.

Jay had heard about the antispasmodic properties of marijuana but preferred his own remedy: careful monitoring of his food intake, combined with the relaxation techniques he learned at a pain management course.

One thing I've been doing in the last five or six months that's really helped my spasms and I see a correlation now is having a banana every day. I don't know what it is; I guess it's the potassium or whatever, but if I don't have my daily banana—like if I skip a couple of days—I can start feeling my muscle spasms getting worse again.

Indeed, research has indicated that working out when dehydrated or with low levels of potassium can predispose individuals to muscle spasms (National Institutes of Health 2005).

Jeremy reported that prescription medications—especially painkillers—had been his primary means of dealing with his disability. He saw his substance abuse as a carryover of the treatment he received while in rehabilitation. "For my rehabilitation part, they had me on some real heavy medication, you know, Class A, and so I more or less turned to drugs and alcohol," he reported. Jeremy has since kicked this habit, however: "I haven't done any drugs like that in about eight years."

## Suicide and Health

Previous research has revealed a heightened tendency toward suicidal ideation among individuals with spinal cord injury (Asch 1970; Dijkers et al. 1995; Kishi, Robinson, and Kosier 2001; Stewart 1988), with some estimates ranging as high as 60% (Dias de Carvalho et al. 1998). Age- and sex-specific suicide rates among individuals with SCI are five times as high as those in the general community, and up to 21% of deaths among individuals with SCI can be attributed to suicide (DeVivo et al. 1989, 1991). These rates may actually be higher if one also considers the role of passive suicide (neglect of health), a tendency that Seymour (1955: 692) calls "physiological suicide." Among individuals with SCI, the risk factors for suicide include poor health; pre-injury depression; post-injury depression; expressions of shame, apathy, and hopelessness; post-injury family disruption; alcohol abuse; and destructive behavior (Charlifue and Gerhart 1991; Hopkins 1971; Kishi and Robinson 1996; Kishi, Robinson, and Kosier 2001). The suicide rate diminishes after the first post-injury year, however, and drops off considerably by the fifth year (Dijkers et al. 1995).

Studies of the relationship between suicide and level of injury have yielded mixed results. Kishi and Robinson (1996) contend that quadriplegics have a higher frequency of suicidal plans than paraplegics. Likewise,

Charlifue and Gerhart (1991) report a suicide rate of 65 per 100,000 for quadriplegics versus 54 for paraplegics. At the same time, however, other authors have concluded that suicidal tendencies are most pronounced among those with complete paraplegia (DeVivo et al. 1991) or incomplete paraplegia (Dijkers et al. 1995). These last reports are consistent with the idea that individuals who are less seriously injured feel more pressure to compete or to keep up with their able-bodied counterparts. It is also possible that the complete care and observation necessary in many cases of quadriplegia reduce the likelihood of a suicide attempt (Hopkins 1971).

Approximately half a dozen study participants—mostly quadriplegics with high-level injuries—stated that they had contemplated suicide at some point. Among these individuals, suicidal ideation is closely linked to the challenges of receiving adequate care, and to the sense of helplessness that results from very limited mobility or chronic pain. Derrick described his suicide attempt approximately a year before the interview, in which he

> ate 80 Valiums. And my sister found me laid back in the chair just unconscious, blue-faced, not breathing and called the ambulance. They came and pumped my stomach and took me to the hospital. And I spent two weeks in the hospital and the doctor said then that he thought I'd probably be a vegetable. But thank God again, I'm back again so he's not done with me yet.

When I asked him why he had attempted suicide, he replied,

> I was so sick of fighting the system. The health care system here is so terrible. They are supposed to have agencies in place to help me stay out of a nursing home. . . . I've had such a problem keeping people in here to work that I have spent all my Social Security Disability income and my mom and [her] husband have had to add to that every month.

Indeed, the sense that one is "fighting the system" has been identified as a key factor detracting from the quality of life among individuals with SCI (Hammell 2004b; Russell 1998). In spite of these challenges, Derrick felt as though suicide was no longer an option:

> I survived that and I feel like I've got a reason for [living]. I'm doing my best to try to figure what that is.

Meanwhile, Meghan's struggles to obtain adequate health care were pushing her closer to the brink. She said that in her 21 years of having a disability, things were at an "all-time low":

> I've never been this close to suicide. I think I'm realistic. I can't afford it. That's not how I feel; I know I can't afford it. I'm gonna be in a nursing home or I'm gonna have to commit suicide. Well, I'm not gonna go to a nursing home and then you smell feces all day and I'm not gonna do that.

Meghan insisted that she was not in immediate danger of hurting herself, however.

Like Meghan, many disabled individuals complain about the challenges of finding reliable attendant care. Attendants are often described as unreliable, lazy, unqualified, not punctual, and sometimes even drug- or alcohol-dependent (Cockerill and Durham 1992). Meghan said that she sometimes spends nights in her wheelchair because no one shows up to transfer her to the bed. When I asked Fred, also a high-level quadriplegic, if he ever had suicidal thoughts, he replied, "All the time, not all the time but I'm too big of a coward to do it myself."

Jeremy said he had contemplated suicide initially ("at the beginning") when his accident occurred, but not since then. (He jokingly told me that if he were found dead, I should "call the police!") He knew a disabled man who had attempted suicide, however:

> He said, "Well, tonight I think I'm gonna do it. I think I'm gonna kill myself tonight." And everybody understood. Everyone went and hugged him and everything. . . . And so I think he took like about maybe 90 [Valiums]. He tried to kill himself. The next day about two or three o'clock he come rolling up, was so pissed off. [I] said, "What happened?" "It didn't work, I woke back up." Come to find out our bodies had become so immune to taking that kind of medication.

## Summary

Individuals with SCI encounter a wide range of health problems that complicate their lives. The secondary complications of SCI are both caused by and result in psychosocial distress, and they frequently interfere with individuals' social, vocational, and recreational lives. Because many of the physical difficulties associated with SCI cause social anxiety, physical discomfort, or a reliance on bed rest and inactivity, individuals who suffer these complications may become preoccupied with health concerns and withdrawn from society. In order to minimize or avert these conditions, the integration of problem-solving training into SCI rehabilitation may help individuals with SCI to attend better to their self-care regimens. The acceptance of responsibility for one's body has been viewed as a prerequisite for adapting to the physical changes inherent in spinal cord injury, and rehabilitation programs can play a key role in instilling healthy habits long before discharge (Trieschmann 1988, 1980).

Unfortunately, some of the individuals struggling with SCI are physically unable to care for their bodies on their own. In fact, several study participants—quadriplegics with high-level injuries—felt suicidal because they lacked the ability to manage their own health regimens and had encountered difficulties obtaining adequate caregiving services. Because the provision of attendant care services can be quite costly, some authors have argued in favor of group living programs that rely on shared attendant care (DeLoach and Greer 1981). Although independent living centers are emerging and beginning to receive government funding, individuals with chronic disabilities must become strong advocates for independent living (Staas et al. 1988). Ultimately, of course, most individuals with serious physical impairments simply want good-quality services that will allow them to live independently in their homes (Morris 1991). This chapter underscores the pressing need for effective responses to the challenge of providing affordable and quality attendant care for those with severe impairments.

# 3
# Psychological Adjustment and Rehabilitation

Adam is a white, 26-year-old quadriplegic man who uses a manual wheelchair. He and his brother Josh live in a four-bedroom house in a working-class neighborhood. Adam's six-year-old daughter Jessica also stays with him about five days each week. Their living room has a big television and two cages—one with a snake and another with rats. Adam told me that Josh periodically kills the rats and feeds them to the snake.

Adam is lanky and has reddish-orange hair, a bushy beard and a moustache. He is soft-spoken, with a somewhat reserved demeanor. He is politically liberal and tells me he is "a really open-minded person" who "likes to see proof." He considers himself somewhat of an atheist, and he told me that he admires Darwin and believes in evolution. "It always makes me nervous trying to explain that to people 'cause they usually try to argue with me."

When he was 20 years old, Adam was injured in a car accident when a large bale of hay fell off a truck and hit his car. The driver of the truck was cited for excessive speed and improperly containing his load; Adam received a settlement of approximately $175,000. He invested most of the money, but he also purchased the house where he currently lives. Adam described his initial reaction to his injury:

> I went through the whole, you know, "This shouldn't be happening to me." I was angry [at] the guy that put me in this position. I was upset because he hadn't taken the time to do what he should have done and I went through a lot of anger over that. But it only lasted about a week and I realized that being mad about it's really not going to change anything.

When I asked him if he experienced phases of denial, anger, and depression, he responded,

> No, I really didn't. I was pretty lucky with that. When I was in rehab we would have weekly sessions with a neuropsychologist. And he told me all of the stages that most people go through, but I really didn't feel that I went through any of 'em.

Adam told me that while alcoholism and suicide are rampant in his family, he had managed to escape these problems. In explaining how his injury affected him emotionally, he reflected,

> I would get more frustrated than angry. Just things that used to be simple everyday tasks that were now taking me half an hour to do, and there was a lot of frustration but I really wouldn't say anger.

Adam considers himself a happy person. He has many hobbies and especially enjoys watching movies and using his computer ("I kind of turned myself into a computer nerd"). He also relishes the time he spends with his little girl.

## Psychological Factors Influencing Adjustment

The sudden onset of disability is a major and unexpected challenge. "You're suddenly thrust into it, with all your able-bodied beliefs, attitudes and misconceptions" (Hammond et al. 1992: S13–3). In the case of spinal cord injury, individuals find that "they must learn to physically navigate a new world—one in which the erstwhile taken-for-granted world of everyday life becomes a burden of conscious and deliberate action" (Bury 1982: 176). The onset of disability often has a strong negative impact on subjective well-being, and some individuals with SCI lack the psychological resources needed to cope effectively (Bonwich 1985; Hampton 2004).

At the same time, however, each person's response to SCI is largely an individual matter. Those who were better at dealing with difficulties prior to their injuries tend to have greater success coping with their disabilities as well (Elliott and Frank 1996; Trieschmann 1980, 1988). Likewise, the capacity to adjust to a major disability is likely to depend on whether the change can be incorporated into the individual's worldview (Crewe 1997; Hammond et al. 1992; Stern and Slattery 1975; Wortman, Silver, and Kessler 1993). For some, spinal cord injury is a challenge to be circumvented—a facilitator of personal growth. For others, disability is an insurmountable barrier—evidence that the world is fundamentally unfair (Mayer and Kessler 1993; Wortman, Silver, and Kessler 1993). Still others accept their situations while making no attempt to minimize the significance of the disabilities they have incurred (Safilios-Rothschild 1970).[1] The individuals most successful in adjusting to their disabilities are often those who are best able to alter the criteria they use to assess their quality of life—those who are able to devalue less attainable goals while emphasizing those goals that remain (or have become) within reach (Drew-Cates 1989; Kemp and Vash 1971; Weitzenkamp et al. 2000).

A number of personality characteristics encourage a positive adjustment to spinal cord injury. These include a strong sense of self, determination, inner drive, independence, interpersonal assertiveness, aggressiveness, intellectual orientation, creativity, optimism, high ego strength and resilience, and the ability to pursue several goals simultaneously (Boekamp 1998; Dew et al. 1983; Drew 1997; Fox 1999; Livneh 2000; Trieschmann 1980; Tucker 1980). Sense of purpose is also a powerful predictor of adjustment to SCI (Thompson et al. 2004), and individuals who are adventurous and risk-taking seem to have energetic traits that assist in the adjustment process (Craig et al. 1990). Each person's history of exposure to stressful life events may also be important, since individuals who are repeatedly exposed to uncontrollable outcomes initially respond with anger or invigoration but also tend to become increasingly helpless over time (Silver and Wortman 1980).

Various indicators of neuroticism, including anxiety, hostility, and self-consciousness, are positively correlated with emotional distress and negatively associated with adjustment (Krause and Rohe 1998). Individuals who experience a weakened sense of coherence following their injuries tend to have greater problems adjusting (Lustig 2005), and those who make internal, stable, and generalized attributions for failure (e.g., inability to secure employment) are more likely to be depressed (Swanson 2000). As might be expected, individuals who place high value on bodily integrity, strength, and physical attractiveness tend to view their physical disabilities in especially negative terms (Safilios-Rothschild 1970).

Numerous studies demonstrate that individuals who feel in control of their lives have an easier time adjusting to SCI (Boschen 1996; Bracken and Bernstein 1980; Carroll 1999; Chase 1998; Craig et al. 1998; Craig, Hancock, and Dickson 1994; Crisp 1990; Dinardo 1971; Frank, Umlauf, et al. 1987; Fuhrer et al. 1992; Krause, Stanwyck, and Maides 1998; Livneh 2000; Livneh and Antonak 1997; Nunchuck 1991; Rodriguez 1991; Shadish, Hickman, and Arrick 1981; Smith 1984). There are a few contrary findings, however. Pelletier, Alfano, and Fink (1994) reported that the locus of control was unrelated to psychological health, and May (1999) found no relationship between perceived control and quality of life. Ferington (1986) concluded that locus of control is related to depression following SCI only if the individual perceives control to be an important element in his life. As might be expected, individuals with SCI who experience greater levels of helplessness are more likely to be depressed (Shnek 1995; Shnek et al. 1997), perhaps because of their inability to alleviate their own suffering (Seligman 1975). Attitudes toward uncertainty and appraisals of danger and opportunity are also closely linked to emotional well-being (Wineman, Durand, and Steiner 1994).

The ability to cope with stressful life events is more important than functional independence as a determinant of psychological well-being in the aftermath of spinal cord injury (Kennedy et al. 1995). Good problem-solving skills reduce the risk of depression and psychosocial impairment as well as the likelihood of secondary physical complications (Elliott 1999; Elliott, Godshall, et al. 1991; Godshall 1989; Herrick, Elliott, and Crow 1994a). Individuals who rely on positive cognitive reappraisal and engagement-type strategies (e.g., seeking social support) also show evidence of more favorable psychosocial adjustment (Barone 1993; Carroll 1999; Coca 1990; Livneh 2000). Overall, problem-focused coping (dealing with problems directly) is more effective than emotion-focused coping (dealing with the emotional reactions that accompany those problems) (Thoits 1995). While emotion-focused coping has been positively associated with sexual adjustment, it may hinder adjustment in the vocational, economic, and social arenas (Pollets 1975; Song 2005). Finally, the least effective coping strategies—behavioral disengagement, escape avoidance, and substance use—have been linked to depression and poor psychosocial adjustment (Kennedy et al. 2000; Livneh 2000).

## Demographic Factors Influencing Adjustment

Previous research has revealed few clear relationships between demographic variables and psychological adjustment to spinal cord injury. In at least some studies, however, the rate and effectiveness of adjustment have been linked to four demographic variables: gender, age at injury, severity of impairment, and time since injury.

## Gender

Many authors have found no association between gender and adjustment-related variables such as self-esteem, quality of life, life satisfaction, subjective well-being, perceived health, or rates of anxiety, depression, and denial (see, for example, Bombardier, Richards, et al. 2004; Carroll 1999; Cook 1979; Hampton 2004; Judd et al. 1989; Marini et al. 1995; Patterson 1989; Post, de Witte, et al. 1998; Post, Van Dijk, et al. 1998). Some research suggests, however, that females adjust better than males (Fitzgerald 1983), report less distress (Laatsch and Shahani 1996), and are more accepting of their disabilities (Woodrich 1982). At the same time, other studies have reported contrary results: that women may be more vulnerable to depression (Fuhrer et al. 1992; Fuhrer, Rintala, et al. 1993) and that they report lower satisfaction with health, more poor mental health days, and lower subjective well-being related to home life (Krause and Broderick 2004). Fuhrer and associates contend that women's poorer psychological well-being may be related to lower levels of mobility within the home and the community (Fuhrer et al. 1992; Fuhrer, Rintala, et al. 1993).

It is likely that gender influences quality of life chiefly through its interaction with other variables. For example, male quadriplegics tend to have higher quality-of-life scores than female quadriplegics, while male paraplegics score lower than female paraplegics (Carroll 1999). Although minority-group males report better emotional adjustment than minority-group females, Caucasian females report higher adjustment scores and fewer problems with physical discomfort (Krause and Anson 1997b). While African American women with SCI report more depressive symptoms and greater difficulty coping than their male counterparts, African American men report greater problems with pressure ulcers and sexual issues (Krause, Broderick, and Broyles 2004).

## Age at Injury

Most research suggests that individuals who become disabled at younger ages tend to have higher levels of well-being, possibly because the young are more flexible in their coping strategies and find it easier to alter their lifestyles (Brenner 1990; Cecka 1981; Craig et al. 1990; Decker and Schulz 1985; Kemp and Krause 1999; Oliver et al. 1988). Younger age at injury has also been positively linked to survival rates (Samsa, Patrick, and Feussner 1993). Contrary findings have also been reported, however. For example, Tate and associates (2004) concluded that those injured at younger ages are more vulnerable to alcohol abuse, and Fitzgerald (1983) found that older persons tend to adjust more effectively, perhaps because they have an established identity, a sense of self, and the maturity and ego strength to accept what happens to them. Another study comparing childhood-onset and adult-onset disability groups found no significant differences on any of the psychological measures examined (depression, self-esteem, etc.) (Kennedy, Gorsuch, and Marsh 1995).

## Severity of Impairment

Most authors report little or no association between severity of impairment (quadriplegia versus paraplegia, for example) and intensity of reaction or psychological well-being (Bombardier, Richards, et al. 2004; Carroll 1999; Cook 1979; Coyle, Lesnik-Emas, and Kinney 1994; Craig, Hancock, and Dickson 1994; Dias de Carvalho et al. 1998; Fox 1999; Fuhrer et al. 1992; Fullerton et al. 1981; Judd et al. 1989; Kemp and Krause 1999; Kennedy 2001; Kennedy, Gorsuch, and March 1995; Kishi, Robinson, and Forrester 1994, 1995; Marini et al. 1995; Shnek 1995; Shnek et al. 1997; Trieschmann 1980, 1988; Vash 1981; Ville et al. 2001; Zirpolo 1986). Ville and associates (2001) looked at individuals with quadriplegia and concluded that the degree of disability and the resulting loss of autonomy had no direct impact on feelings of well-being. Certain variables—the need for help in writing, for example—were linked to self-rated well-being only through their impact on other, social, variables.

Meanwhile, some researchers have documented more severe psychological impairment and a lower quality of life among paraplegics than among quadriplegics. (See, for example, Clayton 1992; McColl and Skinner 1996; Radnitz, Hsu, Williard, et al. 1998; Schultz 1985). While this may seem counterintuitive, it is possible that paraplegics occupy a marginal status between able-bodied and more severely disabled individuals—a difficult role to reconcile with decreased functional abilities (Schultz 1985). Paraplegics may also be more likely to cling to previous life aspirations—to find themselves frustrated with their inability to realize their pre-injury goals (McColl and

Skinner 1996). Individuals with different degrees of impairment tend to emphasize different aspects of their lives. For example, males with complete paraplegia tend to emphasize work and learning, whereas men with quadriplegia tend to emphasize socialization (Weitzenkamp et al. 2000).

In contrast, other studies have revealed a negative correlation between severity of disability and various quality-of-life measures (Clayton and Chubon 1994; Decker and Schulz 1985; Dinardo 1971; Evans et al. 1994; Judd and Brown 1992; Kasprzyk 1983; Krause and Dawis 1992; Pennell 1969; Tucker 1980). Some evidence suggests that more seriously impaired individuals exhibit more depression, higher anxiety levels and discomfort, more irritability, less satisfactory socialization, and greater use of denial as a defense mechanism (Dinardo 1971; Judd and Brown 1992; Melendez 1992; Tucker 1980). Those with more severe motor impairments are less likely to meet their goals and to develop positive coping strategies (Meyer 1998). Similarly, individuals who receive more instrumental support—those who depend most on others—tend to be less satisfied with their lives (Post, Ros, and Schrijvers 1999).

## Time Since Injury

Quite a few authors have found no association between time since injury and variables such as psychological distress, adjustment, or life satisfaction (Buckelew et al. 1990; Cook 1979; Coyle, Lesnik-Emas, and Kinney 1994; Craig, Hancock, and Dickson 1994; Crisp 1990; Dinardo 1971; Elliott, Witty, et al. 1991; Frank, Elliott, et al. 1987; Godshall 1989; Mackelprang 1986; Nagumo 2000; Post, de Witte, et al. 1998; Post, Van Dijk, et al. 1998; Putzke et al. 2004; Schultz 1985; Scivoletto et al. 1997; Whiteneck 1993).

There has been some debate about psychosocial adjustment in the period immediately following discharge from the hospital, however. Some authors have found that the transition from hospital living to community living is associated with psychosocial difficulties (Marini et al. 1995; Povolny 1993; Scivoletto et al. 1997). For example, Tate, Maynard, and Forenheimer (1993) reported that psychological distress is higher one year post-injury than during the period of inpatient rehabilitation. Povolny (1993) asserts that many individuals with SCI experience a decline in self-esteem and perceived social support as they make the adjustment from hospital living to community living. In the rehabilitation hospital, the individual is likely to have visitors and to receive attention and reassurance from hospital staff. Once discharged, however, the reality of disability becomes more apparent. Marini and associates (1995) found that self-esteem is lower in the second post-injury year than during the period of hospitalization but that it increases in subsequent years.

Meanwhile, several authors have reported that subjective quality of life and well-being improve over time (Bracken and Bernstein 1980; Dijkers 1996; Duggan and Dijkers 2001; Fitzgerald 1983; Kemp and Krause 1999; Kennedy et al. 2000; Krause and Crewe 1991; Krause and Sternberg 1997; Livneh and Martz 2003; McColl and Skinner 1996; Richards 1986; Shadish, Hickman, and Arrick 1981). As time passes, individuals with SCI are more likely to seek information about their conditions (Buckelew et al. 1990), to accept their disabilities (Livneh and Martz 2003; Woodrich 1982), and to find renewed satisfaction in their lives (Boekamp, Overholser, and Schubert 1996; Crewe and Krause 1990; Gerhart et al. 1997; Livneh and Martz 2003; Oliver et al. 1988). They are also less likely to experience emotional distress, feelings of disbelief, confusion, depression, or anger (Krause and Sternberg 1997; Livneh and Martz 2003).

Some researchers have found that the association between time since injury and psychosocial well-being varies with the indicator used. For example, Elliott and associates found that time since injury is associated with psychosocial adjustment but unrelated to depression or the likelihood of being assertive (Elliott, Godshall, et al. 1991; Elliott, Herrick, et al. 1991). Likewise, Krause (1998a) reported that duration of injury is positively linked to objective measures of well-being (employment, education, etc.) but not to subjective measures of well-being (positive feelings, etc.).

## Environmental Factors Influencing Adjustment

Individuals' adjustments to disability are based not only on internal factors such as gender, age, self-efficacy, and coping style, but on external factors such as prevailing attitudes and the level of social support (Galvin and Godfrey 2001; Kennedy 2001). An increasing number of authors in the field of disability studies argue that hardship results not from functional limitations, but from the disabling characteristics of the physical, psychological, and social environments (Barnes 1990; Barnes, Mercer, and Shakespeare 1999; Linton 1998; Oliver 1990, 1993c, 1996a, 1996b, 1996c; Susman 1994; Swain et al. 1993; Trieschmann 1980, 1988; White 1983).[2] According to

Trieschmann (1980: 161), there is no evidence that the onset of spinal cord injury leads to psychological problems *per se*. Rather, the major difficulties are "problems of learning to live in an environment designed for able-bodied people." An effective response to disability therefore requires at least three kinds of adjustments: adjustments to changes in physiological functioning, adjustments to changes in others' perceptions, and adjustments to changes in the social and economic opportunities available (Linton 1998).

The interaction between individuals' characteristics and the environment is also important, since a number of situational factors (including economic resources, access to education, adequate help at home, satisfaction with employment status, independent living, mobility, transportation, and community integration) have been linked to the likelihood of a favorable psychological response (see, for example, Duggan and Dijkers 2001; Hammell 2004a; Whiteneck et al. 2004). As Finkelstein and French assert, external conditions should "be seen as providing the context for personal mood states and psychological reactions" (1993: 32).

## Stages of Adjustment and Recovery

*Stage theory*—the idea that individuals cope with the transition to disabled status through a series of defined and predictable stages—is well-established within the literature on spinal cord injury (Dunn 1975b; Parrott, Stuart, and Cairns 2000; Singleton 1985; Weller and Milller 1977a; Wortman and Silver 1992; Wortman, Silver, and Kessler 1993). Although there are several different formulations of the model, the most often identified stages include (1) shock, (2) anxiety/depression, (3) denial, (4) anger, and (5) adaptation. Not all reactions are present in every individual, and the phases may overlap and fluctuate as well as vary in order and length (Livneh and Antonak 1997; Weller and Miller 1977a). Most stage theorists also acknowledge that the nature, structure, pace, and duration of the adaptation process is conditioned by both personal characteristics and situational factors (Bracken and Shepard 1980; Livneh and Antonak 1997).[3]

At the same time, however, other authors view stage theory as an oversimplification. They underscore the impact of individual differences in perception, coping, and adjustment (Allden 1992; Barnes 1990; Cairns and Baker 1993; Cunningham 1986; DeLoach and Greer 1981; Elliott and Frank 1996; Frank, Elliott, et al. 1987; Frank, Umlauf, et al. 1987; Galvin and Godfrey 2001; Hayes, Potter, and Hardin 1995; Hohmann 1975; Kennedy 2001; Oliver 1983; Silver and Wortman 1980; Trieschmann 1980, 1988, 1989; Wortman and Silver 1992; Wortman, Silver, and Kessler 1993). As Bracken and Shepard (1980) and Kennedy (2001) point out, there has been little empirical validation of the sequence, duration, or existence of the various stages; little evidence that they are helpful in promoting adjustment; and even less consensus about what each stage represents. Moreover, the expectations associated with stage theory may cause unnecessary stress among individuals with SCI by suggesting that certain responses are inappropriate or abnormal (Kennedy 2001).

Stage theories (also called *personal tragedy theories*) have come under further attack for failing to pay heed to the economic, political, and social factors that shape adjustment, and for ignoring disabled individuals' subjective interpretations of impairment (Barnes 1990; Barnes, Mercer, and Shakespeare 1999; Oliver 1983, 1993b, 1996b). Both health care providers and the general population tend to have negative and unrealistic impressions of how most individuals with physical disabilities respond to their impairments. In particular, they tend to underestimate the coping abilities of people in times of crisis (French 1996; Taylor 1967; Trieschmann 1980, 1988; Weinberg 1988). As Linton notes, "Explicating the neutral, ordinary, and even the positive aspects of the disability experience that many disabled people have expressed is akin to debunking the myth of penis envy" (1998: 100).

While stage theory has been at least partly discredited in recent years, the five most characteristic responses to SCI—shock, anxiety/depression, denial, anger, and adaptation—have nonetheless provided a useful framework for many of the scholars who have written on this topic.

## Shock

The transition from physical ability to total or partial paralysis has been described as "among the most shocking of all human experiences" (Bracken and Shepard 1980: 77). Heightened rates of psychological distress are common, and serious psychological morbidity is a reality for many during the acute period of rehabilitation (Judd and Brown 1992). During the early phase of disablement, many individuals with SCI experience an intense sense of disorganization, dependency, and loss (Ducharme and Ducharme 1985; Duggan and Dijkers 1999). The sense of grief and loss may be comparable to how one feels upon losing a close friend or family member (Hammond et al. 1992; Safilios-Rothschild 1970). Shock reactions to SCI may even be triggered years after the injury, often in response to major life changes (Martz 2004).

## Anxiety and Depression

Individuals with SCI have relatively high rates of psychological distress and depression, as well as lower levels of subjective well-being in comparison with the general population (see, for example, Boekamp, Overholser, and Schubert 1996; Coyle et al. 1993; Craig, Hancock, and Chang 1994; Decker and Schulz 1985; Fuhrer, Rintala, et al. 1993; Hanson et al. 1993; Kemp and Krause 1999; Leduc and Lepage 2002; Mattlar et al. 1993; Schulz and Decker 1985; Tate, Kewman, and Maynard 1990). They also show elevated rates of phobic anxiety, obsessive-compulsive disorders, and somatization (Tate, Kewman, and Maynard 1990) as well as feelings of inadequacy, devaluation, insecurity, distress, tension, helplessness, and ruminative self-introspection (Dunn 1975a; Mattlar et al. 1993).

During the first post-injury year, many individuals with SCI show evidence of maladaptive coping styles, low self-esteem, and an external locus of control (Hancock, Craig, Tennant, and Chang 1993). One first-year study revealed that 25% of individuals with SCI were anxious, compared to just 3% in a nondisabled control group (Hancock, Craig, Dickson, et al. 1993). Several authors have documented elevated rates of depression in the acute phase of traumatic SCI (Frank et al. 1985; Fullerton et al. 1981; Judd et al. 1989), and approximately 20% to 45% of individuals with SCI become clinically depressed within the first year of spinal cord injury. This can be compared to an annual rate of 5% to 10% within the general population (Boekamp, Overholser, and Schubert 1996; Hancock, Craig, Dickson, et al. 1992).[4] One year post injury, 23% of individuals with SCI have no depressive symptoms, 35% have minimal depressive symptoms, 20% have mild depressive symptoms, 22% have moderate or severe symptoms, and 11% show signs of major depressive disorders (Bombardier, Richards, et al. 2004).

There is considerable debate about the extent to which disability-related depression extends beyond the acute phase of treatment. However, depression that lasts beyond the rehabilitation phase is generally considered pathological (Cook 1976; Knorr and Bull 1970).[5] While an early study of individuals with SCI revealed rates of anxiety and depression no higher than those found within the general population (Cook 1979), later research has documented elevated rates of denial and mild depression (Craig et al. 1990; Fuhrer, Rintala, et al. 1993). Recent work suggests that between 12% and 50% of those with SCI suffer from depression, with most estimates hovering between 20% and 45% (Coyle et al. 1993; Craig, Hancock, and Chang 1994; Kemp, Krause, and Adkins 1999; Livneh and Antonak 1996, 1997). While these figures are considerably higher than the rates reported for the general population, most individuals with SCI do not feel that depression is a major problem (Elliott and Shewchuk 2002).

Although some authors have asserted that depression and grief are necessary for healthy adjustment to severe disability (Woodbury 1978), this notion has never been substantiated (Frank, Elliott, et al. 1987; Sullivan 1990b; Trieschmann 1980, 1988, 1989). While situational depression in the acute phase of treatment is not unusual (Cook 1976; Knorr and Bull 1970), some evidence suggests that this depression may be attributed at least partly to the expectations of rehabilitation professionals (Schweinberg 1995).

## Denial

Denial is a common responses to spinal cord injury. It may be viewed as a stage in the mourning process, or as a defense mechanism used to ward off anxiety. In the immediate aftermath of SCI, denial may also be associated with the sensory deprivation (monotony, inadequate sleep, etc.) that sometimes accompanies hospitalization (Trieschmann 1980, 1980, 1989). Some authors have found that denial is associated with poorer adjustment outcomes, including post-traumatic distress symptoms (Lude et al. 2005; Zirpolo 1986) whereas others have argued that denial is an adaptive strategy important to survival (Livneh and Antonak 1997).

While early researchers believed that failure to face the consequences of injury slowed down the rehabilitation process (Nemiah 1957), a number of scholars have suggested that denial plays a positive role in helping individuals cope with the immediate effects of trauma. Individuals with SCI who adamantly claim they will walk out of the hospital may be expressing hope rather than denial (Trieschmann 1989), and some forms of denial may enhance rehabilitation outcomes by motivating disabled individuals to "get well" (Langer 1994; Safilios-Rothschild 1970). The accompanying danger, however, is that these individuals will ultimately lose interest in rehabilitation once they realize they cannot fully reclaim their previous levels of functioning and fitness. Denial can also become a negative factor when it extends beyond the rehabilitation period, since it is then often accompanied by severe depression (Bracken and Bernstein 1980; Bracken and Shepard 1980).

## Anger

Anger is a common, but by no means universal, response to chronic disability. It can be internalized, externalized, or both. Internalized anger may be viewed as a manifestation of self-directed resentment and bitterness, whereas externalized anger may be viewed as an attempt to retaliate against imposed functional limitations (Livneh and Antonak 1997). Externalized anger is directed at persons, objects, or aspects of the environment believed to be associated with the disability. In some cases, externalized hostility may represent a struggle for self-determination (DeLoach and Greer 1981).

## Adaptation

Most individuals with SCI adjust to their injuries and do not experience long-term psychological difficulties (Kennedy 2001; Kennedy, Hopwood, and Duff, 2001). Over time, they are likely to accept their disabilities and to express positive attitudes toward their life goals (Cook 1982; Hammell 2004b; Livneh and Martz 2003). Although the average psychological well-being indices are lower among individuals with SCI than their nondisabled counterparts (Whiteneck 1993), the overwhelming majority of individuals with SCI are satisfied with the quality of their lives, hold optimistic views about their future prospects, and have relatively high levels of self-esteem and well-being (Charlifue and Gerhart 2004; Reitz et al. 2004; Roessler 1978; Whiteneck 1993). Many individuals with SCI present lighthearted or even comical narratives about their disabilities, and relatively few seem to hold hopeless or negative attitudes (Crewe 1997). On some indicators, individuals with SCI exhibit even better psychological well-being than the general population (Green, Pratt, and Grigsby 1984). This is especially true of military veterans with spinal cord injuries (Radnitz 1996; Radnitz, Hsu, Tirch, et al. 1998).

## Adjusting to Life with a Spinal Cord Injury

The narratives of my study participants are consistent with much of the previous research in this area. For most of the people I interviewed, the period immediately following their injuries had been fraught with turmoil, and several described how they had entered a state of disbelief upon learning about their disabilities. Walter, who reportedly had been thrown out of a three-story window after he had passed out one night, described how he had responded to learning he was a paraplegic:

> I was in a coma for 21 days. And I came out, after the heavy medication I was on, I tried to get out of bed and it's like, "No, you're paralyzed," and I'm like, "No, what? No!" I was in denial for a long time. I thought that there was a plot. [*laughter*] But eventually I came to and I figured I can lie here and die or I can get better.

Meghan, who had been injured in a car accident, responded in a similar manner:

> I always thought it would have to be a phase. It just couldn't go on . . . so I guess I was in some sort of in denial. . . . They kept telling me in rehab, "You're gonna be like this for the rest of your life; you better get used to it." And I kept saying, "Well, I'm gonna walk."

In most cases, the goal of walking is gradually replaced with the objective of making small, feasible gains toward independence (Morse and Doberneck 1995).

Many of the people I spoke with described periods of intense emotional turbulence immediately following their injuries. For example, Stacy reported,

> I freaked out at the beginning. I definitely went through the five stages of grief. I can just picture them of how, like first I was just in denial and then I got really mad, then I got really depressed, and I was there for a while. I was on a lot of depression medication. . . . I was just like, "Why me?" And I was mad at God sometimes. I would be upset that it happened to me and not someone else.

The "Why me?" phase is routine among patients with spinal cord injury (Bulman and Wortman 1977; Dunn 1975a; Hammond et al. 1992; Stewart and Rossier 1978), and quite a few of those I spoke with described how they had asked the same question after realizing they were permanently disabled. Paul, who had been injured in a swimming accident, described his reaction:

> I got a little depressed when it first happened. Not really [right away] but maybe after I got out of rehab. Because when it first happened there were all these people around, you had nurses and doctors, and you really didn't have time to think. And in rehab they kept you busy, but when I got back home . . . I didn't really like to sit in the house . . . so I would go outside and be by myself out there. I went through a little period of "Why me?"

Conversely, a few had made a conscious effort to avoid questioning why they had sustained their injuries. Travis, who had been injured as a result of a motorcycle accident, described the advice his father gave him:

> My dad told me early on, "You can ask 'Why me?' all you want to, but you're not ever gonna get a satisfactory answer even if you do get an answer." And he said, "I don't know who you thinks gonna give you an answer." He said, "You got to figure out what you're gonna do with your life."

Travis seemed to be taking his father's wisdom to heart. Stan, who had been injured in a diving accident, also felt that it was counterproductive to question the root cause of his injury. "You start going down that road, you don't have answers," he said.

## The Process of Recovery

While no single trajectory of recovery characterizes all the study participants, most reported that they had gone through one or more stages of grief and had experienced varying degrees of sadness, isolation, and frustration. For most of them, the frequency and intensity of this emotional turmoil waned over time, yet for many the ongoing challenges associated with SCI continued to cause considerable stress. For example, when I asked Fred if he had gone through the various stages of grief, he replied, "I've hit every one of 'em. I still have 'em." Similarly, Harry stated, "I wouldn't wish this on anybody. That's how bad it is." When I asked Travis about the stages of grief, he reflected,

> I've talked to numerous people about this and most people would like to claim that they don't, but I think every person I've ever known very well has gone through it. And it's really weird to think that somebody sat down in a laboratory and said, "Okay, this is what people go through and these people go through these stages." And you know that you're going to go through these stages but you still go through 'em. It's like an inevitability. You can't stop it. . . . Some people stay in one stage longer or shorter or to varying degrees.

Stan, like a number of the other participants, had sunk into depression when he fully realized that his impairment was permanent. His diving injury had occurred during the summer, and he became very depressed when school resumed in the fall.

> School started and I wasn't in school with my classmates—now that's when I kind of realized that this may be a permanent situation. And that's when I, you know, hit bottom. I felt real bad. Did a lot of crying and stuff like that. Never was angry.

Jennifer reported that she had experienced only some of the stages of grief:

> I don't think I really went through the denial part. I did go through I guess you would call mourning. I had days when I was angry, like when it was a really bad day and something had happened but I never really had it for more than one day. . . . I don't think I'll ever really accept it. I just deal with it.

Leonard said that he had experienced anger, depression, and an acute sense of helplessness in the immediate aftermath of his injury. "It was stressful for sure," he said. "It put me out of control, 'cause I was always kind of a control-type person."

After returning home from rehabilitation, several of the participants in the study—particularly those who had been injured in their early teens—

described how they had become withdrawn and uncomfortable with the prospect of interacting with others. For example, Jennifer said,

> For a while I was, I wouldn't say depressed, but I didn't want to go anywhere and I didn't want to see anybody and I think it got better when I eventually went back to school and started interacting with people again.

> EIW: And in terms of going through the mourning, how long do you think that lasted?

> I think the major part of it at least a year and then it wasn't until I got out of high school and started going to college that I started to want to do stuff and get out in public.

Adolescents who return to school may be particularly sensitive to role changes and especially self-conscious about their image (Mulcahey 1992).

Many of the people I interviewed reported ongoing emotional struggles, which they attributed to a variety of physical and social factors, including limited mobility, physical complications, socioeconomic conditions, and psychosocial disruptions. For example, when I asked Edward how his disability affected his life on a daily basis, he responded:

> Depends on my mood. I'm in a happy mood, it don't bother me too much. If I'm not, then I get depressed. I guess you could say I'm probably depressed every day but sometimes it ain't as bad as others.

He reported that his depression was related to

> not being able to do what I used to do—get up and walk across the room. . . . Just little stuff. Everything. Playing volleyball. Going to the creek, walking around, whatever.

Similarly, Shannon reported,

> I'm sure I got angry every now and then because I couldn't do the things I wanted to do. It really changes your life. . . . Just your physical limitations—like I can't go visit you because I can't get up steps. . . . Just getting around in the world is a lot harder.

Several of those I spoke with were depressed as a result of all the secondary physical complications they had experienced. For example, Fred was battling recurrent pressure sores and struggling with his weight. He described his mood:

> I've got depression. My aunt knows me, what's going on with me: "You're too quiet, you're not eating. You're irritable." And I try not to be irritable with anybody, especially her. She's a very special person taking me on. . . . These last two years were miserable.

Jay, who as a child had been able to "walk" with crutches by swinging his legs back and forth, felt that his mood had changed as he gradually lost his physical stamina. When I asked him if he ever felt as though he was depressed because of his disability, he responded:

> More so in the last couple of years since I've been in the wheelchair. I'm depressed about it, but still try to make the best of what I can. There's a possibility of me getting back up into crutches like I used to, but even that's looking not that great.

A few study participants who seemed depressed also appeared to be neglecting their health. Self-neglect is prevalent among approximately 10% of individuals with SCI and may be symptomatic of a major depressive disorder or reflect a clear and rational desire to die (Macleod 1988). It commonly manifests itself in self-destructive and noncompliant behavior (Craig et al. 1990). For example, Travis had several open wounds on his feet and seemed almost oblivious to them. At one point during our interview, his dog came over and licked at the blood on his feet, but Travis seemed unfazed. Travis also seemed to feel that his disability had "brought him down a notch." It wasn't that he was seriously depressed; he just wasn't contented:

> Overall, my disability has probably caused me to be a little bit less happy in certain situations and aggravated with certain situations, but overall I don't think my disability's made me an unhappy person. I'm just not real giddy.

Meanwhile, several of the people I spoke with described how they had successfully overcome various disability-related episodes of depression in the past. For example, Vibha had experienced particular problems when she had gone home to India:

> I had a problem to cope with my disability at one time and as a consequence of that I was in a deep depression. I felt like I couldn't go anywhere, couldn't do anything on my own, and I felt very stagnant in my situation.

Similarly, Meghan described how she had fallen into a depression shortly after she graduated from college:

> I went into a depression so I had to go back to the rehab center. . . . The doctor who I initially had when I went there when I first broke my neck said, "Meghan, you're not the same." And I wanted to talk to somebody. . . . [I told the doctor], "I don't plan on doing anything but these thoughts have been coming in my mind like . . . 'You can pull that heater over and burn this house down.'"

Both Vibha and Meghan reported that they were able to work through their depression with support from counselors.

## Smooth Transitions

A substantial minority of people are able to deal with SCI and other physical impairments without psychological turmoil (Cairns and Baker 1993; Martin and Gandy 1990; Wortman and Silver 1992). It may be that such people have something in place beforehand—perhaps a religion, a philosophical orientation, or a certain worldview—that mitigates the effects of loss (Wortman and Silver 1992). Over half a dozen individuals in my sample—primarily those who had been injured at young ages—reported that the transition from ability to disability had been relatively free of emotional turmoil. Ryan, who had been injured in a car accident when he was seven, reported,

> Emotionally, it didn't hurt me at all. . . . There were times when I realized, "Oh wait, I can't do the same things other kids do," but I lived in a small town and so all the kids at school got used to me and so after a while it was just like, "Oh, it's just Ryan. He's just an

everyday person." I knew there were still some limitations, but I was just ready to get on [with] life. I was happy. I'm glad the accident happened to me at a younger age. Had it happened when I was in my teens or older, even in my twenties, there would have been a depression stage afterwards. Had I been older or had a girlfriend or been a football star or anything it really would have depressed me.

Ryan felt that it was easier to adjust to a disability acquired at a younger age because children have not "yet had time to establish themselves." Likewise, Jonathan (also injured in a car accident at age seven) reported a smooth adjustment: "I might not be any happier if I wasn't in a wheelchair."

In addition to those who were injured as children, a handful of study participants who had become disabled as adults felt that their adjustments were relatively free of emotional turmoil. Most of these individuals appeared to be optimistic individuals with a positive outlook on life. Cody, who had been shot by his wife's boyfriend, reported:

> I can't say I was depressed but I guess I'm sort of a go-with-the-flow kind of guy so I don't think I was dep[ressed]. I don't think it really affected me in that [way].

Similarly, Shannon, who had been injured when she lost control of her car and drove into a culvert, said that she had "handled it very well" and never went through a depression.

A few participants who were very pragmatic also reported that their injuries had minimal emotional impact. When Ben sustained a spinal cord injury in a motorcycle accident, he became focused on the practical aspects of adjustment to his disability:

> I wasn't angry and I don't think I was depressed. I was mainly just concerned with, "How you gonna get yourself out of this one?" [*chuckle*]

Likewise, Brad felt that it was more important to get on with his life:

> I never really remember being real sad or anything like that. I thought, "Well, that's just what's happened, that's what dealt with me and I'll go on." I'm not gonna cry. Well I did cry. [*laughter*] That's

silly not to say that. But I don't recall dwelling on it or feeling sorry for myself.

## Happiness and Life Satisfaction

While it is commonly assumed—even among health care providers—that individuals with SCI have a very low quality of life, there is considerable evidence that challenges this assumption (Bamford, Grundy, and Russell 1986; Bristo and Burgdorf 1998; Duggan and Dijkers 1999; Frank, Elliott, et al. 1987; Karp and Klein 2004; Weinberg 1988). Only 19% of the study participants disagreed with the statement "I am a happy person," while 81% agreed either *strongly* or *somewhat.*

Similar proportions of men (80%) and women (86%) agreed that they were happy. Those with paraplegia and high-level quadriplegia reported the lowest levels of happiness, while quadriplegics who used manual wheelchairs tended to be the happiest. These results suggest that quadriplegics who rely on manual wheelchairs do not occupy the marginal status that paraplegics do. They are fully cognizant of the need to adjust their goals and aspirations in response to their injuries, yet more independent than quadriplegics who rely on power wheelchairs. Within my sample, those injured within the past five years were the least happy, but there was little variation in happiness after five years. This is consistent with Krause and Crewe's (1991) assertion that individuals with SCI reach a plateau of adjustment after two years.

The high levels of happiness reported here reinforce earlier research showing that 75% of individuals with spinal cord injury rated their quality of life as either *good* or *excellent* (Whiteneck et al. 1992). At the same time, these results are somewhat surprising in light of the complaints about depression and frustration that so many of them registered. Nonetheless, my study participants confirmed that by and large, they are at peace with their disabilities and contented with their lives. In discussing how his disability had affected his life, Jeremy reported,

Everybody [says], "Well, what do you do to cope with being on disability or something?" I don't do nothing. It's a different life. It's something that you say, "Well, that part of my life is over. This is a new part.". . . . Time is the best therapy. Because time goes on and on and you very seldom think about it. Maybe three times a year as opposed to every single minute of the day, okay. [*laughter*]

In general, the individuals who registered the lowest levels of happiness seemed most preoccupied with how their lives had changed in the aftermath of their injuries. For example, Edward reported that he is not a happy person, attributing his unhappiness wholly to his disability:

> I don't see how anybody can be happy with a spinal cord injury. It totally changes your life around—totally and completely. Breathing's different. My chest is still partially paralyzed. I can't take a normal breath. I only sweat on one side and if I overheat it takes a long time for me to cool down. I can get real bad headaches and it just drains me to be out in the sun. Just everything. I love to swim, I haven't been swimming . . . because I never had the real opportunity to and my legs are so skinny I don't like anybody to see. I mean, friends and family, that's OK. But I'm not gonna go out in public.

Derrick was also "not happy being disabled," and Roger felt that his spinal cord injury had negatively affected his disposition:

> I used to have people comment, "You laugh all the time." [*chuckle*] And I still laugh, but it's very short and far and few between. The things that I used to do that make me happy I can't do anymore. I used to love to build something and when I was finished with it, turn around and look at it and say, "I did that." I can't do that anymore.

Race and ethnicity have also been identified as key factors in understanding adjustment to spinal cord injury, but the low minority representation in my sample (three blacks, one Asian, two American Indians, and one Latino) precluded an in-depth analysis of this topic. Nonetheless, the minority members of my sample were more likely than whites to indicate high levels of happiness; all seven agreed either *somewhat* or *strongly* that they were happy people. Meanwhile, previous research suggests that whites report higher subjective well-being with regard to finances and employment (Krause and Broderick 2004). While some evidence suggests that minorities are at increased risk for specific SCI-related health problems (see Chapter 2), other research has revealed no relationship between health variables and race/ethnicity (Johnston et al. 2004; Krause and Broderick 2004).

A number of minority individuals told me that discrimination on the basis of race/ethnicity was more salient to them than discrimination on the basis of disability. Meghan expressed this view, adding that

If I hadn't the experience of being African American, I never would have survived being disabled. . . . It prepared me for being isolated, for being thought of as ignorant, stupid. It prepared me for all of that.

While Jeremy initially told me that being black was associated with more prejudice and discrimination than being disabled, he later revised his statement and said that this depended on where one lived.

## Therapeutic Intervention and Rehabilitation

Effective therapeutic interventions for spinal cord injury should facilitate the management of emotional concerns, maximize rehabilitation potential, and minimize general psychosocial disruption (Kennedy 2001). While the appropriate course of rehabilitation is different for each individual, the techniques of traditional psychotherapy, group psychotherapy, behavior therapy, psychiatry, hypnotherapy, biofeedback, and behavioral medicine have all been shown to be effective (Jubala and Brenes 1988; Kennedy 2001).

Many scholars in the field of disability studies have argued for a distinction between the medical and educational models of rehabilitation (Trieschmann 1988, 1989; Vash 1981). The former emphasizes the organic physiology of individuals and looks at the role of personality problems (e.g., depression, anger) in generating organic complications. Meanwhile, the educational model of rehabilitation emphasizes the need to teach individuals to adjust to living with their disabilities. The medical model emphasizes counseling and therapy while the educational model focuses on active participation in the rehabilitation process. According to Trieschmann (1989), the medical model is appropriate during the acute-injury phase, but the learning model, which emphasizes environmental influences, is more appropriate during rehabilitation.

Researchers have also stressed the importance of cognitive therapeutic approaches that emphasize personal empowerment and are goal-oriented (Boekamp, Overholser, and Schubert 1996; Craig, Hancock, and Dickson 1994; Frank, Umlauf, et al. 1987; Frost 1993; Galvin and Godfrey 2001; King and Kennedy 1999; Roessler, Milligan, and Ohlson 1976; Trieschmann 1989; Vash 1981). Strategic approaches that focus on problem resolution and capitalize on the strengths and assets of each individual are likely to be especially effective (Cunningham 1986).[6] It is also important that each rehabilitant be actively involved in the rehabilitation process and act as an agent of change rather than a passive object in the hands of the rehabilitation team (Fordyce 1976; Safilios-Rothschild 1970, 1976; Trieschmann 1988). Just as behavioral therapy techniques may help promote physical rehabilitation, training in social skills and assertiveness may help individuals with disabilities to cope with a frequently hostile world. Ellis (1997) recommends that individuals use Rational Emotive Behavior Therapy (REBT) techniques—anti-victimization, unconditional self-accepting philosophies—to cope with disability.

While some favor behavioral therapy over group therapy (Trieschmann 1989), many people, including both patients and therapists, find group therapy to be a valuable means of promoting adjustment, leisure satisfaction, and improved quality of life (Daniel and Manigandan 2005; Fow and Rockey 1995; Jubala and Brenes 1988). Vash (1981) argues that group approaches are often especially effective within the educational model of rehabilitation. Other authors have found that structured group therapy is effective in promoting social connectivity and self-esteem among individuals with SCI but that it has a less meaningful impact on productivity, social functioning, locus of control, or life satisfaction (Frank 1992; Galvin and Godfrey 2001). Individual psychotherapy remains the method of choice when treating depression among individuals with SCI (McAweeney, Tate, and McAweeney 1997).

Along with therapeutic services for individuals with SCI, there is often a need for family counseling, independent living training, vocational training, recreation and leisure training, and physical fitness training (Roessler, Milligan, and Ohlson 1976). Other treatment modalities may also be helpful. Meditation, for example, has been shown to promote a sense of calmness and contentment (Trieschmann 2001) and to reduce the incidence of muscle spasms and mobility impairments (Anthony 1985). Exercise and participation in sports have been linked to independence in self-care activities, the avoidance of secondary complications (e.g., decubitus ulcers, pain, and muscle atrophy), reduced rates of depression and pain, and improvements in physical self-concept and overall quality of life (see, for example, Anderson 1982; Dallmeijer and van der Woude 2001; Ginis et al. 2003; Glaser et al. 1996; Katz et al. 1985).

Today, many researchers agree that optimal management of SCI requires a multidisciplinary approach that addresses the patient's physical, psychological, social, educational, vocational, financial, and recreational needs (Ragnarsson and Gordon 1992). The process of team collaboration is critical in establishing strong links in the continuum of care and in producing successful outcomes, including community reintegration (Fox, Anderson, and McKinley 1996; Ragnarsson and Gordon 1992). Moreover, exposure to people with similar disabilities is considered beneficial in terms of modeling and emotional support (see Chapter 8). For example, peer mentoring is associated with greater occupational activity among individuals with SCI (Riggin 1976; Sherman, DeVinney, and Sperling 2004). Cadre network programs, in which individuals who have been successfully integrated into the community provide guidance and support for those more recently injured, are another possible strategy for promoting social integration (Riggin 1976; Wilson and Thompson 1983).[7]

## Counseling and Support

The majority of study participants reported that they had received some form of therapeutic intervention. This intervention was almost always based on the medical model, with its emphasis on counseling and discussion, and most often occurred during rehabilitation or shortly thereafter. (For a discussion of sexual counseling, see Chapter 4.) Several reported that counseling had been a waste of time, largely due to the perceived incompetence of the therapists. For example, Shannon said,

> I don't have a lot of faith [*laughs as she says "faith"*] in psychologists, psychiatrists, or whatever they call themselves. The very beginning when I'm in the hospital and still healing and not really well, a psychologist or whatever he was would come in and he would just sit there, and not even ask me questions. . . . I got real angry at him for not even trying to do anything! I mean, he didn't speak. One day I just said, "You might as well quit coming because I don't like paying for something I'm not getting." I mean, I got nothing from him.

When I asked Shannon what might made the counseling worthwhile, she responded, "If he had talked, it would have been helpful. [*laughter*]"

Many individuals with disabilities report that they spend too much time educating their counselors about the challenges they face (Withers 1996). Perhaps as a result of this, approximately half a dozen study participants emphasized the importance of having a counselor with SCI. As Derrick said,

More counselors need to be paraplegics and quadriplegics. That's what needs to happen. . . . My God, you have to be in this position to understand.

Derrick was considering become a counselor himself. Indeed, individuals with disabilities who are employed in the health and caring professions often believe that being disabled helps them to empathize better with their patients and understand the social and psychological implications of disability (French 1993b). Like Derrick, Jeremy felt he was unable to connect with his counselor:

It was a complete joke. . . . 'Cause I sat and I talked to this counselor and you're sitting there and she's walking around and stuff like that so she can't relate. She didn't have a clue what was going on. They think they do but they don't because they're not [in a wheelchair].

Todd reported,

I think if you could hook up with somebody in a chair, regardless of what they're doing, it helps out. You sure don't want someone able-bodied telling you, "I can understand." [*laughter*]

Leonard said that the best counselor he'd encountered had a spinal cord injury and had been "in a chair" for fifteen years, so he spoke from experience.

Of course, counselors with disabilities can also be unhelpful. Andrew described his experience with a counselor at the rehabilitation center:

It seemed like she was upset or something because I was handling everything on the surface pretty well. And she was also in a wheelchair and she had more of a bitter chip on her shoulder kind of attitude and so she started telling me that I couldn't have that many family members come to visit me at the rehab center. . . . She said that it was bringing other patients down because they didn't have anybody coming to visit them.

Andrew felt she may have been jealous of the attention he was receiving.

At the same time, several individuals described positive experiences with able-bodied counselors. Those who reported favorable results emphasized that their therapists had provided support and helpful advice. In describing his counselor, Brad said, "He was a nice guy, I liked [him] and I came by to shoot shit with him." Likewise, Edward felt his rehabilitation counselor was someone who "relaxed you and put you at ease, and he was pretty cool." Vibha's counselor had helped her work through some of the psychological turmoil she had encountered in the immediate aftermath of her injury:

> She helped me realize one thing: that it's something I cannot blame God for. I was full of blame at that time. And I was pretty hard on myself. My self-esteem was very low.

She said her therapist had helped her to let go of the anger and self-hatred, and to "see things in a different perspective."

The majority of the people I interviewed reported minimal or no contact with psychological counselors in the post-rehabilitation period. By that time, many had learned to draw upon other sources of emotional and instrumental support such as family, friends, and the local SCI association. The SCI group also provided a safe haven for individuals to share their concerns, participate in social and recreational activities, and learn ways to overcome the challenges of living with SCI.

## Summary

Most study participants first responded to their disabilities with emotional turbulence. They experienced episodes of denial, anger, depression, and social anxiety. Many linked these reactions to a sense of mourning over the physical and social losses associated with SCI. Although the conventional stages of recovery appeared in varying sequences and were not present among all individuals, they did occur with relative frequency. Given the wide variation in individual responses to SCI, however, these stages may best be used in a descriptive sense and should not be viewed as deterministic. Moreover, several individuals—particularly those who were injured early in life or who had very easygoing attitudes—reported minimal or no psychological turmoil during the process of recovery. It is also noteworthy that the overwhelming majority of study participants characterized themselves as happy people, and most seemed contented with their lives.

While developmental perspectives on disability (stage theories, for example) have proven useful as descriptive frameworks, the rehabilitation process may be better served by behavioral models that identify the problems to be addressed as well as the adaptive behaviors needed to overcome them (Albrecht 1976). Previous research has shown that the most effective therapeutic approaches for individuals with disabilities tend to have an educational rather than psychotherapeutic orientation.

Many of the participants in the study had received psychological counseling to assist them in adjusting to their disabilities. However, several reported negative experiences with therapists who seemed out of touch with the challenges they faced. In particular, several participants expressed a need for counselors who themselves have physical disabilities. Because both internal and external variables influence the quality of life and psychological adjustment of individuals with SCI, effective interventions need to proceed on several fronts. As Marks (1999) notes, effective psychotherapists must move out of the consulting rooms and begin to act as allies to individuals with disabilities.

# 4

# Sexual Identity
# and Sexual Intimacy

Meghan is a slender and attractive 42-year-old African American woman
with delicate features and a warm smile. As a result of a car accident that
occurred when she was 21, Meghan is a high-level quadriplegic who uses
a power wheelchair and requires daily attendant care. She lives alone in an
immaculate one-bedroom, wheelchair-accessible apartment. There is a fish
tank in the living room and a computer in her bedroom. At the time of
the interview, her niece was staying with her and helping with her personal
care. While Meghan has a law degree and is very articulate, she has grown
weary from her repeated but unsuccessful attempts to secure a job.

Meghan is an activist who has little tolerance for society's mistreatment
of individuals with disabilities. She lamented, "There are so many people
who think we're asexual, we're not pretty, and we're creeps or weirdos." In
response to this perception, she envisioned a fashion show with women
parading down the runway in wheelchairs, that

> would put a theme in people's minds that women in these wheel-
> chairs are attractive and they are beautiful. They are sexual. And so
> where do you start to dispel the myth? You start with the glamour.

Meghan has been involved in a number of sexual relationships since sustaining her injury. While she doesn't think her disability has diminished
the pleasure she derives from sexual relations, she feels that it has affected
her sexual performance:

> Well, you can't move it, Esther. You can't move! [*chuckle*] You can't,
> like, bump and grind kind of thing.

71

EIW: "Bump and grind." That's gonna be a great quote in my book. [*laughter*] Can I use your real name when I quote you for that?

I'll track you down and kill you. [*laughter*]

She also expressed some concern that her disability might dissuade potential partners:

At some point in time you say, "I won't be able to give him the same pleasure he's giving me" . . . because a woman with a disability can't move.

EIW: You think that they want to be with someone who can move her legs and things like that?

Yeah, they want to do acrobats. Y'know men—they're selfish, for the most part.

While Meghan told me that she valued emotional connections to her partners, she also remarked, "I never had a one-night stand or anything until I broke my neck." She also reported that her erogenous zones had shifted in the aftermath of her injury: "I always did like my neck touched. I like it being touched more now. But people don't get that. They don't understand."

## The Sexual Arena

The sexual arena is fraught with difficulty for individuals with spinal cord injury. While the impact of SCI on sexual functioning depends upon several factors, including the level of injury and the severity of damage to the spinal cord, most individuals with SCI are confronted with restricted mobility, reduced sensation, and impaired sexual functioning. As a direct result of having a body that functions in different and frequently bewildering ways, what was once a spontaneous act of erotic pleasure now becomes an orchestrated event. Old sexual positions may no longer be viable, and precautions must be taken to prevent against bladder and bowel accidents. Men may turn to medications or artificial devices to produce erections sufficient to penetrate a partner, and women may have to rely on jellies to promote vaginal lubrication. It can be a challenge to find sexual positions that maximize comfort, minimize spasticity, and compensate for a lack of mobility.

For some individuals with spinal cord injury, "SCI is experienced as sexual death" (Tepper 1997b: 183). As Stewart and Rossier (1978: 77) assert, "The capacity to gratify and to be gratified is altered with a sense of being left out." Individuals with SCI may need to rebuild self-esteem that has diminished in response to altered sexual functioning (Cole 1975; Drench 1992). Concerns about sexuality and a perceived lack of attractiveness create major obstacles to the development of intimate relationships, particularly among women with disabilities (Bogle and Shaul 1981; Yoshida 1994b). Moreover, individuals with SCI must confront the prejudices and stereotypes of the able-bodied world. As Neumann (1978) and Schwartz (1988) note, there are limited opportunities for individuals with disabilities to assert their claims to sexuality.

Many individuals with SCI find that they are no longer competitive in the dating market—that they are passed over as "damaged goods" and unsuccessful at winning the affection of those they find attractive (Quintiliani 2000: 278). People often fail to recognize that disabled individuals have sexual desires and are capable of performing sexually. Consequently, it is commonly assumed that they are not desired by others (Comfort 1975; Cunningham 1986; DeLoach and Greer 1981; Farrow 1990; Hahn 1988a, 1988b; Halstead 1985; Hammond et al. 1992; Hanna and Rogovsky 1993; Kallianes and Rubenfeld 1997; Lifchez 1983; Nemeth 2000; Neumann 1978; Palmer, Kriegsman, and Palmer 2000; Romano 1978; Sidman 1977; Thornton 1979; Tighe 2001; Wada and Brodwin 1975). Even college students characterize sex between an individual with SCI and a nondisabled partner as dysfunctional, incomplete, and unsatisfying (Stiles, Clark, and LaBeff, 1997). On the other hand, some myths portray individuals with disabilities as having excessive or perverted sexual needs (Cole, Chilgren, and Rosenberg 1973).

While the civil and social rights movements of the 1970s helped to eradicate the myth of asexuality among disabled individuals (Knight 1989), stereotypes persist and there is a pressing need to present more positive sexual images of individuals with disabilities. While a quadriplegic woman posed for *Playboy* magazine in 1987, the portrayal of women with disabilities in films and television programs has been predominantly asexual (Hwang 1997). A movement equivalent to the "Black is Beautiful" phenomenon might allow disabled individuals to redefine their identities in a positive manner, although it must be admitted that "'disability is beautiful' hardly flows trippingly from the tongue" (Hahn 1988a: 27).

## The Physiology of Sexual Functioning in the Aftermath of Spinal Cord Injury

The impact of SCI on men's sexual functioning is one of the most widely studied psychosocial aspects of spinal cord injury (Sipski 1997a). As Table 4.1 shows, completeness of injury (discussed in Chapter 2) is a primary determinant of sexual capability in men with SCI. For all five aspects of sexual functioning shown in the table—reflexogenic erection, psychogenic erection, ejaculation, coital success, and orgasm—men with incomplete injuries (those with some sensation or motor function below the level of the injury) are better off than those with complete injuries.

In discussing the sexual functioning of men with SCI, it is also important to distinguish between upper motor neuron (UMN) and lower motor neuron (LMN) injuries. Upper motor neuron injuries are those that damage the nerves responsible for voluntary movement but not the nerves responsible for reflex activity. Lower motor neuron injuries are those that damage the nerves responsible for reflex activity. As Table 4.1 shows, men with UMN injuries tend to experience reflexogenic erections (those produced by direct stimulation of the penis) but not psychogenic erections (those produced by erotic stimuli). Conversely, men with LMN injuries are more likely to experience psychogenic erections but less likely to experience reflexogenic erections (Bors and Comarr 1960; Eisenberg and Rustad 1974; Hanak and Scott 1983).

Much of the literature on spinal cord injury and sexuality has been critical of the lack of attention to women (Althof and Levine 1993; Becker 1978; Bérard 1989; Bogle and Shaul 1981; Bonwich 1985; Hwang 1997; Quintiliani 2000; Sipski and Alexander 1993, 1995; Smith and Bodner 1993; Thornton 1979; Waxman 1996; Westgren et al. 1997; Zwerner 1982). While erectile and ejaculatory dysfunction have been studied extensively, the pathways for vaginal lubrication and female orgasm have received far less attention (Smith and Bodner 1993; Whipple, Gerdes, et al. 1996; Whipple, Richards, et al. 1996). It is often assumed that women's sexuality is less seriously affected by SCI since women often play a more passive role in sexual activity (Eisenberg and Rustad 1974; Fitzgerald 1983; Griffith,

Tomko, and Timms 1973; Romeo 1992; Sandowski 1976; Sidman 1977; Singh and Magner 1975; Teal and Athelstan 1975; Turk, Turk, and Assejev 1983). Over the years, this assumption been widely challenged as a "myopic and narrowminded heterosexually biased viewpoint" (Perduta-Fulginiti 1992: 116).

While the evidence is limited, most studies suggest that erectile capabilities in men have their parallel in vaginal lubrication among women (Bérard 1989; Bielunis 1995; Ducharme et al. 1988; Hammond et al. 1992; Perduta-Fulginiti 1992).[1] Women with SCI may have insufficient vaginal secretions during intercourse, a problem that can be remedied with artificial lubricants (Bérard 1989; Donatucci and Lue 1993; Senelick with Dougherty 1998).[2] (See Table 4.2.) Techniques including manual and audiovisual stimulation have been shown to help women with SCI increase their potential for orgasms (Sipski, Alexander, and Rosen 2001). A recent study revealed that the use of anxiety-provoking stimulation may also improve sexual responses among some women (Sipski et al. 2004).

Spinal cord injury seriously interferes with the orgasmic responses of both men and women (Cole 2004; Donohue and Gebhard 1995; Jackson et al. 1995; Sipski, Alexander, and Rosen 2001). Nonetheless, a significant proportion of individuals with SCI report "orgasms"—physiological events that result in a variety of sensations, often with a reduction in spasticity (Althof and Levine 1993). Both men and women talk about *psychological orgasms* or *para-orgasms,* which have been compared to a "rush" or "high" experience (Ducharme and Gill 1997). These orgasms may include a combination of physical sensations, memories, and emotional responses.[3] Women, in particular, report a variety of psychological and physio-psychological sensations (e.g., affection for their partners) during orgasm, and some evidence suggests that women are better than men at using fantasy to enhance their sexual experiences (Bregman 1978; Comarr and Vigue 1978a, 1978b).

Although the nature of sexual excitement may change in the aftermath of spinal cord injury, sexual identities remain important. The majority of individuals with SCI continue to have a strong interest in sexual activity (Berkman, Weissman, and Frielich 1978; Eisenberg and Rustad 1974; Higgins 1979). While some authors have reported that sexual excitement declines after spinal cord injury (Alexander, Sipski, and Findley 1993; Bérard 1989; Charlifue et al. 1992; Hohmann 1966; Phelps et al. 1983; Singh and Sharma 2005; Sipski and Alexander 1991, 1995; Westgren and Levi 1999), others have found no change, or that sexual interest returns

**Table 4.1** *Spinal Cord Injury and Male Sexual Functioning*

| Injury type | Reflexogenic erection | Psychogenic erection | Ejaculation | Coital success | Orgasm |
|---|---|---|---|---|---|
| All types combined | 71–90%[1] | 23% | 9–24% | 25–35% | 25–75%[2] |
| Complete UMN | 70–95% | ca. 0% | 1–6% | 53–70% | 1% |
| Complete LMN | 0–25% | 25% | 15–20% | 23–70% | 15% |
| Incomplete UMN | 95–100% | 25% | 25–32% | 63–85% | 25% |
| Incomplete LMN | 90%[3] | 80–85% | 70% | 80–90% | 50%[4] |

[1] Between one-third and two-fifths of men with SCI report that sexual stimulation often causes penile erection. About the same proportion report that erection occurs *sometimes*, one-eighth *rarely*, and one-tenth *never* (Donohue and Gebhard 1995).

[2] Between 25% (complete injury) and 75% (incomplete injury) of men with paraplegia report orgasmic potential. Among quadriplegics, the respective percentages are 50% and 66% (Alexander, Sipski, and Findley 1993).

[3] This figure is from Halstead (1985). Sipski (1997a) reports that reflexogenic erections are partially present in men with incomplete LMN injuries.

[4] This figure of 50% is based on a sample of two individuals (Comarr 1970). Halstead (1985) reported that orgasms are "common" among men with incomplete LMN injuries.

UMN: Upper motor neuron; LMN: Lower motor neuron.

Reflexogenic erection: Produced by direct stimulation of the penis.

Psychogenic erection: Produced by erotic stimuli.

Coital success: Percentage able to sustain an erection sufficient for coitus.

Sources: Alexander, Sipski, and Findley 1993; Bors and Comarr 1960; Comarr 1970, 1973; Courtois et al. 1993; Geiger 1979; Griffith et al. 1973; Halstead 1985; Sipski 1997a, 1997c; Talbot 1955; Tepper 1992.

# Table 4.2  Spinal Cord Injury and Female Sexual Functioning

| Injury type | Sexual arousal | Ejaculatory equivalent and orgasm |
| --- | --- | --- |
| All types combined | 61% respond physically when sexually aroused; 18% sometimes respond physically. Of those who respond physically, 70% notice their nipples becoming erect and 65% report vaginal lubrication similar to that experienced before their injuries.[1] | 79% experienced orgasm before their injuries; 37%–59% experience orgasm afterward.[2] |
| Complete UMN | Reflex lubrication; no psychogenic lubrication. | 4% experience the ejaculatory equivalent of males. |
| Complete LMN | No reflex lubrication; psychogenic lubrication among 25%. | 25% experience the ejaculatory equivalent of males. |
| Incomplete UMN | Reflex lubrication; possible psychogenic lubrication. | 32% experience the ejaculatory equivalent of males. |
| Incomplete LMN | Reflex and/or psychogenic lubrication among 95%. | 70% experience the ejaculatory equivalent of males. |

[1] A study by Donohue and Gebhard (1995) revealed that somewhat over half (55%) of females reported vaginal lubrication during coitus and foreplay. A quarter (26%) said it occurred *sometimes*, and 19% were *uncertain* whether it happened.

[2] Only 44% of women with SCI were orgasmic (indicated by genital vasocongestion) under laboratory conditions, compared to 100% of able-bodied controls (Sipski, Alexander, and Rosen 2001).

UMN: Upper motor neuron; LMN: Lower motor neuron.

For females, the "ejaculatory equivalent" of males is characterized by smooth muscle contractions of the fallopian tubes, uterus, and paraurethral Skene's glands, followed by contraction of the striated musculature located in the pelvic floor, perineum, and anal sphincter (Griffith and Trieschmann 1975).

All figures based on "ejaculatory equivalent" are drawn from Sipski (1997a).

Sources: Bérard 1989; Donohue and Gebhard 1995; Geiger 1979; Jackson et al. 1995; Kettl et al. 1991; Sipski 1991, 1997a; Sipski, Alexander, and Rosen 2001; Tepper 1992.

to pre-injury levels after an initial adjustment period (DeLoach and Greer 1981; Ducharme et al. 1988; Fitting et al. 1978; Romeo, Wanlass, and Arenas 1993; Singh and Magner 1975; Sjögren and Egberg 1983; Talbot 1955). Mackelprang and Hepworth (1990) note that approximately half the individuals in their sample reported no change in sexual interest after their injuries. Approximately a quarter reported reduced sexual interest, and a similar percentage reported increased interest in sex.

Although many individuals with spinal cord injury have very active sex lives (Smith and Bodner 1993), a reduction in the frequency of sexual *activity* is not uncommon (Alexander, Sipski, and Findley 1993; Coates and Ferroni 1991; Charlifue et al. 1992; Donohue and Gebhard 1995; Ferreiro-Velasco et al. 2005; Jackson et al. 1995; Kester et al. 1988; Kettl et al. 1991; Kreuter, Sullivan, and Siösteen 1994a; Mackelprang 1986; Mackelprang and Hepworth 1990; Sipski and Alexander 1991; Sjögren and Egberg 1983; Tepper 1992; Westgren et al. 1997; Zwerner 1982).[4] The most common explanations for reduced sexual activity include physical problems (spasticity, catheter interference, etc.), lack of opportunity, impaired sexual functioning, and sexual dissatisfaction (Charlifue et al. 1992; Kreuter, Sullivan, and Siösteen 1994a; Mackelprang and Hepworth 1990; Phelps et al. 1983; Trieschmann 1988; Westgren et al. 1997). Individuals with more limitations in their daily activities tend to report lower levels of sexual satisfaction (Kasprzyk 1983), and locomotor impairment is frequently cited as a cause of reduced sexual pleasure (Sjögren and Egberg 1983). Sexual activity may also stimulate bladder-emptying, which can contribute to sexual frustration and embarrassment for both individuals with SCI and their partners (Bardach and Padrone 1982; Bérard 1989; Comarr 1973; Donohue and Gebhard 1995). A decline in the frequency of masturbation is also common among those with SCI (Comarr and Vigue 1978b).

A significant number of individuals with SCI report problems or dissatisfaction with their sex lives (Alexander, Sipski, and Findley 1993; Bérard 1989; Berkman, Weissman, and Frielich 1978; Fuhrer et al. 1992; Hohmann 1966; Krause 1992b; Mackelprang and Hepworth 1990; May 1999; McCarthy 1991; McColl and Skinner 1996; Noreau and Fougeyrollas 2000; Phelps et al. 1983; Post, Van Dijk, et al. 1998; Ray and West 1983, 1984; Reitz et al. 2004; Romeo et al. 1993; Sipski 1997b; Sipski and Alexander 1991, 1993). The inability to engage in comfortable sexual activity is a significant factor in the reduced level of self-esteem among men with SCI, particularly among those who experience pain during intercourse (Coates and Ferroni 1991). Among women, the sexual problems of greatest concern include urinary and bowel accidents and inability to satisfy a partner (White et al. 1993). While the majority of partners of women with SCI report that they have satisfying sexual relationships, fewer than half (45%) consider their sex lives to be as good post-injury as pre-injury (Kreuter, Sullivan, and Siösteen 1994a). In sexual relationships between disabled and able-bodied individuals, the sexual satisfaction of the nondisabled partner is linked to the disabled partner's level of genital sensation (Knight 1989; Kreuter, Sullivan, and Siösteen 1994a). Those who feel in control of their sexual behavior are more likely to have high levels of sexual satisfaction (Linton 1985, 1990). A number of variables have been linked to sexual adjustment, including severity of injury, internal personal control, optimism, and self-esteem (Mona et al. 2000).

The relationship between severity of impairment and sexual satisfaction is difficult to assess reliably, however. Some evidence suggests that higher-level SCI is associated with decreased "sexual excitement" (Hohmann 1966), and quadriplegics are more likely than paraplegics to report feelings of sexual inadequacy (Phelps et al. 1983). While sexual satisfaction does not necessarily require full sexual functioning (Reitz et al. 2004), the loss of genital sensation is an important factor in sexual depression (Donelson 1997). Similarly, individuals without hand control face special challenges in the sexual arena (Donohue and Gebhard 1995).[5] At the same time, however, sexual functioning is not necessarily less problematic for paraplegics than for quadriplegics (Romeo 1992; Romeo, Wanlass, and Arenas 1993). Among males, the ability to achieve and maintain erections is more common among those with higher-cord lesions (Alexander, Sipski, and Findley 1993; Hanak and Scott 1983; Singh and Magner 1975; Willmuth 1987), and paraplegic men—especially those with complete injuries—are less likely to experience orgasms during post-injury coitus (Donohue and Gebhard 1995). As a result, paraplegics may be more likely to face physiological problems involving intercourse itself. Quadriplegics more often struggle with related issues such as physical maneuvering and social stigma.

Among women, there is an inverse association between level of injury and frequency of sexual intercourse (Jackson et al. 1995); one study revealed a significant post-injury decline in sexual activity among those with cervical lesions but no difference among those with lower-level lesions (Westgren et al. 1997).[6] While some evidence suggests that quadriplegic women are just as likely as paraplegic women to experience vaginal lubrication (Donohue and Gebhard 1995), other research indicates that women with quadriplegia (60%) are more likely to report orgasms than those with paraplegia (40%) (Charlifue et al. 1992). Significantly, one study revealed that nearly a quarter of women with SCI (22%) reported that their ability to achieve orgasm as a result of petting or foreplay *increased* in the aftermath of their injuries. This was just slightly lower than the percentage (27%) who indicated a decline in post-injury orgasms from noncoital sex (Donohue and Gebhard 1995).

Rehabilitation professionals may overestimate the importance of loss of sexual functioning (Trieschmann 1980, 1989). Several studies reveal that this loss is regarded by those with SCI as less important than other functional losses such as mobility and bowel/bladder control (Bonwich 1985; Estores 2003; Hanson and Franklin 1976; Isaacson and Delgado 1974; Phelps et al. 1983; Richards, Tepper, et al. 1997). At the same time, the level of interest in sexual functioning tends to increase over time (Echols 1978). Sexual reintegration seems to lag behind other forms of reintegration, and the reestablishment of a positive sense of self in other areas (work, study, parenting, etc.) often precedes the reestablishment of a positive sexual self-concept (Richards, Tepper, et al. 1997).

## Sexual Activity and Sexual Performance

Overall, 74% of the participants in the current study agreed *somewhat* or *strongly* that their injuries had affected their sexual performance. Men (79%) were more likely than women (57%) to agree. Those with complete injuries were also more likely to report that their disabilities had influenced their sexual performance, and the highest level of concurrence could be seen among paraplegics with complete injuries.

Most of the individuals I interviewed—88%—had been involved in at least one intimate relationship since their injuries, and most felt that sexual intimacy remained vital to their lives. Harry's view was typical:

> The whole sex thing is still important, whether I enjoy it as much as the other person or not. But I want to be able to have sex as close as I can to normal with the other person enjoying it.

Many of those I spoke with, especially women, felt that limited mobility was a key factor hindering their sexual performance. For example, Shannon said,

You're not able to do the things you want to do. In your mind you can do 'em, but you physically can't move. It makes it harder. I think men have to be a lot more understanding of what you are capable of and aren't, but I think you can still have a very fulfilling and satisfying [*pause*] sexual relationship.

When I asked Shannon what she couldn't do, she replied, "Gosh, I don't get on top. [*chuckle*] That's hard. It doesn't work well." Likewise, Adam explained, "I'm not going to be hanging from the ceiling or anything."

Adam further stated that SCI affected not only his ability to maneuver in the bedroom, but how his partner responded to him. His girlfriend

was really, really nervous. She was afraid of hurting me or not knowing what to do or how to please me because I have no sensation below the chest. She was kind of worried about me being satisfied as well.

The situation Adam described—when a sexual partner approaches intercourse with a high level of anxiety—has been referred to as "the fragile partner syndrome" and constitutes one of several obstacles to intimacy for individuals with SCI (Lemon 1993: 77). The response of female partners—fear of hurting, pity, or disgust—is among the most common sexual complaints of men with SCI (Donohue and Gebhard 1995).

Meanwhile, many of the women emphasized their diminished enjoyment of sexual intercourse. Rosa put it bluntly: "There's no more orgasm after you're paralyzed." When I told her that many women with SCI do experience orgasms, she responded, "Oh, that's wonderful. They must not be as injured as the rest of us." Stacy described a similar problem:

My feeling is weird, like I don't know how to explain it. It's not the same, but I can still feel it. It's not as pleasurable, but it's still pleasurable.

Stacy also reported that she was uncomfortable telling people about this.

While Andrew reported that his disability does not affect his sexual performance, he also admitted that he had quite a bit of anxiety about his ability to perform sexually when he first arrived home from the hospital:

At first you have to deal with the fact that okay, I can't walk, I've got this halo, can I even get an erection?. That's the first major block that you have to go through. It's like, okay if I do get an erection, will I be able to please a woman with my erection staying up long enough? I had those worries whenever I first got out of the hospital and I told [my partner] about 'em and we talked about 'em and we pretty much started having sex before I even had my halo off. . . . She was like, "Look, we've been through this, we've been through that. I'm here for you and I'll help you any way that I can." And I was like, "Okay, well basically you're gonna have to do everything." And she did. She didn't have a problem with it.

At the same time, Andrew experienced another problem while lovemaking:

When we would be making love, she would be on top of me and I'd get to a certain point after the lovemaking where I would get a terrible headache—kind of like the ones that threw me into seizures. And they would hurt so bad that she could tell that I was in pain so she would stop. Once she would stop, then the pain would start to subside and it would go back down. Well, then of course I'd be like, "Okay, come on, I can't climax but at least you can. So get back up here. We're gonna finish this." . . . And one time I just decided, "Look, if I'm gonna die, I would like to die making love." [*laughter*]

Andrew's condition was diagnosed by his physician as a dysreflexic reaction (see Chapter 2). While it is generally recommended that individuals who suffer from this reaction remove all sources of stimulation and seek medical attention (Bielunis 1995; McDonald et al. 1993; Mooney, Cole, and Chilgren 1975; Sipski 1997a), Andrew reported that he would continue to engage in intercourse up until the point of orgasm, at which time the pain "went away."[7]

Lack of control over sexual functioning is a source of stress among many men with SCI, and complaints about difficulties achieving and maintaining erections are widespread. Harry explained:

I couldn't even get a normal erection because of my paralysis. That right there in itself is—if you can go a step further than a humbling experience, that's past humbling, that's degrading. Let's put it this way: I don't hate anybody, but sometimes there's people I'd like to suffer for that little small time—people worse than [a professor at the university]. I just get mad at people like that, but there are certain people that I'd just like to suffer for a while, [but] I wouldn't wish this on anybody.

Brad also focused on erectile difficulties when explaining why he agreed *somewhat* that his disability had affected his sexual performance:

That's a fact. . . . Because of the level of injury for a quadriplegic that it affects whatever nerve it is down in the groin area to allow blood into the penis and stuff like that, I cannot keep and slash maintain the erections I had when I was 18 and stuff. So they're there, just not as long.

Several individuals—mostly men—expressed frustration about the ways in which sexual intimacy had changed after their injuries. For example, Roger said that his SCI had become a "huge issue":

Me and my wife tried to be intimate with each other a couple of times, but it played with my head so bad that I turned into an idiot. Said and did things that I should have never done because you get totally frustrated because there is nothing there—no erection. So sex is more of feeling than emotion, than it is anything else. But when you're used to having the other type of sex and you can't do that anymore, I became very angry. And instead of funneling it or trying to figure out who to take it out on, I took it out on my wife.

He explained that he and his wife are heading in different directions: "I'm married to a very healthy, vibrant woman, and I'm half dead."

While some participants in the study felt that their disabilities meant the end of sexual intimacy, most reported otherwise. Still, individuals who can no longer engage in "conventional" sex often feel a sense of loss. As Nathan stated, "I can't do the regular sex stuff." Ironically, however, in describing his ideal partner, Nathan reported, "I probably would want to be able to have sex with her all the time." Meanwhile, Jonathan neither agreed nor disagreed that his disability affected his sexual performance. While he acknowledged that many men with SCI suffer from erectile dysfunction, he also emphasized that there are able-bodied men who "before they took Viagra, they couldn't have sexual relations either as far as intercourse is concerned." For Jonathan, intimacy remains closely tied to intercourse:

> My wife is always getting on me about this. Just cause we have to kiss we have to go have sex and stuff? But if I'm with a woman and we are intimate, I always feel like it's gonna lead to the big Kahuna. I don't know if all men are like that, but I have that tendency. And if it doesn't, if we don't go the whole way then I'm going like, "Man, what I do wrong in this?"

He told me that his wife's "requirements or needs" in terms of sexual activity are considerably less than his.

Al's lack of control over his sexual functioning causes him considerable stress, not because he can't perform as he wishes, but because he frequently experiences erections at inopportune times:

> If you were to take my foot off [the wheelchair], it'd sit there and just jump, jump, jump, jump, jump. And it's the same way with the sexual organ. A lot. I'll tell you an embarrassing story. I've gone to school and I try to pull my shirt down and I'll hit bumps and stuff, and I get to school and it's there! . . . Oh, it's really embarrassing.

Frequent reflex response of the penis to slight stimuli (reflexogenic erection) has contributed to the myth that paraplegics are especially sexualized in their activities or interests (Cole, Chilgren, and Rosenberg 1973). At the same time, spontaneous erections are generally of little importance in sexual activity since they cannot be controlled (Hanak and Scott 1983).

## Obstacles to Intimacy

While the overwhelming majority of the participants in the study expressed no reservations about entering into intimate relationships, over half (57%) the women and one-third of the men agreed either *somewhat* or *strongly* that they were hesitant to engage in intimate relations. A few of them expressed discomfort about revealing personal information about their daily bowel and bladder regimens. For example, one female was very self-conscious about her colostomy as well as her catheterization regimen:

> It's just like explaining what that is and that's just not normal. I think if I just told people, they'd just be like, "Oh." But I just make a huge deal out of it; I'm like *ooohhhhhhh*. That's one of my biggest problems right there. Like other than that, I would have no problem at all. . . . I feel abnormal about it, y'know? It's just kind of different. Most college guys don't know what a colostomy is. They just assume I do everything normally and that's 'cause they're idiots. [*laughter*]

Adam also expressed reservations about opening up about his personal routines:

> I'm a little more nervous about getting involved in an intimate relationship because I know that it's gonna have to be something pretty serious because there are certain things that are involved in my routines that you can't bring just a perfect stranger into. It has to be somebody you feel fairly comfortable with.

Meanwhile, Vibha reported, "Because I leak permanently, I would hesitate to let [my boyfriend] get into me," she said. "We don't have sex as often as I would say a normal person has." She told me that she preferred activities like hugging and kissing as opposed to coitus, and felt she would enjoy intercourse more if she had more sensitivity. Meanwhile, Ryan attributed his hesitancy to get involved in an intimate relationship to discomfort with his sexual functioning:

> You probably know that a person in a wheelchair has problems with erection, has problems with ejaculation and that sort of thing. And that makes me feel a little bit less of a man, so that's one of the reasons I'm hesitant to get involved.

Interestingly, individuals with greater impairment were less hesitant to engage in intimate relations. This may be related to the fact that quadriplegics often experience less sexual dysfunction than paraplegics. It is also possible that the requirements of attendant care for bathing and bowel/bladder management make some quadriplegics more comfortable exposing their bodies to others. Indeed, Soliz (1981: 113) characterizes the relationship between an attendant and a person with a disability as "an intimate one."

Within this sample, 34% agreed (somewhat or strongly) with the statement, "My disability makes me undesirable." The fact that 38% disagreed and 28% neither agreed nor disagreed with this statement suggests that most individuals with SCI do not internalize society's sexual and social stigma of disability.[8] The extent of agreement with the statement did not vary based on gender or level of impairment, and additional analyses revealed that neither education nor length of time since injury had an impact on perceived desirability or willingness to engage in intimate relations.

Several participants in the study who felt that their disabilities made them undesirable stressed the ways in which they failed to the meet the "ideal partner" standard. For example, Stacy stated:

> When I picture a guy's dream wife or their fantasy—like tall, dark, and handsome for a woman—you don't really picture it like, I don't know if I find people, if I would find me as desirable as I would have if I were [able-bodied]. I feel like if they had like a choice of me, like if they had a choice of someone like a replica of me—the same personality, everything—why wouldn't anybody pick the person that's standing up? It's less complicated.

Todd expressed a similar sentiment:

> I just think that a lot of people are not interested in people in wheelchairs. If you have a girl and you put her up against me and some real nice able-bodied guy, who is she gonna go for first? And I'm not saying this is true with all women, but I'd say the majority.

Many individuals with indwelling catheters complain of the inconvenience and unattractiveness of the device (Miller 1975). Fred described the challenges he faces in the bedroom:

> Even to me [the catheter]'s probably a turn-off—to try to have sex with a tube sticking out of your penis. I haven't dated much, and it threw me off. Making love or sex was, always thought was the biggest part for a man to satisfy his spouse or [partner]. . . . And I can't

perform like that no more. [My girlfriend and I] tried other things, went to "Eden's Fantasy" and stuff like that and bought little gadgets. A couple of times it might be fun, but you know I'm not going to ever give up on it, but it's just not the same.

An indwelling catheter may be removed prior to coitus, although some physicians recommend that the patient instead fold the catheter tube along the penis and use a condom (Halstead 1985; Miller 1975; Sandowski 1976; Webster 1983).

## Treatment of Erectile Dysfunction

There are a variety of techniques available to treat men with SCI who experience difficulty getting and maintaining erections. Some examples include penis rings, vacuum devices, penile implants, penile injections (Papaverine or prostaglandin injections), topical pharmacological therapies, and prescription medications such as Viagra.[9] Most pharmaceutical interventions work by dilating blood vessels and increasing blood flow. The effectiveness and safety of each of these techniques varies considerably. For example, while Papaverine has a 90% satisfactory erection response rate (DeForge et al. 2004), overuse may result in long-term erections that have potentially serious side effects (McCarren 1990).[10] Topical vasoactive agents applied to the penis are less dangerous, but they are also less effective (DeForge et al. 2004). Recent studies indicate successful erectile function ranging from 75% (Derry et al. 1998) to 79% (DeForge et al. 2004) among men with SCI who use Viagra. Meanwhile, men who use penile implants are at high risk (10%) for serious complications and should therefore be advised to consider alternative treatments (DeForge et al. 2004; Montague and Lakin 1994).

Viagra was by far the most common remedy used by the men in my sample, although many had experimented with other products and techniques. While most reported that Viagra was effective, a number expressed ambivalence about the drug. For example, Brad told me that his girlfriend didn't like it when he used Viagra. When I asked him why, he responded, "We had had sex slash relations before I got the Viagra and she was just as happy with me then than after." Brad said his girlfriend reported that his erections were "better before the Viagra than after," but he wasn't certain whether she was telling the truth.

Some men with SCI are uncomfortable with the idea of using any substance or "artificial" technique to enhance their sexual functioning. While Ryan believed that Viagra works great, he was uncomfortable with the fact that he *needs* to use the drug. Likewise, Edward had tried Viagra by himself with positive results but was nonetheless "scared it won't work" during intercourse. Chris had never used his prescription for Viagra because neither he nor his wife were particularly interested in coitus. Similarly, Leonard felt that the techniques used to treat erectile dysfunction detract from the pleasures of lovemaking. "There's no spontaneity," he said. "It's almost like it's scripted."

Leonard had tried both Viagra and injections. While he didn't have a strong preference for either, he felt that Viagra wasn't quite as "intrusive as the needle." In contrast, Harry reported that his girlfriend was oblivious to the fact that he was using injections:

> I could do it without her knowing about it. We'd have sex and she didn't know any different. . . . There was these times when [*clears throat*] I'd ask her to leave the room and I would either go to the bathroom or do something and she'd never really ask any questions. It was really odd, it was like I didn't know if she knew. I was at a point where if she knew and she was living it, I don't give a shit.

Eventually, when she moved in with him, he told her "everything" about his sexual functioning and she was "cool with it." Meanwhile, Harry spoke quite favorably about his experience with injections:

> Whereas it wasn't a normal sexual relationship—there's a lot of things I couldn't do but yet, as a man on my side I was like, "we can have sex for three or four hours if you want." So I was, "I'm cool with this." You gotta take what you can get. . . . I went through a period to where I kinda abused it, and that medication quit working for various reasons . . . At one time when they were first starting to try it out on me, I had one for like nine hours. It was like really uncomfortable. I had to go to a hospital and they had to take you and fix it with medication. I was at a point where I was definitely trying to experiment.

Some evidence suggests that the misuse of Papaverine injections has been widespread among individuals with SCI and multiple sclerosis (McCarren

1990). The more recently available prostaglandin injections, while more expensive, are less likely to result in priapism and discomfort (DeForge et al. 2004).

## Secondary Erogenous Zones and New Sources of Sexual Pleasure

In the aftermath of SCI, areas at or above the level of injury sometimes become sexually hypersensitive (Bardach and Padrone 1982; Becker 1978; Bérard 1989; Bregman 1978; Mooney, Cole, and Chilgren 1975; Phelps et al. 1983; Robbins 1985; Sipski 1997a; Trieschmann 1980, 1989). Spinal cord injuries result in the disinhibition of spinal reflexes, which in turn may lead to stronger somatic sensations in the unaffected parts of the body (Bermond et al. 1991). For example, many individuals with SCI report that activities such as kissing, nibbling of the ears, and light touching of the chest, back, and arms are especially arousing (Donohue and Gebhard 1995; Mackelprang and Hepworth 1990; McCarthy 1991; Sipski and Alexander 1991, 1993; Trieschmann 1980, 1989). Moreover, individuals with SCI can often experience sensual arousal in other parts of their body even if they have no sensation in their sex organs (Becker 1978; Mooney, Cole, and Chilgren 1975; Perduta-Fulginiti 1992; Teal and Athelstan 1975; Thornton 1979; Whipple, Gerdes, et al. 1996). It is not uncommon for individuals with SCI to experience phantom sensations of genital awareness by erotic stimulation of other erogenous zones (Cole, Chilgren, and Rosenberg 1973).

Several participants in the study described new sources of sexual arousal that had emerged in the aftermath of their injuries. For example, Adam reflected,

> To me just a little kissing or nibbling on the neck was, y'know, a lot more arousing than it was before my injury. I don't know if it's because of sensation shifts or just because I couldn't feel the other stuff. I don't know what caused that to be more important, but it was a lot more sensual than it was before.

Likewise, Rosa said, "You're more sensitive to everything from the waist up that's not paralyzed—your breasts, your neck, the hugging, the kissing, all of it." Stimulation above the level of injury is frequently mentioned in sexuality education programs (Sipski 1997a). Kevin said that when he was in rehabilitation, the counselors emphasized the importance of finding a new spot that served as a source of pleasure. Had he found that spot?

> Not really. If I was with a girl, I'd like to have her play with my hair, run her fingers through my hair and stuff like that. I don't see that being a big turn-on or anything.

Meanwhile, Todd said that he would like to learn more about his sexual functioning:

> I haven't had any practice. I really feel like we need sexual surrogates. . . . I'd like to have one just to kind of experiment. . . . I would like to have a girl that I could not necessarily have to get super serious, that we could have fun. And I'd like to have sex to experiment things and try things—just to see what's going on.

A number of the people I interviewed, especially the men, said that oral-genital sex increased in importance after they became disabled. This finding is consistent with previous research.[11] When I asked Jeremy whether intimacy had changed in response to SCI, he responded:

> Yeah, like oral. [*laughter*] See, I would never do that when I was able-bodied. Maybe, you know, birthdays or . . . [*laughter*] But now . . . I find that real; I like it a lot now. . . . Let's put it this way. Now I know a lot more about a woman's body than when I used to.

Travis expressed a similar change in his view of oral sex:

> It's gonna sound funny, but I got good at it. . . . And, probably the reason I got good at it was to compensate for what I couldn't do. To say that that's true of everyone, I don't know if I could say that. It just depends on the person.

Then there's Derrick:

> [My former girlfriend and I] had numerous sexual encounters. And, like tying *that* with my tongue [*gestures to a string he tied with his tongue*], tying cherry stems with my tongue in less than a minute,

that helped things a lot at that time. And that was before Viagra came out.

Now that Viagra is available, Derrick sees endless possibilities "when the right lady comes along."

When asked whether his disability had affected his sexual activities, Todd said that he hadn't had much recent experience; he had not been involved in a sexually intimate relationship since his injury more than ten years earlier. He added,

> I think that I could still please a woman very well. Maybe better! [A bisexual woman] wrote this article. She said that paralyzed men she'd been with were better partners than able-bodied males, but not quite as good as the women. [*laughter*]

Todd was referring to an article in *New Mobility,* a popular disability life-style and cultural magazine. In the article, Roberta Travis (1997: 39), an able-bodied woman, claims that the best lover she ever had was a paraplegic man who was "incredibly responsive and seemed to never get enough of making me feel wonderful." She reports that he made love "like a woman" and was "not, like so many men, primarily penis-oriented and in a hurry to climax."

## Sexual Counseling

There has been considerable research into sexual counseling for individuals with SCI (see, for example, Chicano 1989; Chipouras 1979; Cole, Chilgren, and Rosenberg 1973; Farrow 1990; Levitt 1980; Miller 1975; Miller 1988; Pervin-Dixon 1988; Schuler 1982; Tepper 1992, 1997b, 1997c, 1997d; Zwerner 1982). The general consensus is that sexual rehabilitation is part and parcel of total rehabilitation. Some have even argued that sexuality is one of the most important aspects of rehabilitation since it is so closely related to self-esteem, body image, interpersonal attachment, and motivation (Ducharme et al. 1988). While individuals with SCI disagree about who should take responsibility for providing advice and information on the sexual aspects of rehabilitation, there exists an unmet need for health professionals who have specialized training in this area (Northcott and Chard 2000). Tepper (1997b) recommends a multidisciplinary approach that includes all the patient's team members.[12]

Although there have been significant improvements over time, research conducted in the United States and Europe reveals that many individuals with SCI receive inadequate or unsatisfactory sexual counseling during their rehabilitation programs (for examples, see Ferreiro-Velasco et al. 2005; Gatens 1980; Isaacson and Delgado 1974; Morgan, Hohmann, and Davis 1974; Oliver et al. 1988; Sishuba 1992; Tepper 1992; Webster 1983; Yoshida 1991; Zwerner 1982). This seems to be especially true among women (Charlifue et al. 1992; Ferreiro-Velasco et al. 2005; Fitting et al. 1978; Gatens 1980; Sipski and Alexander 1993). Although I did not ask study participants about the sexual counseling they received in rehabilitation, several volunteered complaints that are worthy of attention. For example, Jennifer reflected that her counselor

> told me that the injury, even though it would affect the feeling, it wouldn't affect me being able to do anything. . . . I was 14 years old and she gave me that talk and I was kind of like, "I don't even want to think about that right now."

Meghan described a similar situation:

> I didn't want to talk to a white man who was walking around. Besides, what the hell can he tell me? I even asked him, I said, "You're a white male; you're walking around; what are we gonna talk about?" He's like, "Well, do you want to talk about sexual issues?" I said, "Not particularly." I said, at this point I'm worrying about how I'm gonna feed myself because I couldn't hold a fork or anything at the time. So all I ate was sandwiches. And I thought, "Man, that's the last thing on my mind."

Chris expressed disappointment with the sexual counseling he and his partner had received. When he was newly injured, one of the first things the counselor told him was he'd "never have sex again," and he was devastated:

> On the list, that's just one of the things in adulthood that's part of your life. . . . We were animals [*chuckle*] when it comes to that. So that's just like cutting your gut open because you're never gonna do one of the main things that you enjoy in life so that tore me up, that first day. That was the only time I really broke down crying.

Chris also said that his counselor had been "real negative" on a wide range of issues. The counselor stated that Chris would be getting divorced within six months, and that he'd "rot" in his wheelchair if he didn't get a job and a car.

While some authors have argued that individuals with SCI do not start thinking about the sexual implications of their disabilities until several months after their injuries (Isaacson and Delgado 1974), other research suggests that an interest in sexual information and counseling is often highest among those in acute care and rehabilitation programs (Miller 1988). Rehabilitation counselors have been encouraged to initiate discussions on topics dealing with sexuality, since individuals with disabilities frequently want such information even though they may be uncomfortable broaching the subject (Underwood and Atwood 1983). Although many women agree that counseling should include information about altered sexual response, some think this should be discussed before the first pass or home visit, whereas others think it should be presented whenever the woman has begun to understand the permanency of the situation (Gatens 1980). These findings suggest that the timing and content of sexual counseling are best determined on a case-by-case basis.

## From Sexual to Emotional Intimacy

While Dunn (1975b: 210) asserted more than two decades ago that "the young, unmarried SCI male is more concerned with his ability to seduce than with his ability to maintain a close, emotional relationship," considerable research indicates that the emotional component of intimacy often grows in importance after spinal cord injury (Chicano 1989; Krause 1998b; Westgren and Levi 1999). As many as one-third of men with SCI report that their relationships have improved in the aftermath of their injuries (Donohue and Gebhard 1995). This can be attributed to a number of factors, including better communication, longer foreplay, more sensitivity to a partner's needs, and the overall emphasis on emotional intimacy in conjunction with sexual intimacy.

Quite a few study participants suggested that their injuries had led to a closer alignment of sexual intimacy and emotional intimacy. Several men stated that they had become much less "orgasmically" focused and that they now place greater importance on their partners' sexual satisfaction. Travis summarized this transition:

I think that if you can't feel it, it becomes a lot more mental, it becomes a lot more where you look at it as pleasing your partner. It's less of a situation of reaching ejaculation being the important part of it. Because your feeling changes, I think your view of sex changes.

While much of the older prescriptive literature suggested that individuals with SCI should focus on satisfying their partners, this is no longer the case (Farrow 1990). At the same time, however, many studies have reported a tendency for men with SCI to be especially concerned with their partners' satisfaction (Comarr 1970; McCarthy 1991). Todd's remarks are consistent with this idea:

If I was with a woman I would receive my pleasure from her being pleasured. Her ecstasy would be my ecstasy. . . . I would spend a lot more time in taking time with the woman—no need to rush into anything, I guess. This is one of my sayings: "You're naive because you can feel your penis." [*laughter*] And that's a true statement because I remember when I [*pause*], it took over. It has a mind of its own.

Through pleasing their partners, individuals with SCI may vicariously enjoy sexual pleasure or experience empathetic gratification (Hohmann 1972; Trieschmann 1980). Indeed, some men with SCI report experiencing a sort of "para-orgasm" when their partner achieves orgasm (Hohmann 1972).

When I asked the study participants whether activities such as kissing, hugging, and touching had increased in importance, the overwhelming majority agreed that they had. For example, Brad said that he valued just being close to a woman:

Laying in bed, just sitting next to each other is fine. Very good. It doesn't have to be sex every time you get together. . . . [I] try to be sensitive and give my partner what she wants and needs more than before.

Roger, who had been experiencing problems with sexual intimacy with his wife, expressed a yearning for more emotional depth in his relationship:

I've become more of a caring person since my disability. I want us to sit down and talk more, I want to share more. Before it was, "I got to go." But now I feel more opened—more share and care than before.

Roger also added that his approach toward physical intimacy had changed in the aftermath of his injury: "Cuddling means a lot to me right now," he said.

A number of individuals indicated that sexual and emotional intimacy were inseparable. For example, Jennifer said, "I don't see sex as a physical thing. It's more on the emotional level for me." She told me that one of the ways she enjoyed expressing intimacy was through cuddling, something her fiancé wasn't very enthusiastic about. His lack of interest in being affectionate "is really the only thing that makes me feel unfeminine," she noted.[13] When I asked Stacy if her values regarding intimacy had changed as a result of her injury, she responded that an emotional connection was vital before she would engage in intimate relations:

> I was 16 at the time of the accident so it wasn't anything that had happened before, but I think it made it a lot more personal and it's a lot harder to just come to that. . . . I couldn't just do a one-night stand now. I don't think I would have [before], but that wouldn't be anything I'd ever consider.

Indeed, casual sexual activity is relatively rare among individuals with SCI (Mackelprang 1986; Mackelprang and Hepworth 1990).

Unlike many others, Tonya adamantly disagreed that activities such as hugging and kissing had increased in importance since her injury. "I'm not a huggy, kissy, touchy type of person. I never have been, so no."

## Perceptions of Masculinity and Femininity

Spinal cord injury may have a stronger bearing on the masculine identities of men than on the feminine identities of women. "Some of what it means to be a man in Western culture—physical strength, sexual prowess, and range of influence—is threatened by the loss of physical function that accompanies SCI" (Hutchinson and Kleiber 2000: 32). In mass culture, sports and masculinity are closely tied together (Connell 1995), and the loss of the ability to participate in various sports activities often has a demasculinizing effect on men's identities (Sparkes and Smith 2002). For men, SCI also frequently results in a variety of functional losses, including erectile capability, ejaculation, and fertility (Drench 1992; Teal and Athelstan 1975). In contrast, the physical changes associated with SCI are more congruent with society's view of female sexuality (Cole 1975). Although women with SCI lose both mobility and sensitivity, they retain their ability to bear children and to engage in intercourse without medical intervention. In addition, the expressive characteristics commonly associated with the female gender role (emotional connectivity, passivity, submissiveness, and dependency) are perhaps more consistent with disabled status.[14]

While the majority of men with SCI (52%) agreed either *strongly* or *somewhat* that their spinal cord injuries made them feel less masculine, only one female respondent concurred with the statement, "My disability makes me feel less masculine/feminine." Individuals with less severe impairments and those with complete injuries were especially likely to report that their disabilities influenced their masculine identities. The strongest concurrence was expressed by male paraplegics with complete injuries—those most likely to suffer from the sexual complications associated with SCI.

When asked to explain why their disabilities made them feel less masculine, men focused on a variety of issues, but especially on sexual functioning and the ability to perform stereotypical masculine tasks. For example, Cody stated, "The most predominant one is because I can't get an erection when I want one." He added that the woman he was dating would occasionally criticize him for being unable to perform sexually. In explaining why he agreed that his disability affected his sense of masculinity, Ryan reflected, "Well, sexually—the problem with erection, but I've been to a urologist and issues of having kids come into play." Ryan had seen two physicians who gave him contradictory information about his ability to father children.

The link between masculinity, self-worth, and sexual function is especially strong among lower-class men (Lovitt 1970; Trieschmann 1980), who are more likely to view impaired sexual functioning as a complete trauma because they have fewer alternative resources on which to base their self-respect and self-esteem (Lovitt 1970). While my results reveal no clear relationship between economic status and the extent to which male participants agreed (or disagreed) with this question, those with postgraduate education were the most likely to disagree that their disability made them feel less masculine. This finding supports the view that higher education is associated with a more multifaceted conception of masculinity.

Changes in appearance (e.g., wasting of leg muscles or flabbiness of abdominal muscles) may also affect sexual identities in the aftermath of SCI (Allden 1992). In explaining why his disability made him feel less masculine, Edward reflected on the "sexual thing" but also added that his body was "not near what I used to have" in terms of muscle tone. Similarly, Kevin said, "Well, when you look at my little bitty skinny arms and legs and my fat gut, that tells it all. . . . Self-confidence, man, has gone down the drain." I asked Kevin if he associated masculinity with self-confidence, and he responded, "Yeah, and being pretty muscled up and all that stuff."

A traditional conceptualization of masculinity, characterized by physical strength and power, has been reinforced by magazines such as *New Mobility*, which are aimed specifically at individuals with disabilities. Representations of men with SCI in these magazines promote an image of "heroic masculinity"—aggressive action and stoic perseverance in the face of overwhelming challenges (Hutchinson and Kleiber 2000). This standard may be inspiring to some, but it is more likely to be discouraging for many men who cannot live up to the heroic ideal. A number of the men I interviewed spoke of their inability to perform stereotypical masculine tasks. For example, Leonard said he just couldn't do "masculine things":

> Can't change the oil on the car anymore! . . . mow the grass or any physical things like that. I never worked really at an inside job; I always worked outside and did a lot of physical labor—construction, worked in the oil field. Physical work. I kind of learned that from my dad and my brothers. But things like that you can't do anymore.

Two other participants focused on their lack of physical strength. For example, Nathan agreed strongly that his disability makes him feel less masculine. He explained, "I can't get up and kick around now. If I wanted to whop somebody, I couldn't." Jeremy had a similar view:

> Oh, man. Sometimes you just want to kick some guy, you know what I'm saying? People wouldn't act that way toward you if you were standing up. The only reason why they mess with you is because they know that you can't do nothing.

When I asked him how people "messed" with him, he described a recent encounter he had had with a cleaning lady at a restroom in Wal-Mart:

This lady was in there cleaning, which I understand. I said, "Miss." I had to; I can't hold my urine. So I said, "Please, just let me in there," I said. "You can just stand right outside for a minute. I just want to use the bathroom." And this lady just jumped right here in my face, "No, you can't come in!"—screaming and everything. And I mean she was really rude! Man! You don't know how bad I wanted to just bust her in the face.

Although disability appears to have a more limited impact on women's socially defined gender roles, women with disabilities sometimes feel as if their femininity or femaleness is not noticed by others (Henderson, Bedini, and Hecht 1994). Rosa reflected,

I always thought it must be harder on a man—to feel less of a man being in a wheelchair. But a woman; she feels less of a woman being in a wheelchair, too. You don't feel sexy in a wheelchair.

Meanwhile, most of the women in the sample listed only minor ways in which SCI influenced their femininity. Tonya's response was typical:

The only thing I have a problem with is I used to wear dresses all the time to church and I still do, but I won't wear panty hose because they're too constrictive and too difficult to get on now. They're not worth it to me so I just wear a dress so long that it covers up my legs. About ankle length is good with me, and then you can just wear sandals and not have to worry it.

Tonya further explained that the panty hose were uncomfortable and pressed against the tubing of her catheter.

## Summary

Individuals with SCI confront a number of challenges in the sexual arena. They must overcome the physiological constraints of their disabilities while contending with a social world that frequently views them as asexual and undesirable. In spite of these challenges, the majority of individuals with SCI have meaningful sexual lives. While both men and women with SCI agree that their disabilities affect their sexual performance, women are more hesitant to engage in intimate relations, largely owing to the physiological changes that have resulted from their injuries—the loss of bladder and bowel control, for example. Individuals with low levels of impairment—especially males with paraplegia—are also somewhat hesitant to engage in intimate relations. This may reflect their relatively high rates of sexual dysfunction.

The influence of SCI on gender roles is strongest among men, and the majority of male participants in the study indicated that they feel less masculine as a result of their disabilities. This may be attributed to a wide range of factors, including erectile difficulties, changes in social roles, and altered body images. For some disabled men, gender can be an oppressive social construct (Morris 1993a), and rehabilitation services that teach men how to broaden their conceptualizations of masculine identification may be especially important (Farrow 1990; Hutchinson and Kleiber 2000; Loughead 1983). Tepper (1997a: 141) offers a number of concrete suggestions in this regard, emphasizing the need to replace old messages with new ones (that good sex does not have to be spontaneous, that orgasm is possible without ejaculation, etc.).

The sexual difficulties and challenges faced by individuals with SCI are rooted in both physiological conditions and environmental conditions, and in the interaction between the two. Griffith and Trieschmann (1976) argue that sexual dysfunction has two components: primary and secondary. Primary dysfunctions are those problems rooted in organic impairments—neurological, endocrinological, urological, etc. In contrast, secondary dysfunctions are those unrelated to organic impairment. Their etiology is behavioral, rooted (for example) in the attitudes and anxieties that interfere with sexual satisfaction. Consequently, new social scripts that define individuals with disabilities as sexual and aesthetic beings should be developed and disseminated among the nondisabled population (see, for example, Knight 1981).

# 5
# Religion and Spirituality

Harry is a 34-year-old college student studying philosophy, with aspirations of going to law school someday. He lives alone in a small, university-owned, wheelchair accessible apartment. There is a big television in the living room, a flyswatter on the couch, and videos, cassette tapes, and books strewn all over. The kitchen smells of tomato sauce, and there are bags of food on the countertop. Harry broke his neck playing high school football when he was 15 years old: "I tackled somebody and I hit him hard, and he was bigger than I was. Something had to give, and the weakest point was my neck."

Harry has quadriplegia. He is able to move his arms and hold things, but his gripping power is limited. He has light brown hair, a beard and moustache, and is in good physical shape. Harry is also very warm and friendly, and he spoke openly and freely about a wide range of topics. At one point during my visit, one of his neighbors (who is legally blind and nearly deaf) stopped by to ask Harry to order a pizza for him since he has difficulty communicating on the phone. Harry kindly agreed to help out. During the interview, Harry would periodically wipe his face or put his arms together on his lap while stretching.

Harry says he is a nondenominational Christian. When I asked him if religion was important to him, he replied,

> Yes and no. I wasn't raised up in church, but when I was like eleven
> or twelve years old . . . my mom would send me and my brother to
> my aunts' for the summer. I'd go to one aunt's house and he'd go to
> a different aunt's house. And my aunt was a diehard Pentecostal. I
> mean, no TV. You've got to be covered from the wrist to the ankle.

So I got some experience there with some really highly spiritual, you could say the far radical, extreme spiritual side of the church.

Following his injury, Harry began exploring religion on his own:

There was a period of time from like 1985 and '86 that I took a Bible study course. I was really confused about what religion was and what the right religion was. I was pretty sure I believed in God, but I didn't know who God was and I wanted to know if God even cared and if we needed to know who God is.

His involvement in religion was also motivated by a desire to avoid going to hell:

I know God's probably real and I'd like to get to know him but I like drinking beer and running around and chasing women and doing things like that, too. [Pentecostals] were fire and brimstone and hell preachers: "You're gonna go to hell for this crap." And I struggled with that for years. And I was like scared to death of going to hell. So, I didn't so much want to be a Christian as much as I wanted to miss hell, you know. [*laughter*]

Moreover, Harry thought there might be some perks to being religious:

I was really scared about what the truth was and if there was really a hell and if there was really a God and what he wanted me to do about it, about life, and I thought, well, hell, one of the fringe benefits is I was going to a church that believes in faith healing. So man I went into it deep. I studied faith healing. I studied Oral Roberts, studied Kenneth Hagin—any faith healer, Kenneth Copeland, a lot of faith healers back then. Jimmy Swaggart. I used to listen to Jimmy Swaggart music and it made the hairs stand up on the back of my neck. . . . And I felt like God could heal me.

Harry told me that his religious involvement had subsequently waned. He is no longer actively involved in the church. He said he had "fallen off the wagon" in 1988 when he started to hang around with "the wrong people" and wasn't living the way a good Christian should. When I asked him if he thought being a "good Christian" might expedite his healing, he responded,

> I don't know. . . . If I do believe in God, and I do believe God is gonna heal me, then maybe my attitude is, well, God would have healed me back then if I would have been faithful but since I wasn't faithful and God knew I was gonna go off on this tangent, maybe he's gonna wait and when I get my act together maybe it will happen. Sometimes I think about stuff like that.

Harry also said that he expected this healing to occur because he had seen a "vision of it." "One time I had a dream that God healed me," he said. "It was like in a church setting." He also told me that he had "seen my accident happening before it happened."

## Religion and Spirituality

The lives of individuals with disabilities are strongly influenced by the medical establishment. The Western biomedical perspective locates disability within the individual, tracing its origins to microlevel natural and etiological agents such as genes, germs, accidents, and physiological stress (Zola 1982a). Consequently, rehabilitation tends to focus on the body, which is treated without reference to spirituality, community, or family (Belgrave and Jarama 2000). The neglect of nonmedical components of rehabilitation may be linked to discomfort among health care workers with expressions of religious and spiritual identification among their patients (Craigie et al. 1988; Freijat 2000) and to fear of intruding into clients' religious beliefs (Trieschmann 2001).

At the same time, however, religious and spiritual beliefs can provide frameworks for the understanding and acceptance of disabling conditions. Among other things, a strong personal faith can promote self-esteem and confer a sense of meaning onto what sometimes appears to be an irrational world. Religious communities also provide both emotional and instrumental support (see, for example, Bennett, DeLuca, and Allen 1995; Ellison et al. 2001; Horton 1999; Idler 1994; King 1998; Rogers-Dulan and Blacher 1995; Selway and Ashman 1998; Treloar 1998; Weisner, Beizer, and Stolze 1991; Wrigley and LaGory 1994). Certain aspects of religious involvement and spirituality, including faith in God and participation in organized religious activities, have been shown to promote better health and subjective well-being among the general population (Byrd 1997; Craigie et al. 1988; Ellison et al. 2001; Idler and Kasl 1997a, 1997b; Koenig et al. 1994; Levin 2001a, 2001b, 2002; Levin and Vanderpool 1987, 1989; Selway and Ashman 1998).[1] The relationships between private religious beliefs, participation in organized religious activities, and subjective well-being are especially pronounced among individuals with disabilities (Idler and Kasl 1992, 1997a, 1997b). The internalization of religious norms and moral messages may serve a regulatory function by reducing exposure to chronic and acute stressors, thereby encouraging healthy behaviors (Ellison et al. 2001; Idler and Kasl 1997a). There is considerable debate, however, concerning the particular health outcomes that can be influenced by religious involvement (Ellison et al. 2001). The direction of causality is especially difficult to determine (Levin and Vanderpool 1987).

Many disabled individuals find solace in prayer and religious activities (Nosek and Hughes 2001). In particular, individuals with high levels of life-event stress may derive considerable benefit from perceived spiritual support—perceptions of God's personal love, presence, constancy, guidance, and availability (Byrd 1997; Houston 1999; Maton 1989; Treloar 1998). Previous research has shown that individuals who draw on religious and spiritual resources in adapting to physical disabilities are more likely to feel divine companionship, a connection with the universe, and a determination to persevere (Houston 1999). Among individuals with SCI, religious faith and spirituality have been linked to human fulfillment (Freijat 2000; McEver 1972) and life satisfaction (Brillhart 2005). Strong spiritual beliefs may serve as an important adaptive mechanism among ethnic or cultural groups that maintain strong family and religious ties (Rogers-Dulan and Blacher 1995). These same beliefs appear to promote the recovery of individuals with chemical dependencies (see, for example, Borman and Dixon 1998; Sherman and Fischer 2002; Warfield and Goldstein 1996).

## Religion as a Source of Comfort and Strength

Eighty-eight percent of the participants in the study reported some form of Christian religious identification, and the most commonly reported denomination (Baptist) accounted for 40% of them (Appendix shows the religion of each person). Overall, the religious profile of the sample corresponds with that of the Heartland region in general. The individuals I interviewed, like their neighbors, were especially likely to identify as Southern Baptist. Church of Christ, Methodist, Pentecostal, and Holiness groups are also especially common throughout the American Heartland, while mainstream Protestant, Catholic, and Jewish denominations are underrepresented. While 13% of the study participants listed no religious affiliation, many had strong spiritual beliefs nonetheless.[2]

It is sometimes assumed that spinal cord injury might shake one's faith in God. While such reactions to disability do occur (Weisner, Beizer, and Stolze 1991), most study participants maintained strong religious convictions and spiritual beliefs. For example, Rosa told me she "never questioned [God] at all" and Cody said he had never doubted his religious faith. In fact, many study participants became *more* religious in the years following their injuries. Critical life experiences such as disabilities can provide the impetus for individuals to experience personal growth, and "experiences of dissolution and decay can precipitate people into entering into a process of 'wholing' in which they move toward rediscovering their true selves and their relationship to the world" (Do Rozario 1997: 33). Similarly, parents' spiritual commitment often increases when their children become disabled (see Rogers-Dulan and Blacher 1995 for a review). For many study participants, religious involvement and spirituality gave a sense of meaning and coherence to what had been a very disruptive event in their lives. For example, Ryan reflected,

> I think there was a need there for something and I tried to fill it
> with going to church. And it was good for me. I enjoyed it and I
> still do. I believe heavily in God and believe that I'm gonna go to
> heaven afterwards. . . . I'm not gonna lie. There were times it was a
> little depressing when I saw other people having girlfriends and other
> people playing football and I didn't, or stuff like that. And so this
> gave me hope.

Several seemed to feel that their religious beliefs had helped them to maintain a healthy state of mind and to withstand the emotional and physical stresses of their disabilities. For example, Roger reported,

> I became closer to God because of this. I talk to him a lot more than
> I used to. I pray more. It has basically kept me sane. My religion
> has kept me sane. If I [hadn't] had God, I think I might have lost it

because I have thought suicide, but because of my religion I won't do that.

Similarly, Derrick told me that his religious convictions were an important element in his recovery and in his constant striving to better himself. "I could not possibly have gone as far as I have without religion. Every day I pray and meditate and I believe God has a reason I'm still here." Likewise, Andrew reported that his religious convictions and his belief in God served as "a coping mechanism for everything." A number of the people I interviewed reported that they had always had strong religious beliefs, which they continue to hold. For example, Tonya said that she "just never questioned it."

For other study participants, the beneficial effects of religion were closely tied to participation in organized religious activities. For example, Al told me that he was actively involved in a Christian fellowship at his university:

I have a lot of friends that go to school and we usually get together a fellowship. It gives you more energy. I just get like a tingle in me. I just feel better after the fellowship.

Likewise, Walter told me that he had become more religiously involved in the aftermath of his injury. He and his girlfriend now regularly attend church, and he is an active member of the choir.

For a few, the church has been a source of both spiritual comfort and material support. For example, Roger described how members of his church had helped him and his family:

When I first became paralyzed, the church stepped up and really helped the family. . . . People from church came by and helped financially. The church gave money, food, support, did things for [my wife]. . . . And people from the church would come and take the kids so that [my wife] could come to the hospital. One lady would come over and say, "Here, take my credit card, go fill the truck up with gas. Go see Roger." They cut us a huge break on tuition for the kids to go to Catholic school. There's a woman that lives in our neighborhood that goes to our church that has become like a grandmother to the children. Um, has become like a mother to my wife. And just has helped in as many ways as she possibly could.

Likewise, Stacy commented, "My church helped out a lot; they brought food to my family all the time; they were really great."

## Making Sense of Spinal Cord Injury

Previous research has shown that personal efforts to understand disability and illness tend to be either *theories of natural causation* or *theories of supernatural causation*. Natural causation theories emphasize the relationships between illness and causative agents such as viruses, infections, aging, accidents, homicides, and stress. In contrast, theories of supernatural causation often involve factors such as mystical retribution (punishment by God for violating rules), animistic causation (soul loss or spirit aggression for violating rules), and magical causation (witchcraft, "the evil eye," etc.) (Belgrave and Jarama 2000).

Individuals with a strong religious orientation following SCI are more likely to believe that their disability was predestined, that it contributed to their becoming better people, and that they will be compensated for their suffering and sacrifice in this world in the next (Schultz 1985). The notion that "there is a Grand Design—and that the design for each of us holds nothing but good" (Blatt 1985: 122) may be a source of considerable strength. Individuals with SCI who ascribe meaning to their disabilities have fewer symptoms of psychological distress (Brenner 1990), and those who believe that their disabilities happened for a reason may be motivated to develop their potential more fully, to find ways to help other people, or to revitalize connections with family, community, or religious institutions (Palmer, Kriegsman, and Palmer 2000).

In trying to make sense of their spinal cord injuries, many study participants found meaning in religion. None reported that their injuries were symbolic of any kind of retributive justice or malevolent force, however. While some individuals believe that certain people have the power to cause illness or disability through a hex or a spell (Belgrave and Jarama 2000), none of those I spoke with reported such beliefs. Vibha, who had immigrated to the United States from India, said that the situation is different in her home country:

Unfortunately, in our country people are very superstitious. You could hear comments like, "Oh probably sins of the past birth," and stuff like that.[3]

At the same time, however, many of the participants do attribute religious meaning to their disabilities. Several described how they had been specifically selected as part of God's greater plan. For example, Ryan reported,

> I believe that God has a will for everybody. And he has a reason for everything. There was a reason for me being put in the wheelchair. Maybe I've already fulfilled that reason. Maybe that reason's gonna come in the future or maybe I'm in the middle of fulfilling that reason. But God has a reason for me being in a wheelchair. Maybe my reason is to show other people that, "Hey, y'know, you can go on and live life."

Jay also felt that the reason he had sustained his injury was "probably just to show other people how to get around, what's possible." Although injured as a child, he reported that he had become an Eagle Scout when he was 18.

Overall, 47% of the study participants agreed either *somewhat* or *strongly* with the statement, "My disability has given me a purpose in life." Just over 25% disagreed, and 28% neither agreed nor disagreed. Women (72%) were considerably more likely than men (40%) to believe that their disabilities had given them a purpose in life, as were participants with lower levels of impairment. Most of those with strong religious beliefs agreed with the statement, and even half of those with no religious affiliation felt that their disabilities had given them a purpose.

Participants reported three major purposes or goals: to educate others, to advocate for disability rights, and to have a positive impact on the lives of others. Tonya agreed strongly that her disability had given her a purpose in life. When I asked her what that purpose was, she responded:

> I think to educate people that we don't have something that's contagious and that we don't bite or we're okay to be around. I always try to encourage people to get involved, to not be so scared. Like in church and things, I try to socialize with people and let them know. If you can meet 'em and get to know 'em, they'll realize that you're not that different, that you're still a person.

Several participants described how their disabilities have motivated them to fight for disability rights or to carry a message to able-bodied people. For example, Travis said,

I've done a lot of educating about disability. . . . Most Christians believe that God controls the world—things that happen, happen because he wants them to happen or allows them to happen. The only thing I could tell you that has come about from my wreck that's been a positive, really, is probably my ability to get a message out to the able-bodied community about disabled people and to make it more acceptable. And that's something I've done since early on when I got hurt. I did it through racing, I did it through fighting for handicapped parking rights, I've done it here at Flagship University.

Ryan had a similar perspective:

I have hopes and aspirations of going into sports broadcasting or just going into broadcasting in general. If this happens, I will be in a wide audience and my belief is that if this happens, part of God's reason for me being in a wheelchair is that I can show people that you can do anything you want.

Quite a few felt that they have a responsibility to educate others and to advocate for the rights of individuals with disabilities. Derrick distilled the sentiments of many when he stated,

If [God] doesn't heal me, I believe that he's got me here for a reason and hopefully I'm doing what he wants me to do to fight for the disabled to get some rights for people that are not able to fight.

Not all of the participants in the study were so motivated, however. While Andrew initially felt a missionary zeal to fight for disability rights, he later decided that he could earn a better living doing other things:

I felt like, "All right I'm going to go out and I'm gonna campaign for people in wheelchairs, especially Hispanic people in wheelchairs because not only do they have to deal the discrimination of being in a wheelchair they have to deal with the racial discrimination." But the more I thought about it, I was like, "Well, I kind of like an income." [*laughter*]

Jeremy believed that his disability has provided him with a purpose in life—namely, to inspire others. He said,

I inspire people sometimes. Like one time I was just getting in my car and this Asian lady walked up to me and she said, "I am so inspired—the way you do so and so." And she said, "You just really made my day," and I said, "God, what's up with this?" I don't understand it, but it happens all the time.

While Leonard neither agrees nor disagrees that his disability has provided him with a purpose in life, he nonetheless tries to raise children's awareness of the importance of safety precautions:

If somebody wants to sincerely ask me like, "Hey, well what happened to you?" I'll tell them . . . and I'll be sincere about it. And those little kids ask—they're curious of course, and I'll tell 'em, "Hey, wear your seatbelt." If I had a seatbelt on I wouldn't have been like this.

Several study participants felt they were "chosen" for SCI because it was unlikely that their other family members could have handled such an injury. For example, Jeremy said,

Not that I'm a religious person, but the first [thing] you ask is you say, "Man, what did I do? What did I do to end up feeling like this? . . . I didn't think I really been that bad." And I say, "I didn't kill no-body." But then after a while you get to thinking and say, "Wow, well God chose me to carry this load." Out of all the family members he chose me. If he had chose some of my other brothers . . . or people in my family, I don't think they probably would have handled it.

Harry expressed a similar sentiment:

God has a purpose for some people's lives. . . . Had this happened to my brother, there's no way in hell he could've lived through it. He has a hard time not killing himself now much less being through something like that.

Several of the men who agreed that their disabilities had given them a purpose in life told me that their injuries had prompted them to refocus their energies on the things that really mattered—education, family, and children. For example, Paul explained that his disability motivated him to do something. Just to contribute some way. . . . Before I was happy with do nothing, goof off. I had no plans, no nothing.

Paul intended to get his degree in architecture and "hopefully" to start a family. "Simple stuff now," he said. Meanwhile, Cody felt that his disability had prompted him to slow down and to forge a closer emotional bond with his children:

> Before my disability, I really didn't connect with my children that much and after my disability—I guess maybe it's because I needed someone or something—I started focusing. I think I was probably there financially for them, but I was not probably there emotionally for them before. . . . We created a better bond. . . . I probably tried to help them more than they wanted me to help them.

Several of the individuals I interviewed told me they had become better people because of their disabilities. For example, Vibha reported,

> I feel maybe if I was a normal person, my personality would have been different. I may not have been so empathetic toward people who are disabled.

Other respondents saw their disabilities as challenges. For instance, Roger felt that

> it's given me another obstacle to overcome—to be able to defeat this. To be able to continue on, to be able to help support my family, raise my kids, and just be able to do it out of a chair. That's a huge, in my eyes, accomplishment. I don't want to become one of these people that, "I'm in a wheelchair, I'm gonna go sit in that corner and just fade away and disappear."

Similarly, Chris said that before his injury, his purpose in life was "to have a family, have a job, retirement, stuff like that." After his injury, however, his life trajectory had shifted:

> When you get in this predicament your purpose in life is to survive the day and maybe make it past the forecasted life expectancy. And then in between have as much fun and satisfaction as you can have.

As Todd explained, "My purpose in life now is to carry on."

Some felt confident that their disabilities had occurred for a reason but were uncertain what that reason might be. As Al said, "I heard that there's a purpose for everything, but I'm trying to find it." Similarly, Jennifer reported that God had caused her injury for a reason. When I asked if she knew the reason, she responded, "No. But I wish he would let me know," and laughed. Likewise, when I asked Tonya if she had any sense as to why her injury had occurred, she replied, "My preacher at church says we may never know. And I may never know until I die. I may never know, so I don't question it."

A few seemed to resent the notion that their disability might have provided them with a purpose in life. For instance, Shannon disagreed strongly with the idea that her disability had given her a purpose in life. Nathan said "It's all negative; no positive," and Fred reported, "There's nothing that is good that has come out of this accident." Likewise, Brad expressed little understanding of those whose disabilities have given them a purpose in life:

> Why do they need a disability to have a goal? They should be able to have a goal in life besides their disability and have their life focus around something other than their disability. I try to put my disability in the background. I forget that I have these problems most of the time.

When I asked Brad whether he thought that God had selected him to have his disability for any particular reason, he responded, "No. Just bad luck, I guess." Similarly, Edward reported that the purpose of his disability was

> to screw up my life. 'Cause I hear that all the damn time: "It happened for a reason." And I don't agree with that. I say the only reason why it happened was to screw up my life, and that's that.

## Making Peace with Religion

Although none of the participants in the study indicated that they were presently angry at God, several reflected upon earlier periods in their lives when they had experienced such feelings. For example, Vibha told me that she had been angry toward God when she was younger. Over time, however, those feelings had dissipated:

There was a state in my life when I was questioning God's ways, especially in terms of my disability. . . . There are times which is quite natural when you wish you could walk and that's the time you say, "Why did God do this?"

EIW: Right.

But that, I would say, very rare moments.

Likewise, Stacy reported,

I woke up a lot of times with people praying around me and my preacher was there. When I was like really getting upset, he came and talked to me and he told me that it was okay to be mad at God, it was okay to have these feelings and it was a confusing time. He brought me some passages and I definitely became a lot more religious.

As Stacy's experience demonstrates, religious leaders may assist individuals with disabilities by providing acceptance and reassurance, promoting adjustment, and helping individuals commit to positive goals and challenges (McEver 1972). Kevin also described how his religious beliefs had fluctuated in the years following his injury:

For about a year after I got hurt, I was exercising all the time, trying to get back in shape and everything but things never got any stronger. Then for about a year I got real pissed off at God and everybody else . . . and that didn't work!

Later, his friend's mother started visiting Kevin and influenced him to become more religious:

She'd come over and talk to me about all kinds of stuff. And she'd always throw in stuff about God and all that. And then I got real religious for a couple of years and that didn't work. It just made me miserable.

EIW: Why did it make you miserable to become really religious?

Well, every time I'd think about doing something, I'd think, "Well, would God like this or not?" I ended up not doing a lot stuff that I would have thought was fun [like] going out drinking with my buddies or whatever. I guess I finally figured out kind of a little happy balance in there somewhere.

A number of study participants had turned to religion for meaning and solace in the aftermath of their injuries. For example, while Chris was living at home after his injury, he was visited by some Mormon boys who inspired him to start reading the Bible. Shortly thereafter, he joined a local Baptist Bible study group and decided to become baptized. In order to be baptized in the church, however, Chris would have had to be carried up several flights of stairs. Since Chris was uncomfortable with this scenario, he ultimately opted for a baptism in the swimming pool of the parish's music director.

Paul has never been religious and considers himself an agnostic. He nonetheless understands the search for meaning within a spiritual context:

It would be nice if there is a god or a higher power. Right now about the only thing I believe in is myself. Because right now if I can't do or if I don't do it, it usually doesn't get done.

## Faith and Healing

Although they realize that the likelihood of a medical cure is uncertain, quite a few of the participants in the study believe that God might someday heal them. As Roger stated,

[Religion] is an avenue to take to ask for help, to ask for healing. It is an avenue of hope. I have a lot of hope that one of these days my prayers will be answered and I will be healed. It's one of the things that's in the back of my mind. My belief is that you ask God and you will receive. I believe, I ask for it and if he feels that I deserve it or that I need to be healed, he'll heal me.

Stacy believed in God's healing potential, but she didn't necessarily feel that a recovery was going to happen in her lifetime,

> I think he definitely has the potential to heal me but I'm not relying
> on that. I don't pray for him to heal me, I don't ask for him to heal
> me. I know that many other people, like my church, and they pray
> for that. If he wants to, he will. [*laughter*]

When I asked Stan about the connection between religious beliefs and
healing, he also affirmed God's power to heal:

> The Lord is sovereign. He can do that at any time. . . . He could
> heal me today. I can't wait on with the processing of my life for the
> Lord to come in and heal me. It may not be his will. . . . I don't wait
> around for some godly event, pining for a miracle.

Numerous others—Christians of many denominations—mentioned God's
healing potential. When I asked Vibha if there was any possibility she might
be healed, she responded, "Well, I have the faith." Although Shannon
initially had held a cynical attitude toward those who linked prayer with
healing, she had since changed her mind:

> God wasn't as important to me back then, and I kind of rejected it
> because people would say, "Oh my church is praying for you." And
> I'm thinking, "Prayers aren't gonna help me, y'know. Forget it!" . . .
> Now it would mean more to me today. I would appreciate that. Back
> then I just was like, "I don't care." [*laughter*] "We've been praying
> for you at our church." *I don't care, that's stupid.* I didn't say it, but I
> thought it.

Shannon told me that she believed "strongly in prayer," and that she has
"grown a lot in the church."

Others pointed to "miracles" they had observed as evidence of God's
healing power. For example, Todd reported:

> Well, my dog had evidently eaten something poisonous and the vet
> said, "She's gonna die," and miraculously the next day she was fine.
> That's what made me kind of believe that there's a possibility.

When I asked Todd if there was anything he might do to promote his
healing, he replied, "I think it's beyond my control." Fred described a
similar story:

I pray that I will [be healed]. . . . I hear about people laying there, 99 percent dead and the doctors give up on 'em and the next day they're up walking around there. An Indian girl in New Mexico was in a coma for 16 years in a nursing home and the next day she was talking to her mother on the phone so there's got to be something strong going on there.

The belief in an afterlife may be an important coping mechanism for individuals with SCI (Ellison et al. 2001), and several of the individuals I interviewed emphasized that their spinal cord injuries would not necessarily follow them after death. For example, Chris believed in a noncorporeal afterlife:

This is my philosophy. When you die, you're a spirit. Spirits don't have physical bodies. We live in a whole different dimension.

Ryan also looked forward to a disability-free afterlife:

I don't know what's gonna happen when we go to heaven. We all could be flying around; I don't know, but I'm gonna be like everybody else. . . . I'll be in total joy at that time. . . . In my afterlife I won't have this disability; I'll be walking and doing everything.

Several of the people I spoke with predicted that they will get new bodies when they die. For example, Tonya remarked, "I know that when I die and go to heaven that I'll get a new body and then everything will be okay then. But not before then." Stan said, "I know when I die I will have a renewed body."

A number of participants had faith in God's healing ability but felt that this power would be expressed indirectly, through scientific advancements that would eventually lead to a cure for SCI. For example, Chris said,

There's no major miracles being done on earth by the Lord 'cause it's through each individual where he works. He's put the brains in your head. And you can do what you want to with 'em. It's up to you. That's the free will that you have.

Similarly, Rosa told me that she had faith in God's ability to heal people with SCI, and that she attributed recent scientific advancements to a higher power:

There's more technology going on. I see it all the time on TV where they have people up and they've tested rats. They've severed their spinal cord and they get 'em walking again. . . . I believe it's all from God. If he wants it to be, it'll be. My mind is set that I've adjusted to the condition I'm in and if it was to change, that would be wonderful. But I believe it all has to come from the good Lord up above.

Ben, a walking quadriplegic who had previously used a wheelchair, expressed confidence that religious faith had helped him to walk again:

I'm sort of I guess what they call a lukewarm Catholic. [*laughter*] I don't practice all the time, but my mom's a real devout Catholic and so when I first got injured she'd start all the prayer groups and everything.

EIW: Do you attribute some of your recovery to your religion? All the prayer and everything?

Yes, yes. I can't find any other explanation because all the doctors at the time were pretty negative and they were saying, "Well you'll never walk again. You won't do this and you won't do that."

Others, including many confident in God's healing powers, expressed ambivalence as to whether or not prayer and religious involvement would result in physical healing. For example, Brad told me that although he was confident in God's ability to heal him, he didn't necessarily believe it would happen during his lifetime:

I think it could happen, but what's the old saying, I'm not holding my breath.

EIW: Do you think that your behavior or anything you might do might affect whether or not that happens?

From a religious standpoint, I could certainly be more religious and participate more in a religion. But I don't feel that by not participating fully, that's not going to heal me.

Todd described a period during which he prayed regularly for a recovery, although he later resigned himself to the notion that there was not necessarily a connection between prayer and healing:

> I think it's beyond my control. If it weren't, then I'd be walking right now! [*laughter*] I mean I asked God every night in the beginning, "Please let me walk again." I asked him a lot and it didn't happen. That didn't make my beliefs change any, or anything like that. I don't blame God for this happening.

At the same time, Todd seemed irritated by the notion that people might believe in a strong connection between faith and healing. He said,

> I don't know if you've heard of Dennis Byrd or anything. . . . He broke his neck and he did come back and walk, and they made a movie about it. *The Dennis Byrd Story* or something like that. And of course everybody believes that the only reason that he was healed was through God's hands. And that's not my belief at all. I feel like his spinal cord was at a level that he was able to come back and walk. But that show really bothered me because after I saw that show, I had to listen to people, y'know, I'm sure they were thinking in the back of their minds, "Well, if you believed like Dennis believed, you'd be walking right now." And that's not the fact, Jack. [*laughter*]

Nonetheless, Todd finds it comforting when others offer to pray for him:

> You'll have people come up to you and say, "Do you mind if I pray for you?" And I'm like, "Well sure, go right ahead!" [*laughter*] I need all the help I can get, y'know? [*chuckle*]

Given Todd's cynicism about the Dennis Byrd story, I first thought he was being facetious when he said that he welcomes prayers. This was not the case, however. He genuinely derives comfort from the prayers of others: "I appreciate them doing it. It's nice of 'em to do it. That doesn't bother me at all."

## Disillusionment with Organized Religion

While individuals with disabilities often turn to religious institutions for support and comfort, they are sometimes treated with hostility by churches, synagogues, and other religious establishments. Religious and cultural attitudes vary widely across time and place, and individuals with disabilities have been viewed as saints, sinners, and almost everything in between (Belgrave and Jarama 2000; Hanks and Hanks 1948; Oliver 1990). While ancient Judaism treated many impairments as signs of "uncleanness and ungodliness," Judaism prohibited the killing of disabled newborn children and emphasized the importance of providing charity to those unable to care for themselves (Barnes, Mercer, and Shakespeare 1999: 17). Christianity has historically exhibited a similar ambivalence toward individuals with disabilities. Impairment has been interpreted both as a punishment for sin and as a condition warranting special support and healing (Barnes, Mercer, and Shakespeare 1999). Rose (1997) argues that four central beliefs inherent in the Judeo-Christian tradition account for the reluctance of churches and synagogues to welcome individuals with disabilities: (1) disability is felt to be a sign of punishment, evil incarnation, or disease; (2) disability is seen as a challenge to divine perfection; (3) individuals with disabilities are viewed as objects of pity and charity; and (4) individuals with disabilities are perceived as incompetent and therefore not expected to participate in the usual religious practices. Although instances of a profound regard for persons with disabilities can be found in all religious traditions, many organized religions help maintain erroneous perceptions of disabled individuals (Bryant 1993).

The underrepresentation of disabled persons in religious activities has been attributed to a lack of disability awareness, misguided assumptions about the needs of participants, and outright avoidance by church staff (Treloar 1998). Disabled individuals' interactions with their religious communities sometimes bring on feelings of devaluation due to ambivalence on the part of the churches, a tendency to spotlight individuals with disabilities, and a desire to correct (i.e., cure) such individuals through spiritual means (King 1998). Moreover, the inaccessibility of church buildings and grounds often makes it difficult, if not impossible, for individuals with disabilities to enter the premises where religious rites and activities take place (Bryant 1993).

Several study participants described their negative experiences with organized religion. For example, Andrew described his encounter with a faith healer:

I went a couple of times to my sister's church, and one time we went she told me that there was this really good speaker and he was a miracle worker and she wanted me to go. And I told her, "Well look, if I go, it's not because I want to be saved, it's because I want to see just how good of an orator he is." And she said, "Okay, it's no problem. I promise you nobody will mess with you." So we get there and of course when he starts preaching and talking about all the miracles he's performed, people want to see some of these miracles, especially my ex-wife at the time. And she just kept looking at me and I just looked at her, and I'd be like, "No."

Ultimately, however, Andrew was persuaded to approach the preacher:

Everybody else in the church is just kind of peering at me like, "Now's your chance." So of course they wheel me down there. And I'm just like, "Okay." And he starts preaching in Spanish and he was a pretty good preacher, but the one thing I didn't like is that he said, "If this man has enough faith, the Lord will give me the power to lay my hands on him and he'll get up out of his chair." So of course when I didn't get up out of the chair, it's because I have a lack of faith.

Since this experience, Andrew had been to church just a few times. As his narrative demonstrates, so-called faith healers convey an especially insidious message to individuals with disabilities. Because faith in God is believed to be able to restore good health and overcome the imperfection of disability, disability is "seen as an abomination, an act of punishment or evil that is an unwelcome addition to the lives of the faithful" (Rose 1997: 398). This attitude can be especially hurtful when families and religious figures instill the belief that disabilities are punishment from God for sins in this life or previous lives (Nosek and Hughes 2001).

In a similar vein, Meghan described how she had become disillusioned with organized religion:

It was such a crock. I thought the church would be accepting and open-armed and "this person can participate because they still have a mind," and they treated you like you were just crippled: "What good can you do? Just come on and be saved, let the Lord save your soul." All right, "because you're in a wheelchair you need salvation a lot more than anyone else." Like you wouldn't need as much salvation as I do because I'm in this wheelchair.

Meghan reported that organized religion had been a destructive force in her life:

> I went to church with this girl that I liked a lot . . . and she got mad because I didn't join and everything. She said the reason I wasn't healed was because I didn't believe, and she, her friends would come and pray over my head speaking in tongues and stuff. Like it was my fault because I was in a wheelchair because I didn't believe. And she would come out, I'd be reading a novel—then I was reading novels like crazy: "Well you shouldn't be reading this, you should be reading the Bible." And, well, I was like, "Wait a minute, you know, I don't think it's either/or, I can read both."

Megan makes a distinction between religion and spirituality. "That church stuff is definitely a man-made thing to make money," she said. At the same time, she considers herself a spiritual person. When I asked if she believed in God, she responded, "Of courrrrrse! My lord, how can you not? Look at the trees and the sky and you have to believe in God."

Like Meghan, Leonard was turned off from going to church because he was treated in a condescending fashion:

> [My ex-wife and I] would go a few times a year before I got hurt. But after I got hurt, I don't like being pitied and petted. I mean, it really bothers me. 'Cause I go to a church and this happened several times, they'd come up to me and everyone would put hands on me and I don't want to be pitied.

Unfortunately, organized religion has played a role in constructing disability as a vehicle through which others can gain spiritual status by providing pity and charity (Fitzgerald 1997).

## "My Disability is a Positive Force in My Life"

Many disability scholars have argued that the essential task for individuals with disabilities is to refocus attention away from the negative aspects of disability to the structural causes of victimization. "It is about the subversion of stigma: taking a negative appellation and converting it into a badge of pride" (Shakespeare 1993: 253). Indeed, "simple but iconoclastic thinking—that a disability, of itself, is not tragic or pitiable—is at the core of the new disability rights movement" (Shapiro 1993: 20). Increasingly, disability is being reinterpreted in positive terms (Morris 1991; Nagler 1993a), and disabled individuals "have taken the lead in challenging 'taken for granted' assumptions that an impairment greatly reduces a person's quality of life and devalues them as a human being" (Barnes, Mercer, and Shakespeare 1999: 221).

Overall, 31% of the study participants agreed with the statement, "My disability is a positive force in my life." Forty-seven percent neither agreed nor disagreed, and 22% disagreed either *somewhat* or *strongly*. Women and those who had been injured for longer periods of time were especially likely to agree, as were those with less severe impairments. Interestingly, none of the four participants without religious affiliations felt that their disabilities had been positive forces in their lives.

Many of those who saw their disabilities in a positive light described the ways in which their injuries had encouraged them to become better people, i.e., less selfish and more sensitive to the needs of others. For example, Leonard seemed to think that more good than bad had come from his injury:

> At the beginning, well, you're just devastated, but then when you look back almost sixteen years you can go, "Well, it's really made me a better person." It teaches you to be not so selfish. And you appreciate things whereas before I got hurt, I didn't always do that.

Walter echoed Leonard's perspective:

> There have been more positives. It's helped me get my life going back in the right direction—quit smoking, quit partying as much, got my anger under control. There's really no negatives when I think about it.

Andrew agrees that his disability has been a positive force in his life. Before his injury, he had been "living on the edge." His SCI has caused him to slow down and to treat women better:

Well, I hadn't been faithful anytime before I had my accident, and I don't know, I think at the time that I had my accident maybe, I don't know; feel like I was maybe on a death-wish-type of situation. . . . I was doing crazy things. I was out walking on top of bridges, not very sturdy bridges and driving crazy. I guess at the time I felt invincible. And then after I had my accident, well of course it slowed me down; I wasn't promiscuous like I had been.

Jonathan also elaborated on the positive aspects of his disability:

I think sometimes just being around me is somewhat inspirational to them. "Well gosh, if Jonathan can do blah blah, surely I can. If Jonathan can go raise a family and have a nice job and be involved in the community and do the things that he does, surely I can. Or do even better." I give 'em a little bit of inspiration.

In keeping with this general idea, Jonathan also stated that those with more severe impairments were inspirational to him. "I see someone that's much worse off than I am physically doing stuff, I'm going, 'Man, I gotta work harder.'"

Other research participants described how their disabilities had taught them patience and perseverance and empowered them with the sense that they could overcome whatever adversity might come their way. While Kevin did not think his spinal cord injury was a positive force in his life, he did report at least one positive consequence:

It's given me a sense of, "No matter what, I can take it." Heartbreak, whatever; physical pain, emotional suffering, whatever you want to call it, I can take it.

Ben, who neither agreed nor disagreed that his disability was a positive force in his life, echoed Kevin's sentiments:

It showed me how tough I can be. [*chuckle*] I mean, as far as being thrown in an adverse situation and overcoming it and everything. I didn't think I had it in me, so it's been a source of strength that way. Now whenever anything bad happens to me, I sort of kind of look at it, "Well, it's not any worse than anything else that's been thrown at you, and you overcame that so you can overcome this."

Likewise, Shannon reflected,

> I think it helped me to learn patience, which I had absolutely zero
> patience before, I'm not kidding. I couldn't even sit still and watch
> TV. . . . So I didn't even watch TV pretty much until I got in a
> wheelchair and I had nothing else to do. [*laughter*]

Surprisingly, just a few participants focused on the negative aspects of
their disabilities. For example, Meghan disagreed strongly that her disability
was a positive force in her life. "It's the cause of most of my heartache," she
said. "Anything that causes me pain is a super negative." She had suffered
physical and financial devastation as a result of her injury. Jennifer also
emphasized the negative aspects of her disability:

> Well, [*chuckle*] I don't see it as a positive force anywhere. [*chuckle*]
> I kind of see it as negative because it does make everything more
> difficult. I think it makes me try harder because you kind of have to
> get things accomplished. But I would see that more as negative than
> I would as positive.

Edward felt that his disability was both positive and negative, but mainly
negative:

> I can't say, "Yeah, it's a positive effect," even though it does in some
> cases. But mostly it's worse. Just in terms of the struggles of daily
> living, relationships, all these kinds of issues.

While Derrick disagreed strongly that his disability was a positive force in
his life, he did come up with one positive consequence: "Well, I stand out
when I go to these government meetings. They remember me—especially
with this chair that stands up."

## Summary

Based on his experience living in a Nazi concentration camp, the eminent
Austrian psychiatrist Viktor Frankl (1959: 114–15) argued that "suffering
ceases to be suffering in some way at the moment it finds a meaning." For
nearly all the study participants, strong spiritual convictions rendered the
shift from able-bodied status to disablement a purposeful transition—some-

thing that had existential meaning (even if the participants were not sure exactly what that meaning was).[4] While the people I interviewed readily acknowledged that their spinal cord injuries had occurred because of accidents or physiological complications, a substantial number also believed that they had sustained their injuries as a result of some supernatural force—that is, God had willed it. For a few study participants, religious beliefs also served a regulatory function, helping guard against self-destructive tendencies such as suicidal ideation. Although several of the study participants were actively involved in organized religious activities, these results suggest that the assignment of meaning is founded not in particular activities, but in personal religious convictions and a strong faith in God.

Although some of the individuals in the study had gone through periods during which they had questioned God and felt angry about their injuries, these phases had been generally short-lived. At the same time, pitying attitudes and hostile religious views (e.g., the notion that disability represents a lack of faith) discouraged a few study participants from participating in formal religious activities. Since the negative and destructive experiences endured by some of the study participants appear to be linked to deeply rooted tenets of Judeo-Christian thinking (Rose 1997), it is important for religious institutions to confront their prejudices and assumptions if they are to openly welcome individuals with disabilities into their congregations. Treloar (1998: 225) suggests that churches "reevaluate the positions they have taken toward disability, adequacy of faith, and the judgment of God."

While the medical model has come to dominate the construction of disability in Western societies, a more integrated and holistic view of disability is crucial to promoting the well-being of individuals with disabilities (Fitzgerald 1997). Attention to each individual's religious and spiritual needs may be an important component of the rehabilitation process (Byrd 1997; Houston 1999; Longo and Peterson 2002; McCarthy 1997; Nierenberg and Sheldon 2001; Palmer, Kriegsman, and Palmer 2000; Piedmont 2001; Trieschmann 2001; Wrigley and LaGory 1994). While it should never be assumed that individuals with disabilities need or want religious or spiritual help, rehabilitation counselors should provide a supportive environment for individuals who wish to explore their religious and spiritual identities.

# 6
# Social and Political Beliefs

Nathan lives in a one-bedroom, disability accessible apartment in a city of approximately half a million with his half-brother Harold. The apartment is very messy, with junk and clutter strewn everywhere. When I arrived for my interview, Harold, a lanky man with a moustache, was sitting on the couch in the living room smoking a cigarette. He looked over at us and asked, "Are you guys going to have sex?" Nathan responded that I was there to conduct an interview. As I roamed around the apartment to get a better sense of their living conditions, Harold yelled out, "Are you looking for drugs?" Nathan later told me that Harold is an alcoholic.

After my brief foray into the apartment, Nathan and I decided that it would be better to conduct the interview somewhere else. We left the apartment and decided to talk in the apartment complex's laundry room, but a dryer was making loud noises. With few alternatives remaining, we held the interview in Nathan's car.

Nathan is a 49-year-old white paraplegic man. He was injured at age 27 when he and Harold were involved in an auto accident. Harold had been driving drunk. Nathan has a round face and gray hair that is thinning on the top. He is tall (over six feet) and is slightly overweight with a large belly. During our interview, he wore a t-shirt and long black jeans. He seems a bit awkward socially, and has acquaintances from church but no friends with whom he regularly socializes. He works as a production management specialist at the local Air Force base, where he earns between $25,000 and $35,000.

Nathan is a member of the Assembly of God, a fundamentalist Christian denomination. He became a born-again Christian at age 20, and he tells me he is "saved." His religious beliefs have a strong bearing on his attitudes toward many political and social issues. In describing his views about abortion, he reflected,

> I know the church people don't like it, but I'm all for it.

> EIW: You think women should have the right to have an abortion?

> Well, I don't know about their rights but I think most of the people that are in the world are going to hell anyway so why not kill them before they get in the world? I think the church is really against it. I might change my view if they showed me in the Bible where it says everything. I'll agree with whatever the Bible says, but that's my personal belief.

When I asked him why so many people were going to hell, he told me it's because they haven't accepted Jesus.

While Nathan is a registered Democrat, he considers himself more conservative than liberal and doesn't necessarily vote according to his political affiliation. He does support charitable causes:

> I think [welfare's] a good idea. I guess it's abused and it probably teaches people to live that way, but what would you do without it?

> EIW: Have you ever received benefits?

> I got Social Security Disability 'til I got out of school and for a year after. . . . And some people with disabilities, they're not able to work, or they got a lot of pain or lack of movement and stuff. I think it's a real good deal. In fact, I think they ought to get a lot more than what they get.

He is also very charitable to his brother, who depends on him for financial support.

On the other hand, Nathan maintains strong conservative views about other social issues. For example, he is strongly opposed to euthanasia:

> I think that euthanasia is like giving up, and there's always hope no matter what the situation is.

Paradoxically, however, he told me that he wished he'd never been born:

> I wish I'd have been aborted. . . . I think that there's enough people in the world and enough suffering; I think you're not even supposed to enjoy all this life, anyway. . . . I'd rather not be here myself.

## Social and Political Ideologies

Historically, individuals with disabilities have been persecuted, stigmatized, and excluded. While Oliver (1990, 1993a) blames the rise of capitalism for the segregation of disabled individuals in modern industrialized societies, negative attitudes toward disabled people date back to antiquity. Efforts to eliminate individuals with disabilities have ranged from the abandonment of infants with obvious impairments to the killing of children with deformities (Sobsey 1994). Policies toward disabled individuals have sometimes taken a eugenicist tone. At the beginning of World War II, individuals with physical, mental, and developmental disabilities were targeted for murder in the Nazis' T-4 euthanasia program. Although approaches toward disability in the United States have shifted toward charity, rehabilitation, and medical treatment, the legacy of prejudice and paternalism that defined earlier eugenicist and exclusionary policies remains firmly entrenched (Breslin 2002).

While the social and political treatment of individuals with disabilities has received considerable attention, little has been written about these topics from the vantage point of individuals with SCI. Individuals with SCI share similar physical, social, and environmental challenges that may influence their ideological beliefs. For example, the majority of individuals with SCI navigate the world using wheelchairs. This common experience largely determines where they can live, with whom they associate, and how others relate to them. Although individuals with SCI share the experience of oppression that is common to many minority group members, they are distinctive in that many have entered into minority (disabled) status only after the formation of their fundamental political and social convictions—convictions that are sometimes at odds with progressive political ideologies. Consequently, the political views of individuals with SCI are often more varied (or more subtle) than those of disabled individuals whose minority status was ascribed at birth.

## Political Identification

I asked the individuals I interviewed if they were registered voters, and if so, for which party they had registered. For unregistered individuals, I asked which party they most strongly supported. Altogether, 43% of the study participants identified as Democrat, 40% as Republican, and 17% as independent or unaffiliated. Compared to local residents in the area (of whom approximately 60% voted Republican and 28% voted Democrat in the 2000 presidential elections), the study participants are more likely to favor the Democratic party—a tendency that is especially pronounced among women and minority respondents.

Because my study overlapped with the 2000 presidential elections, I asked the study participants which candidate they favored. Most supported the candidate of the party for which they had registered, although half a dozen said they were not party loyalists. While the overwhelming majority indicated that their political views had not changed as a result of their injuries, approximately half a dozen said they had become more politically oriented and more sensitive to disability concerns. For example, Ben reported,

> When they passed that Americans with Disabilities Act back in 1990—at that time I wasn't disabled and I was "ahhhhgggh"— griping about they're gonna do this and they're gonna do that. I thought there'd be a proliferation of lawsuits and things like that. I just thought it would be taken advantage of. Then once I got in the wheelchair, I thought, "Gee," [*laughter*] "I'm kind of glad they passed it," as far as making things accessible and everything because at the time I hadn't really thought about things like that. But once I was faced with it, it was like, "Ohh."

Similarly, Travis thought his political views had

> changed a lot as a result of my disability. It's stuff I didn't look at before I got hurt. And you can say, "Well, you're a 14-year-old kid, you're not thinking about those things," but I don't think I would have thought about them if I would have continued on this track I was on, because my whole idea was to play pro football, be famous, make money. I don't look at it that way anymore. I think that I've had a lot of interaction with minorities, I've done a lot as far as

advocating for minorities, not just people who have disabilities. I think we live in a society that's really stupid to stratify itself on the basis of sexuality, on the basis of gender, on the basis of race, on the basis of disability, on all these things. I think that we're missing out on a lot of wonderful people that could be participating in our society.

Although he was a registered Democrat, Travis said he didn't really support either party, since "they're both in the business of getting reelected, and that's it."

Meanwhile, approximately half the group—especially those who identified as Republican—maintained traditional conservative views. Some told me that liberals and Democrats pose a serious economic and moral threat to society. For example, Chris commented,

I don't like whiners and stuff like that. . . .

EIW: Do you think Democrats are whiners?

Oooh, man, it's pitiful. Always wanting something—there's a million different subjects you could get into that. Yeah, I'm a conservative—always have been.

When I asked Chris if he supported Bush, he replied, "I don't know much about him. I liked his dad." Jay also described himself as a conservative Republican: "It just seems like the Democrats want to keep people in the lower class so they can support 'em." Cody also had conservative leanings:

I think the Republicans are a little bit better than [the Democrats]. I always think that if you're like dependent on the government, the Democrats are real good, but if you're more of a higher income thing like that, Republicans are. . . . But there are evils with each.

Several of the people I surveyed reported that they had become more conservative over time, although this wasn't necessarily related to their disabilities. For example, Jonathan remarked,

You're born a Democrat and you die a Republican, basically. Isn't that what they say?

EIW: Is that true for you?

That's kinda true for me. I've gotten more conservative as I've gone a little older. I've been voting Republican for a while. . . . I support Bush. And I even kinda liked old Ross Perot until he went off the deep end.

Brad also reported that his views had changed over time:

I believe I've become a little bit more conservative over the years.

EIW: How so?

More regard for life. What stands out immediately is when I was younger I would have permitted and believed a little bit more in pro-choice. I don't any longer.

A few—both Democrats and Republicans—seemed disillusioned with politics altogether. Harry, a registered Republican, told me he was "fed up with both parties." He added,

I voted for Ross Perot the last two elections because that was my none-of-the-above vote. . . . I don't want to vote for Al Gore because he's too liberal. But somewhere inside of me that little voice is still talking to me about God, to where it's telling me that an abortion is not right and we should have our guns and keep the government in check. But don't get me wrong, I'm not [pro-life] to the point where I think that every woman that gets an abortion is going to hell. I think it's abused. I think it definitely needs to be used if it's gonna be important for the life of the woman. But I think that a stripper that goes out, don't know how to protect herself from sex, and has nine, ten, twelve abortions, five of them been paid for by the state, that's bullshit to me. I don't believe in that.

When I asked Edward if his views had changed in the aftermath of his injury, he responded, "Nope, I still hate politicians." Meghan, a registered Democrat, also seemed disillusioned with politics:

Politics is just a bunch of crap. There are people, I think, with lots of money hidden behind the scenes running the show. . . . They're all cut from the same cloth.

She told me that if she were to register again, she would sign up as an independent. When I asked which candidate she favored in the presidential elections, she replied,

What would be the purpose of voting for any of them? They have no vision or imagination. It's the same old malarkey you've heard for years and years and years. And if anybody deserves anything from the Democrats, it's definitely the black vote. . . . They take us for granted and we keep voting for them and I don't understand why. They haven't done a damn thing for us. And neither does the Republican; that doesn't mean I'm gonna vote Republican either, though. But I'm not gonna vote, they're all the same. They just have different names.

Fred seemed especially annoyed by what he perceived as the moral degeneracy of the Clinton administration:

They're all crooks. . . . I have people in my family that were Vietnam vets, fought for our country; Bill Clinton split to Canada, having this affair with this woman, all these women.

Some simply had no interest in politics. For example, Paul said,

I really don't keep up with it—probably not as much as I should. You get this feeling it's your responsibility because they're the ones that are going to be controlling everything but I really haven't gotten involved.

Similarly, Tonya remarked that she was registered, but uncertain for which party. "I'm not political at all," she said. "Whatever I'm registered to vote, if I don't like that person, I won't vote. If I can't vote for the other person, I won't vote."

On the other hand, Derrick has strong political leanings—and the ambition to run for public office:

> I even announced at the Republican headquarters meeting that I was
> going to run for representative. . . . But then the next week, I had
> this chair and my butt just wouldn't even let me get out of bed so
> I wasn't able to go any place to do anything in order to pursue that
> goal. And I hope that I'll be able to get a chair where I'm able to stay
> in it all day, 'cause I think I can make one heck of a good governor.

He even aspires to the presidency:

> When I was in fifth grade, Bob Dole was a senator in Kansas. He
> came to our school and gave us a talk about politics and told us
> that any of us could become President and then he looked at me
> and pointed at me and said, "Even you." And I thought, "That's it,
> President Derrick Walters. Yeah, I'm gonna do that."

## Euthanasia

Euthanasia is a controversial topic among individuals with disabilities. In recent years, many disability activists and organizations (e.g., ADAPT, Not Dead Yet, the National Council on Disability) have come out forcefully against physician-assisted suicide, arguing that euthanasia, "though often described as compassionate . . . is really about a deadly double standard for people with severe disabilities" (Not Dead Yet 2003). It has been argued that any law, procedure, or standard used to regulate euthanasia will be misapplied to prematurely end the lives of people with disabilities (Bristo and Burgdorf 1998).[1] To the extent that individuals with disabilities are devalued or perceived to be burdens on society, social prejudices may pressure them to end their lives (Barnes and Mercer 2003; Coleman 2000; Miller 1993; Russell 1998; Wendell 1996). Consequently, many disability activists have reacted with outrage to "the unquestioned assumption that a physical disability, *in itself,* means that life is not worth living" (Morris 1991: 44). Those opposed to the legalization of euthanasia argue that in order for assisted suicide to be the result of a free and unconstrained choice, society must first rid itself of the constructs that make life with a disability stigmatized and undignified. They also point out that disabled people live in an oppressive environment—that those who want to die may simply be reacting to the societal limitations that have kept them from realizing their full potential (Bristo and Burgdorf 1998; Miller 1993).[2]

In contrast, those who favor physician-assisted suicide assert that euthanasia is consistent with respect for individual autonomy, liberty, and the right to self-determination in one's intimate affairs—values that are prominent within the disability rights movement. They argue that the denial of individual rights is one of the principal factors that has kept people with disabilities from attaining equality and dignity in society (Bristo and Burgdorf 1998). Many contend that the right to assisted suicide is guaranteed under the 14th Amendment of the Constitution, and virtually all disagree with the idea that the right to assisted suicide is premised on society's widespread misperception that people with disabilities have a diminished quality of life (Batavia 1997).

Although support for euthanasia is lower among disabled individuals than among the general population, most individuals with disabilities favor a legally protected right to assisted suicide (Batavia 1997). Of course, support for euthanasia depends on how the question is framed. While the overwhelming majority of study participants expressed some support for physician-assisted suicide, more than half the proponents had serious reservations. Many expressed ambivalence about this option for individuals with SCI, and several stated that physician-assisted suicide should be allowed only for individuals in great physical pain. For example, Stacy explained that she would be reluctant to support euthanasia for a high-level quadriplegic:

> I can understand when you're in pain. But quads, I mean, are they? If someone wasn't in pain, if they just had to live with the daily disabilities and it's just an emotional thing . . . I don't think they should be able to do it, y'know? Kind of help them change their attitudes. But I don't know; I'm not in that position. Like if I was paralyzed from my eyes down, I don't know. . . . That's hard; that's really hard.

Likewise, Shannon reflected,

> I don't know if I believe in euthanasia or not. And the reason I probably don't have strong feelings is I've never been down that road, don't know anybody that has. And I can understand it would be a very tough place to be. . . . But then if you was telling me someone was in a lot of pain and is dying, I'd feel differently and I'd probably say "yes."

While Edward supported euthanasia for terminally ill people (he had watched his grandfather die from cancer in tremendous pain), he did not support it for individuals with SCI. "I've still got a lot of hope that they're gonna find a fix for it. So I would say 'No' for that."

A few said they might support euthanasia for someone with SCI if all other options to improve the person's well-being had been exhausted. They emphasized, however, that this option should never be taken lightly. For example, in describing whether she would support euthanasia for a high-level quadriplegic, Vibha reflected,

> It depends on why they would want to be put to death. Is it that they just cannot function being tetraplegic, or is it that they're so depressed that they want to be out? If they really cannot cope and they're physically suffering and they find themselves useless to themselves and to the people around them, I suppose that's their choice.

Similarly, Ryan described the conditions under which he would agree to giving a high-level quadriplegic a lethal dose of morphine:

> I would support it under the agreement that they had gone through some psychological treatments to determine that this person's never gonna get out of this depressed stage. I would not agree with it if they just said, "Put me out."

A few individuals mentioned quality of life as a determining factor. For example, Jay reflected,

> [Euthanasia]'s good for animals, why not? . . .
>
> EIW: What about for a person with a serious spinal cord injury?
>
> If it was serious enough, I guess.
>
> EIW: And how do you determine whether or not it's serious enough?
>
> There's the quality of life. . . . I'd have to evaluate [it] on a case-by-case basis—not myself personally, but I think there should be the option there.

Derrick, who had watched his grandmother for three months in "excruciating pain," expressed similar sentiments:

> You can kill a dog and put it out of its misery. Why can't you kill a human being to be put out of misery?

Likewise, Leonard described how watching his grandmother die from cancer had led him to reconsider his views on euthanasia:

> She died a terrible, a terrible, just a horrible death from colon cancer—which can make you change your views. [*clears throat*] And ever since then—that was, uh, five, six years ago—we were going, "Well, Dr. Death." [*chuckle*] "Kevorkian—maybe he's right."

Two participants were unequivocal in their support for physician-assisted suicide. When I asked Tonya if she'd support euthanasia for a high-level quadriplegic who wanted to die, she responded,

> If he wanted to, I feel they have every right to choose that. I think that that's something everyone should have the right to do.

The diversity of opinion within this sample is consistent with previous research. Fadem and colleagues (2003) investigated the attitudes of people with disabilities and found that physician-assisted suicide (PAS) was perceived to be a highly complex, difficult, and personal issue. Disabled individuals' personal views often contrast with the position of the organized disability community, which has emphatically opposed PAS (Fadem et al. 2003).

## Deserving and Undeserving Benefit Recipients

Many disability activists have expressed concerns regarding Social Security, welfare services, and charitable endeavors that are "designed to compensate us in some way for the personal tragedy that has befallen us" (Davis 1996: 124). Some have argued that the welfare state has actually compounded rather than alleviated discrimination against individuals with disabilities—by creating stigmatized and segregated residential facilities, for example (Oliver 1996a; Oliver and Barnes 1993). Moreover, individual citizens lack sufficient power to influence decisions about rationing scarce resources (Rummery 2002). While many disability activists would support a market-based solution that gives each individual sufficient economic independence (i.e., a national disability income), most agree that this must be part of a wider package of reforms (Davis 1996; Oliver 1990).

In the United States, one of the greatest challenges confronting the Social Security program is the need to ensure that benefits are provided to eligible applicants but withheld from those who do not meet the eligibility criteria (Fisher and Upp 1998; Leonard 1991, 1986; Wilder and Walters 2005). Increasingly, disability benefits are being awarded to those whose disabilities are hardest to assess—applicants with musculoskeletal disorders, for example (Stone 1984). Consequently, the definition of disability has become an important public policy issue (Mashaw 1991; Parsons 1991; Stone 1984). Limits on knowledge and technology make it difficult to assess the nature or severity of many impairments, and there is not always a direct relationship between the severity of the disability and the ability to work (Weaver 1986).

While most of the study participants feel that government welfare assistance for disabled and low-income individuals is a necessary evil, many think there should be stricter eligibility guidelines for financial assistance, and that benefits should be time-limited or contingent on disability status. Edward distilled the views of many when he stated,

> Welfare is good as long as it's not abused, and there's a lot of abuse around. . . . not abused by people that are really disabled, but abused by people that say they're disabled. And what they say is a disability—like alcoholism, I don't call that a disability; they can go out and work if they wanted to, so make 'em. And I believe in limiting the welfare, like people that have kids and got twelve of 'em and they're still having kids just so they can get more welfare. I think that ought to be stopped. If they're able to work then they should be able to get on welfare for a short amount of time and they may be offered training assistance. . . . They should be geared back into the work force, take care of their selves and not depend upon somebody to pay all the bills. I did it; everybody else can.

Several participants stressed that eligibility for benefits should be more closely monitored. For example, Shannon reflected,

Do we need them? Yeah. Should they be an entitlement? No. Should they get off it eventually? Yes. I don't think it should be something for life necessarily.

Shannon had never received disability benefits in spite of the fact that she had been eligible when she first became injured:

> Gosh, I didn't want to stay at home at 29, and I like working. I mean I did at the time. I'm kind of burned out right now. [*laughter*] I might change my mind. But I was still able to work. I wanted to.[3] . . . And besides, you don't get that much on disability. [*laughter*]

Tonya also feels that "there should be strict guidelines and checks so that people that get it really need it. I don't have a problem with it, because especially in my position, I have limited income so any help we can get is greatly appreciated."

Among those I spoke with, there was widespread frustration with non-disabled individuals who become dependent on the welfare system as their primary means of support. Several participants made a distinction between individuals who deserve welfare benefits (primarily those with chronic disabilities) and those who do not (primarily nondisabled individuals). For example, Adam reported,

> I grew up in a small town and I saw so many people that would have seven kids and no job and they would get more money a month than my family would with two working parents so I think there should be some sort of accountability. I think if you're able-bodied then you're perfectly capable of working and I think that you should try to work. I believe more in welfare as a way for people to get back on their feet than a way to support themselves.

Likewise, Harry stated:

> I don't believe in welfare babies. . . . Well, let's say a woman keeps having kids every year, she's not even married, don't have a job. I don't think there's a problem with the state stepping in and going, "Look, if you want any more money from us, you need to go to school to have a goal to get a job and quit having these damn

babies," or, "We'll pay for you to be fixed if you want to keep your benefits because we're not paying for no more kids."

Like Harry, Al was especially critical of "welfare mothers":

> I don't sympathize for anybody that doesn't help themselves. . . . You got women that are having babies and having babies and having babies. And they're mooching off of the welfare. They don't want to work. . . . I'm not sexist. They don't care about helping themselves. Guys are the same way. All these people that have kids and they're on welfare, I think they should suffer. They shouldn't need help.

In particular, Al stated that welfare should be reserved for "people in chairs." Fred has a similar attitude:

> I hate welfare. If you can walk and use your hands, got a good mind . . . get off your butt and get this United States in order here. . . . I see people that draw a check from the government, they say they have disabilities, there's not a thing wrong. That gets to me.

Fred said that doctors and lawyers are especially reprehensible, since they help undeserving people claim benefits. Vibha feels that welfare benefits are important, although she does see the potential for abuse:

> The disadvantage of having welfare is some people say, "Okay, I've got welfare, why should I work?" . . . In India, people feel that if they can go and beg, why should they work? You'll find able-bodied people just begging [who] just don't want to work.

Meanwhile, however, Ben said that his own experience with disability had made him more sensitive to the fact that everyone may occasionally need help:

> I'm not very strong in favor of welfare, but at the same time I also realize that you get down on your luck and there are times when people do need help. You can't turn your back on them. . . . I'm fairly independent-minded; I do believe everybody should do their best to take care of themselves. At the same time my situation has kind of

opened my eyes up to the point where, you know, "Well, we all need help once in a while."

Many authors have argued in favor of time-limited benefits as a means of reducing the cost of public welfare programs. In 1997, the Temporary Assistance to Needy Families (TANF) program introduced time limits for families receiving welfare. Several study respondents spoke in favor of this kind of reform, especially in combination with job training. For example, Ryan said,

> I think they should get assistance to put them to a spot to where they can provide for themselves but after that, I don't think they necessarily need it. . . . We have vocational rehab to where a person can go to college and get most of it paid for to put them in a situation to where they can provide for themselves.

Jay argued that assistance should be available primarily to disabled people who are enrolled in schools or colleges. While he supports time limits, he doesn't necessarily feel that people should be automatically cut off: "Give a man a fish and you feed him a meal. If you teach him how to fish, you feed him for a lifetime." Meanwhile, Derrick suggested that social welfare programs might be reconstituted as a form of government employment:

> If they're on welfare, they should have to work if they're able-bodied. If they're not able-bodied, they should have a job that, y'know, I mean there's thousands of computer operators working for good salaries under the government. And I can [use] a computer and I'm a quadriplegic. . . . If I can do it with no hands then why can't these women that aren't working and are able-bodied doing computer work or paper work and filing and things like that? It ought to be like it was with the work incentives, or the work projects of America. In order for them to get a check, they should have to earn it.

## Special Treatment

Altogether, 72% of the individuals I polled agreed either somewhat or strongly that people give them special treatment. At the same time, only 28% felt that individuals with disabilities deserve special treatment. Of course, the phrase "special treatment" means different things to different people. When I asked study participants to describe the special treatment they had received, most focused on the ways in which others were especially helpful and superficially pleasant in their day-to-day interactions. For example, Brad reflected,

> I receive special treatment from people that are nice to me. They don't mind doing me favors—picking up something off from the floor or asking me if I need coffee that's at the other end of the building. . . . Someone tomorrow gonna give me a lift from our building over to another so I can get my hair cut. You have to go outside and then there's places where I could not manually push myself.

Likewise, Stacy reported,

> People are—especially girls—they're like, "Hiiiii," y'know, just super sweet to me. And I don't mind that but I'm just like, "If I wasn't in a wheelchair, would you really be saying 'hi' to me and being so sweet to me?" . . . And I don't have a problem with that. If they want to be nice to me, go for it!

Walter described how people sometimes give him preferential treatment:

> I know some people down here at the car wash, they'll give me car washes for free or I'll go places and I get stuff. I get away with things.

Of course, special treatment—even when it is well-intentioned—can be perceived as patronizing and may therefore be unwelcome. Walter, for instance, would prefer that people treat him just the same as anyone else.

While most people with SCI appreciate people's willingness to ask if they need assistance, many are annoyed by individuals who assume they need help, or who try to help without asking first. As Derrick said,

> My mother is really bad and she doesn't do it in a meaningful bad way. She always grabs stuff for me before I have a chance to try. And I'm three years and nine months [post-injury]. I've just finally got her where she doesn't do it unless I ask. Or she'll ask me if I'd like some help. . . . The first year I couldn't do nothing for myself 'cause she

jumped in there and did it for me. And the worst thing that anybody that's disabled, especially newly disabled can do, is have somebody doing it all for 'em. If they don't learn how to do it themselves, what happens when there's not anybody around and they need to do it?

Fred reported that his aunt treated him in a similar fashion,

always asking me if I need this or that or "What can I do for you?" "All right," I'll tell her, "Please, I'm fine. Please go back to reading your book."

Adam noted that even many strangers tend to adopt an overly helpful attitude:

I think people try to do a little too much for people that are disabled. I'll be opening a door and I'll have five people run up to open it for me. I've noticed that I get a lot more attention from the wait staff and stuff. I'm just the same as everybody else in there, I'm paying the same for my food that everybody else is.

EIW: So it bothers you when people do that?

It doesn't bother me, but it's not really necessary. . . . There are a lot of people that are disabled that really like the extra attention. I mean, I'm not gonna say, "Hey, get away from me, I can open the door."

Brad is mildly irritated by overly helpful people:

A lot of times people will offer to do something and it's something I'm already on the way that I'm doing and I can do. "Do you want me to get that for you?" Fine, y'know, I do it every day. But thank you.

In discussing how they received special treatment, many individuals mentioned people's eagerness to open doors for them. Although they generally appreciated this courtesy, most paraplegics indicated that the assistance was unnecessary. As Nathan remarked, "I don't need it, but it's nice." Derrick had mixed feelings about this kind of assistance:

There's a lot of times that I'll be going into a building or something and a lady will be coming in or out or something and they'll grab the door for me. That's special treatment.

EIW: Is that good?

Well it's nice of 'em, but it makes me feel awkward. Before I was always the one that opened the door for ladies.

In contrast, many quadriplegics reported that door-holding was not only appreciated, but necessary. While Edward was grateful for help, he felt that some disabled individuals alienated potential helpers:

Special treatment to me would be like people getting the door. I fight with doors coming in and a lot of people in wheelchairs don't like that. I mean, people want to try to help us. "What the hell you're doin'? I can do that." And that kind of leaves me out. They say, "Well, he's disabled; he don't want no help!" And I need the help because the door will knock me down.

Todd also remarked that disabled people are "crazy" to complain when others provide this kind of assistance.

Many individuals with SCI appreciate it when others provide help in a routine manner, but not when people go to extra lengths to coddle them (Lys and Pernice 1995; Wright 1960). For example, Paul described the "little things" that irritate him:

Just like going into the store . . . and you get the door all the way open and somebody runs halfway across the parking lot to hold it. And you've already got the door open, it doesn't make any sense. I mean, I'm already there; don't break your neck now to help me do it. . . . But if somebody's there and they're going to hold the door for me, it doesn't really bother me.

Paul reported that in general, he doesn't want people going out of their way to help him: "That will bug me, that just draws more attention" to his disability. Meanwhile, Ben—who was able to walk at the time of the interview—described how this used to frustrate him when he was using a wheelchair:

People would knock themselves over to open doors for me. . . . I appreciate all that, but at the time I wanted to be as independent as I could, and so it kind of irked me 'cause I kind of liked the challenge of opening the door from the wheelchair and getting in myself.

Harry described how people's eagerness to help would sometimes put him in a quandary:

Two people will go up to that door at the same time . . . and they'll be a person on this door and a person on this door [*gestures to two doors*], and they'll both open up their door, and there's a bar in the middle. Now which side do I go in? Now both of them know I can't go straight down the middle so I've got pick one of them and the only reason they're both standing there holding the doors is 'cause I'm in a wheelchair.

EIW: Does that bother you when people hold doors for you?

No, no. Whenever I need help, I totally accept it. It doesn't bother me a bit.

Although there were a few exceptions, most of the individuals I interviewed said they genuinely appreciated it when people offered assistance. Jonathan reflected, "I think most people are honest and just trying to be friendly and helpful and neighborly." Likewise, Jeremy remarked, offering help is "showing concern. I think that's the best thing in the world."

While some individuals with SCI prefer to be as independent as possible, others appreciate assistance almost whenever it is offered. The study participants' responses suggest that the distinction between these two outlooks depends on individual, personal attributes more than anything else. However, participants with different attitudes expressed the hope that nondisabled individuals would try to ascertain the real needs of individuals with SCI when offering assistance. As Roger noted,

I appreciate parking spots in front of the stores, but . . . I would rather have my parking spot in the very back of the store because that means nobody would park in it except a handicapped person—because it's not the closeness that I need; it's the room that I need to get in and out of my car.

## "People Push Me Around"

Quite a few of the participants in the study mentioned particular discomfort with people's attempts to provide wheelchair-related assistance. Many expressed a strong dislike of being pushed, picked up, or helped into or out of their wheelchairs. Several of them had come to regard their chairs as extensions of their bodies, so that even the best-intentioned efforts to provide assistance in this area were often felt to be unwelcome and intrusive. While Leonard appreciated it when people did things like holding doors for him, he felt that strangers frequently overstepped their boundaries (and his):

> They want to help me. "Let me give you a push; let me do this and that." I hate that. . . . I don't like people coming up and grabbing me and touching me and hugging me and petting me. I don't like that at all. "Keep your hands off of me."

Complaints about pushing were widespread. As Chris explained, "Most people don't like to be pushed because you're out of control." The participants in the study repeatedly emphasized that if they want someone to push them, they'll request it. For example, Tonya remarked,

> If I didn't ask, I don't wanna be pushed. [*laughter*] . . . Doesn't bother me that they ask, I just tell them, "No, thank you." It's nice that they ask. I'd rather them ask than them just start doing it for me. I don't like it when they do that and when they try to take over and do it for me. . . . I think they assume that you're stupid and you can't do it.

Shannon doesn't mind people asking if she needs help—as long as they pay attention to her response:

> They want to push me. I don't necessarily want 'em to. And then when you tell 'em you don't want 'em to do, they think that you want to anyway. They think they're helping. Or when I'm going up an incline which I want to do because I need to build my strength and I'm not very strong, so I pause, they think they're helping when they push me up it. [*chuckle*] . . . Sometimes they just come up and grab and do it anyway. They don't say a thing, and that scares me when someone grabs hold of me. And I don't like someone just

hanging on my chair. Like when you come talk to me and you're on my chair, *back off.* It would be like me touching you.

Andrew said he was bothered by people who'd try to adjust his chair for him—"like they know where the chair would be better off than I would." Like Shannon, Adam complained that many people don't bother to ask before pushing him around:

> People are always trying to push me up ramps and stuff like that.
> I don't need that extra help and I'm not gonna get mad and yell at somebody for doing it, but I would much rather someone ask me because if they ask me if I need help, I'm usually gonna tell them, "No." And I know they're just trying to be nice. . . . I can count the number of times I've been at the store and going up into my van and had something in my lap and somebody come up and push me and catch me off guard and I'll be off balance so everything dumps off my lap into the floor. And I'm like, "I know you were trying to help there, buddy, but I had everything under control."

Most of the participants described feeling helpless and out of control when unsolicited pushing occurs. In many cases, the pushers either moved too fast or took them where they didn't want to go. Andrew described his experience:

> There's a janitor at work and he doesn't speak very much English. After work I'm kind of dragging so I don't push real fast. Well, one day he saw me kind of pushing down the hall and he just took it upon himself to help me out. I don't like to tell people "no" when they're trying to help you out. That's kind of rude. But he was going really fast [*laughter*] and I thought I was gonna get thrown out of my chair so that was a little scary. The very next day I could see him. He's bird-dogging, looking for me: "All right, where is that guy? I'll help him again." . . . He's an Oriental man and he's a little-bitty short guy. He's always around there, he's always working super hard. And so after that day I'm kind of a little leery about him. And so I'm boogying down the hall and about that time all of a sudden I get this gust of speed behind me and I'm like, "Whoa." And I look back and there he is. "Rrrrrr." He's thinking that I'm his personal bumper car

or something. So the very next day I'm like, forget it, I'm not gonna avoid him this time, I'm just gonna tell him "No, I appreciate it, but no." And so, sure enough, I saw him. He just looks at me and puts his hands like, "You want me to push you?" "No, thank you!"

Chris had a similar experience, losing a toenail when someone pushed him too fast through a doorway:

> [I] said, "There's doors!" . . . I knew she wasn't gonna stop, she was gonna hit 'em. So I hit it with my hand and blocked some of it, the pressure, but that big toe hit that door and you see the blood showing up through the socks. Of course, I can't feel a thing.

Meghan described an incident at her grandmother's funeral:

> This usher grabbed my wheelchair and was gonna push me, 'cause it was time for family to view the body. Course I don't do that; to me that's just so morbid. I go to the mortuary for the viewing. I don't do it at the church. She was gonna push me up there. . . . I couldn't turn around and make eye contact.
>
> EIW: Did she push you up the ramp or no?
>
> No, because an electronic chair will not move, but she was like being persistent. . . . And I'm going, "Uh, excuse me."

Several individuals reported being especially irritated when people try to help them maneuver their wheelchairs, particularly when getting in or out of vehicles. Most of them have established a routine method of accomplishing this task, and the "assistance" of others only complicated matters. As Jeremy stated,

> I run into this all the time. When I'm getting out of my car and I'm taking my chair out of my car, I wish people wouldn't help me do that because it throws everything off. But if you don't allow them to help you, I found this out, you kind of hurt their feelings. I'm serious. Because they feel like they've been cheated of getting their blessing. So you got to let them have their good deed for the day. . . .

EIW: Almost everyone I talk to—that's something they complain about. They say whenever they're going to stores and stuff, someone wants to help them get their chairs out. And they don't want that help, and it complicates matters.

It complicates if they don't know. Like my son, he knows what to do. He just chu-chu [*gestures moving the wheelchair*] and he throws it in the back, but someone who has no experience, it throws you off.

On the other hand, Jeremy acknowledged that there were situations in which he really did need help. One such occasion:

When your wheel pops off and it's rolling across. [*chuckle*] I'm saying, "Please go get that wheel! If you don't, I'm gonna back my car and run over it, all right?" [*laughter*]

Harry seemed concerned that by turning down overtures for assistance, he ran the risk of alienating those who might otherwise assist wheelchair users in need of help. He graciously accepted the efforts of others to push him even when he was just exercising:

I'll go ahead and let them help me just because they were nice enough to ask. I'm not gonna go, "Hell no, I'm exercising." A lot of times I'll go ahead and let people do that for me just because they offered, plus I don't want them to ever go again and not ask somebody if they need help. Maybe they might see me next time and I really need help.

He described just such a situation:

I was getting out of my car and it was real icy outside, and I started to transfer to my chair and the chair started sliding away from my car and it stuck it up against the snow drift. And I was like stuck in limbo here and I didn't have enough function to either go back one way or the other. And there was this guy, he pulled up next to me. He looked at me real funny and he watched me, and he's like, "Can I help you?" And I said, "I really wish you would! My ass is gonna hit snow here in a minute." But he goes, "I wasn't gonna ask you, because I had an experience a couple of weeks ago with a guy in a wheelchair." He said, "I was at a gas station and this guy was pumping gas in his car and he dropped the gas cap and it rolled under his a car a little ways. And I came up and asked him if I could get the cap. . . . And he cursed me out. It was like, 'What do you think, people in wheelchairs can't do things for themselves?' and 'Hell no, you can't help me; I can do things myself, Goddamnit!'" So this guy, he's walking off and he's like, "I'm never gonna help a disabled person again, this is bullshit!"

Meanwhile, Derrick reflected on one of the most annoying things people in wheelchairs experience:

> Patting me on my head. That's one thing that I don't like. In fact, I have said a few times, "You think I'm a dog?" . . . Patting me on the head instead of reaching out to shake my hand or something—that pisses me off.

## Necessary Accommodations

To the extent that the participants in the study favored any kind of special treatment, most expressed a desire for the same opportunities as able-bodied individuals. Regarding accessibility, for example, most of them wanted access to the same establishments that anyone else might visit. This qualifies as "special treatment" in the sense that existing structures (stairways, heavy doors, etc.) might have to be modified in response to the needs of wheelchair users. For example, Ben said he advocated "a level playing field—not so much special treatment but just for people to give you a chance." Similarly, Stacy was a strong advocate for equal opportunity. She described a conference where a "big activist" had spoken:

> She was like, "Well, what makes us different?" And then people said different things and someone said, "We're special." And she said, "Who the hell told you that?" And that clicked, because we're really not. We just have different needs. . . . They just need to accommodate so we can have the same thing. There's nothing special about letting me see a concert just the way someone else could. Other than that, I don't think we deserve any special treatment.

Likewise, Jonathan described the kind of special treatment he thought individuals with disabilities should get:

> Just make the door of the restroom wide enough so we can get the wheelchair in. When you get out of your car, let's have a parking space where you can get the door open and once you get the door open, let's have a way you get up the curb. Once you get up the curb, let's have a way you get into the building besides going through the back door by the trash can. . . . I bet 90 percent or more feel that same way. They don't want special treatment, they just want an opportunity so you can be in the mainstream and be treated like everybody else.

Travis expressed similar sentiments:

> All I ask for is the same opportunity everybody else has. That in our society is not currently the case. That's currently not the case racially, that's currently not the case gender-wise, and it's certainly currently not the case for someone who has a disability.

Several study participants mentioned that time constraints are often especially problematic for people with spinal cord injury. Some need additional time to complete examinations, for example, due to impaired motor functioning. Describing the kind of special treatment he favored, Jeremy said,

> Special treatment to me means like maybe allowing me enough time to write a paper. [*laughter*] . . . Allow me just a little more time to take a test.

A few individuals thought of special treatment in terms of the attendant care that a person with a chronic impairment might require. This kind of care was deemed both necessary and justifiable. For example, when Jay reflected on the question of special treatment, he thought of individuals with high-level injuries and remarked:

> Some spinal cord injuries gonna need special treatment; they need someone to take care of 'em for the rest of their lives.

Similarly, Brad stated:

> Some people would maybe not be surviving if they did not have Medicare or Medicaid, and I don't think that a person should have that indefinitely unless they are severely disabled and cannot work.

Just a handful of the participants expressed a desire for preferential treatment (economic discounts, for example) in their day-to-day lives. For example, Tonya reflected:

> We get discounts on our tags for our vehicles because we're disabled. I think we should get more stuff like that because we're disabled and we have a limited income, most of us. And I think we deserve more things like that. Financial breaks which we don't get. But the other stuff—opening doors and pushing you and things like that. . . most people in wheelchairs, quads or paras are pretty independent and rather do it themselves.

Shannon also agreed that individuals with disabilities deserve preferential treatment:

> Like not having to wait in line sometimes, or getting through; I'm thinking of Disney World where they had a different way to go into some place and you didn't usually wait in line. You just go in the back door or whatever. Or special seating or special prices on tickets sometimes. Or getting in free to different things. So that's what I mean by we get special treatment. Now do we deserve special treatment? . . . Yeah, maybe we should have preferential seating or ticket price breaks of whatever like that or something.

Kevin had a similar attitude:

> I've heard that Disney World is one of the most wheelchair-friendly places in the world. Everything's pretty flat and level and you get around real easy. And I've heard that anybody in a wheelchair, they'll let you right up to the front of the line. And I think that's pretty damn cool. Not to say we deserve it, but I think that's pretty cool. Um, handicapped parking spots. They come in real handy especially

when it's raining or something. Really appreciate that. They can at least accommodate us a little bit so we can get in there and spend some money or whatever.

On the other hand, some feel that special treatment should not extend too far. For example, Andrew reflected,

I guess I'm kind of old-fashioned. I figure if you had the accident, you put yourself in that condition and you better be a little ingenious and figure out ways to fit in. There are some people who are pains in the butts, really. They'll go around thinking, "Woe is me, the world owes me everything because I'm in a wheelchair." Why? I mean why does everybody else have to [*pause*]

EIW: accommodate

you just because you're in a wheelchair? And on one hand, yeah, I think that bathrooms should at least be set up to where somebody in a wheelchair can go in and use the restroom. But as far as beyond setting up ramps where there's nothing but stairs, I don't understand why people are screaming, "accommodations, accommodations" all the time. I think that if you try hard enough, you can overcome pretty much anything.

Likewise, Chris argued that there are limits to what should be available. While he believes that handicapped parking is necessary, he doesn't think every business needs to be wheelchair-accessible:

Just because they're handicapped, Peter over there is supposed to redesign his storefront to accept you. Just because you're wanting to go in his store doesn't mean you're gonna give him any business or you're just gonna come that one time and nobody will ever come again. What right do you have to sue this guy or get angry at him just because of that? Why don't you just take your case and go down the block? That bothers me. I don't like that. A lot of people just raise Cain about things like that. If they don't want our business, go off. And either accept it or go on.

## Summary

Although most of the participants in this study felt that their political views had not been affected by their disabilities, a minority asserted that they had become more socially conscious and supportive of civil rights. At the same time, many are apolitical, and a large number maintain traditional and conservative political views on a wide range of social issues. Finkelstein and Stuart have argued that "the vast majority of disabled people are non-politicised, are marinated in a disabling culture and identify themselves with a repressive, rather than a progressive, model of disability" (1996: 176). My findings provide some evidence for this position, especially among participants who voiced support for welfare programs that define the problems of individuals with disabilities as individual rather than social in nature.

The views of individuals with SCI are sometimes at odds with those of disability activists and scholars in the field of disability studies. While disability activists and organizations have voiced strong opposition to physician-assisted suicide, most of the study participants support the right to euthanasia in one form or another. Moreover, none of the study participants who oppose physician-assisted suicide cited discrimination against individuals with disabilities as justification for their views. Discrimination is one of the more common rationales given by disability activists who believe that the legalization of euthanasia will result in pressure for individuals with disabilities to end their lives.

Among those interviewed, some of the most progressive ideological views were expressed in regard to the issue of "special treatment." Many study participants mentioned their dislike of situations in which others treat them in a condescending way or presume that they need help simply because they are disabled. Nearly all of them are irritated when strangers or acquaintances try to help them maneuver (e.g., push them or help them transfer in or out of vehicles). At the same time, most of them appreciate the good intentions of people who ask whether they need assistance. To the extent that individuals with SCI do want special treatment, most would like what they describe as "a level playing field"—an environment in which they have the same opportunities as everyone else.

# 7

# Dating, Marriage, and Parenting

Derrick is 39 years old. He uses a power wheelchair that gives him the ability to stand upright—a feature he enthusiastically demonstrated to me. Although he is a high-level quadriplegic (C-4/C-5/C-6) and has limited arm control, he works out regularly. At the time of the interview, Derrick had recently had his head shaven. He was wearing jeans and a t-shirt that read, "You can do anything."

Derrick was injured approximately four years ago when he fell asleep while driving home from work. He currently lives in a garage apartment adjacent to his mother and stepfather's house. Shortly after I arrived and told him the purpose of my study, he interjected, "To start with, it sucks. And it sucks more than I could have ever imagined before I got injured." Derrick is especially irritated by the ways in which his disability has restricted his social life:

> Before I got injured, I never went more than a month or two without a girlfriend and I was able to go out and go places where I could meet people. . . . See how my social life's changed? I mean there's ten gorgeous Hooters girls standing around me there, and they wanted their pictures taken with me. [*Derrick shows me a picture hanging on the wall with him in an Elvis suit surrounded by several buxom women*] . . . And girls out the kazoo wanting dates; I mean it was no problem to go home after an evening appearance and to have ten or fifteen phone numbers in my pocket that girls just walked up and gave me.

Since he became disabled, however, his dating life has taken a turn for the worse:

Now they don't have anything to do with me. . . . I've asked quite a few ladies out and I've got phone numbers for quite a few of them and I've asked if they'd be willing to go to lunch or dinner or something to get to know each other—just phone calls and talk or whatever. Call 'em or try to make the date and they don't have time or they're already seeing somebody else now. All the excuses that there [are] in the world, I've heard them. A lot of them will tell to my face, "Yeah, that'd be great. I'd love to. That would be fun." And then they don't.

Even while lamenting his difficulties dating, Derrick told me that he understood women not wanting to go out with him:

I mean, there's thousands of other guys that are able-bodied and can take them out and wine 'em and dine 'em and take 'em and go do anything they want to go do. Go dancing and anything else.

He explained some of the difficulties involved with dating someone with SCI:

It's a pain in the butt. It's a pain in the butt to take me anywhere. I have to have a specialized vehicle that has a drop floor in it or a lift. And then you got to park in handicapped parking and it's hard to find that a lot of times.

## Relationships and Reproductive Rights

Individuals with SCI encounter a number of challenges when it comes to dating, marriage, and fertility. The standards of physical beauty are high in Anglo-Saxon countries, and significant deviations from these standards can lead to social exclusion (Safilios-Rothschild 1970). The "body beautiful" obsession results in the glorification of athletes, movie stars, and sex symbols (Cecka 1981; Henderson and Bryan 1984), while the myth of control—the belief that if you take proper care of your body, you will stay fit until you die—leads to the subordination of individuals with disabilities (Wendell 1996). As a result of functional limitations and aesthetic considerations, many people will not date individuals with disabilities (Vash 1981).

Individuals with disabilities may also be counted among those whose reproductive capacity is met with social resistance (Fine and Asch 1988b; Kallianes and Rubenfeld 1997; Reinelt and Fried 1993; Shaul, Dowling, and Laden 1981; Waxman 1993).[1] Many people fear that individuals with disabilities will produce disabled children (even though most disabilities are not hereditary) or that they will harm or burden the children they raise (Fine and Asch 1988b). The notion that women with disabilities are unfit for mothering has resulted in a number of abuses, including compulsory sterilization and abortion, the use of harmful contraceptives, and the loss of child custody (Waxman 1993). For individuals with disabilities, reproductive rights are not merely about the right to have (or not have) a child. Rather, they encompass the right to be recognized as sexual beings, to conceive children, and to be accepted as capable parents (Kallianes and Rubenfeld 1997).

## The Dating Scene

Over half the individuals with SCI are single at the time of their injuries (Go, DeVivo, and Richards 1995; National Spinal Cord Injury Statistical Center 2004, 2005; Trieschmann 1988), and the difficulty of finding a long-term partner is often one of the greatest challenges they confront (Trieschmann 1988). Individuals who become disabled due to accident or illness tend to date less often after their disabilities (Tepper 1992), and those with SCI tend to experience an initial awkwardness when they resume dating (Yoshida 1991). While both the male and female participants in my study expressed some discomfort in this regard, the sense of distress was more evident among the women. Although 57% of the men agreed either *somewhat* or *strongly* that they felt comfortable dating, only 14% of the women did. Several of the women told me they had little experience dating, and many expressed fears that courtship and intimacy would require them to reveal very personal information (see Chapter 4).

Along with a certain anxiety related to physical issues, concerns about accessibility and accommodations were common among both men and women. Cody typified the sentiments of many of the participants when he stated,

> It just seems like more of a hassle to do things—just like going out to date or dinner, or if you meet somebody you have to say, "Well, does she live on the first floor?" Y'know, little things, little stupid things.

When asked why he felt uncomfortable dating, Travis spoke about accessibility issues as well as others' lack of understanding about SCI and sexuality:

> Most people don't know sexually what can happen. And that's something that at some point if you're dating someone then you're going to have to deal with that. But also if you go to a restaurant you always got to make sure that the restaurant's accessible because I've gone to restaurants before and like, "We're gonna go eat at this place," and you get there and you're like, "Oh shit, there's no ramp . . . uh-oh." And you got to ask your date for help to get up like on the curb. That's like really emasculating! . . . You have to put a little more planning into it for it to work out very well.

The notion that others underestimate their sexual potential was expressed by several study participants. For example, Walter said, "They see somebody in a wheelchair and they think they're dead from the center or from the chest down." Similarly, Adam described how women frequently do not understand what his sexual capabilities are:

> When I've known girls and they have worked up the nerve to ask whether I can still function sexually—it usually takes a pretty good while for them to be able to work up the nerve to ask. So I think that might be one reason that women might have trouble approaching me. . . . They assume you're not capable of sexual function.

Meghan lamented the fact that men rarely hit on her anymore:

> I never had trouble with guys when I was walking around. I mean, they were all over me. But after the disability I became an *it*. And that was very, very disappointing. Guys can come in a room and they never looked at me twice except to look at me like I'm a freak—a sideshow or something. But when I was walking around; I mean I was married and they'd, "Hey, what ya doing? What's happening?" I'm like, "I'm married." And they're like, "I'm not afraid of your husband. Are you?" . . . And I'm like, "My husband wouldn't want that too much." Y'know, the flirting I enjoyed. 'Cause I wasn't gonna do anything but just the play. The banter. I miss that.

Kevin also reported that his disability—and especially his need for a personal attendant—hampered his ability to meet and date women:

> I used to date and stuff before I got hurt. I haven't since. That's one area I really screwed up in. . . . After I got hurt for a while I was concerned about getting myself back to normal. And then that didn't happen. Going to school, I always had somebody with me taking notes and stuff like that—taking me to class and all, and it's kind of a pain in the ass to get to know somebody when you've always got somebody.

Kevin also felt his disability adversely affected his willingness to approach women: "I surely wouldn't feel comfortable going up to a good looking woman and talking to her. Felt pretty much that I'm worthless, what have I got to offer?" Similarly, Leonard lamented the fact that his friends in wheelchairs encountered considerable difficulty in getting dates: "I've got a couple of close friends that are great guys, good jobs, and they couldn't buy a girl's attention."

## Barriers to Involvement with Disabled Individuals

The majority of those surveyed agreed that "people do not want to get involved with someone who has a disability." All of the female and 60% of the male participants agreed either *somewhat* or *strongly* with this statement. Moreover, those with less severe impairments were especially likely to agree. Previous research has shown that disabled women are more likely than disabled men to be viewed negatively, to have poorer self-image, and to internalize society's rejection (Fine and Asch 1985). Many women with SCI also believe that they are unable to fulfill the traditional female roles expected of them (Yoshida 1991).

Nondisabled individuals distance themselves from those with disabilities for at least two reasons: "existence anxiety" (the perceived threat of the loss of physical capabilities) and "aesthetic anxiety" (the fear of others whose traits are perceived as disturbing or unpleasant) (Hahn 1988a, 1988b). Many of the people I interviewed felt that negative attitudes toward disabled individuals are deeply rooted in the psychic structure of the nondisabled majority. For example, Vibha told me, "It's quite natural in human nature to prefer a nondisabled person than a disabled person."

Nearly all the male participants who hadn't been continuously involved in a relationship since their injuries reported that they had been rejected at some point as a result of their disabilities. Females were much less likely to report having been rejected, owing in part to their hesitancy to ask others out. For example, Vibha told me that if she ever liked a man, she just kept it to herself and "didn't do anything about it." She said she'd wait for the other person to show some interest because she was "scared I'd get rejected, being disabled."

A few of the men told me that rejection or fear of rejection had brought their dating lives to a halt. When asked what effect his injury had on his relationships with women, Nathan replied, "I quit going with 'em." He attributed this to his own self-consciousness. Similarly, Edward reflected:

I haven't dated anybody for almost three years. And it's because I don't want rejection. I used to deal with it and just brush it off, but now I don't want to deal with it so I won't ask anybody out.

As Zola (1982b: 63–64) writes, "We the physically disabled withdraw or deny the need for intimate contact not through lack of desire but fear of rejection. A self-fulfilling prophecy has thus been created."

Many able-bodied persons believe that concerns regarding public stigmatization and sexuality are among the most pressing issues that a disabled/nondisabled couple would confront if they established an intimate relationship (Stiles, Clark, and LaBeff, 1997). Indeed, a few study participants reported that able-bodied individuals do not want to be seen in public with those who are disabled. For instance, in explaining people's reluctance to get involved with individuals with disabilities, Edward reflected, "Maintenance maybe. I would say embarrassment of being with them in public, but that depends on the person. That's only part of it, but it's probably a big part of it." Two male participants in the study focused on the challenges they had confronted while dating in high school. For instance, Ryan reflected:

In high school, kids are just all about being socially accepted. And there were instances in high school where I asked a girl out and while they didn't say it to my face, I heard it second-hand that they weren't gonna go out with me because I was in a wheelchair and afraid of how people would look at them because they were dating a person in a wheelchair.

Jonathan, who had been injured when he was seven years old, experienced similar difficulties:

> I didn't date in high school. I drove a jeep, a convertible GTO, and I was a pretty cool guy now that I look back but I didn't think so at the time. And it was all because of the wheelchair. You're self-conscious. You're in a high school and you've got 500 seniors and you're the only person in a wheelchair. . . . And back then, these old wheelchairs, they were big, bulky, and they were big, chrome, silver things. They were behemoths and they weighed 80 pounds.

After high school, Jonathan attended college, where he had an active dating life. He married an attractive woman and remains married.

For several men, the wheelchair remained a barrier to asking women out even in adulthood. Ryan reported,

> There's a big fear on my part of reaching to a woman . . . because of my wheelchair. I'm afraid that they're gonna look at the wheelchair and say, "Oh, he's in a wheelchair, I can't do that. I want a perfect man." Or something like that. . . . I can't see just any girl out on the street and just go up and ask her because of that doubt in my mind.

Similarly, Ben, a walking quadriplegic who had previously used a wheel-chair, said he was timid about asking women out, and that the wheelchair compounded his shyness: "It prevented me from taking any risks."

Several women stressed that a disability is often regarded as a practical encumbrance. For example, Jennifer felt that able-bodied individuals

> don't want to work out all the accommodations that go with it 'cause there's a lot that can't be done. . . . My fiancé knows that I can't cook and I can't clean and there's just a lot of normal everyday stuff that he has to do for me. And I think a lot of people wouldn't either be willing or wouldn't want to go that far.

Likewise, Shannon stated,

> I think they feel it's limiting to what you're able to do or they'd be able to do. And maybe they want to go do all these things and the

person that's disabled wouldn't be able to keep up or do this with them.

Meanwhile, Tonya attributed people's reluctance to get involved with disabled individuals to her belief that "most people are not educated":

> I think they all think we have the plague or something. It's contagious or something—it's gonna jump out and get 'em or something.

Finally, a few disagreed with the statement that "people do not want to get involved with someone who has a disability." As Jay realistically reflected,

> There are some people that wouldn't mind, and there's some people that would mind. Some people might want to purposely find someone with a disability and some people could care less either way.

Still, the majority complained that the tendency to dismiss individuals with disabilities was all too common.

## Disability and Dating Preferences Among Individuals with SCI

Altogether, 19% of the participants in the study reported that they had been involved in intimate relationships with others who had physical disabilities, with slightly more women (29%) than men (16%) indicating this. There was no consistent pattern between the degree of impairment and the likelihood of involvement with other disabled individuals. Meanwhile, individuals who had been paralyzed for longer periods of time were somewhat more likely to indicate prior intimate involvement with other disabled individuals, a finding which may reflect more opportunities (lengthier exposure) or a greater openness to such relationships.[2]

Goffman (1963) asserted that the more individuals with stigmatized identities ally themselves with nonstigmatized individuals, the more they see themselves in nonstigmatic terms. There is, in fact, a tendency for disabled individuals to distance themselves from others with disabilities (Low 1996; Yoshida 1991, 1994b). Disabled men, in particular, have been shown to prefer able-bodied partners (Fine and Asch 1988b). While the overwhelming majority of participants (74%) reported no preference regarding the disability status of their dating partners, it is noteworthy that 26%—including 29% of females and 25% of males—preferred to avoid relationships with other disabled individuals. Of the twelve participants involved in intimate relationships at the time of the study, only one reported that his partner had a physical disability (asthma and Reflex Sympathetic Disorder).

The individuals I interviewed gave a variety of reasons for their avoidance of romantic relationships with others who have physical disabilities (which was generally understood to mean others with SCI). For example, Edward stated,

> I'm the same as everybody else. I don't want to date somebody that's disabled. It's not that I wouldn't like the person, but it just doesn't turn me on. And that's probably another reason why I don't blame anybody for not wanting to go out with me or not showing interest in me. It's just a fact of the world.

He first explained that his reluctance to date women with disabilities was related to two issues: maintenance and the fact that someone in a wheelchair would be a "turn-off." Upon further probing, however, he mentioned that his willingness to get involved in such a relationship might depend on "how much feeling she has in her legs," assuming they were to have sexual relations.

Many felt that bringing together two individuals with disabilities would compound the practical problems that each one experienced—difficulties with mobility, access, etc. Meanwhile, Travis pointed to what he perceived as his own hypocrisy in having a preference for an able-bodied partner:

> That's a hard question because it makes me seem like an asshole. . . . If I'm out there fighting for disability rights and I don't see myself being able to have an intimate relationship with somebody who has a disability. . . . Knowing what I have to go through, I can't imagine how it would work out with two people with disabilities. I just think you would have to overcome so much. . . . I know that I'm really hard to live with because I'm an asshole at times, but I also know that part of that is my disability. And I can't imagine being able to deal with that if both myself and my partner were disabled.

Similarly, Ryan explained his reluctance to date women with SCI by pointing to the challenges involved in accomplishing day-to-day tasks:

> If I date or say that I get married to another person in a wheelchair, those are gonna be a lot of problems that are gonna be put together.
>
> EIW: Can you tell me what problems you have in mind?
>
> For instance, I know this sounds bad [*laughter*] but if I buy a house later on in life and it has a yard or something I can't necessarily go out and mow that yard. But if I have an able-bodied wife who didn't mind, and I'm not saying, "Oh, I have to have a wife who goes out and does all this stuff for me." I'm not that kind of person. But she can go out and mow that lawn. But if you have two people that are in a wheelchairs, how's your lawn gonna get mowed?

Ryan also worried that a disabled woman might be less able to bear children—a statement not supported by medical evidence, at least as far as SCI is concerned. Stacy mentioned the potential difficulty of getting chores accomplished, and the challenges of maneuvering:

> I think I would feel uncomfortable. I feel horrible saying this. . . . Like, okay, we went out on a date, two wheelchairs in one car—nu-uh—not gonna happen, y'know? [*chuckle*] It's just the little things.

Interestingly, when the people I interviewed pictured the problems that might arise in relationships with other disabled individuals, they always thought of partners with disabilities that paralleled their own (paraplegia, quadriplegia, etc.). While those with paraplegia tended to mention the difficulties of accomplishing day-to-day tasks, many of those with quadriplegia focused on sexual relations. For example, Meghan described the challenges she envisioned:

> They can't maneuver, so what are you gonna do? Well, it would be kind of limited to oral sex if we could get positioned in the right way. I don't want to do that.

She also imagined what it would be like to have a personal care attendant assisting with sexual relations:

And we're gonna have an attendant right there or like standing there. We'll be the royalty of all, and have a thing like, "Okay, put me here. All right, move that leg over there. Put this hand here. All right. Put the other. Okay, now go back outside."

She even jokingly described a scenario where she might call the Department of Social Services to request assistance:

"Dammit, I needed my thighs spread. There was no one here to do it." That's a problem.

EIW: [*laughter*]

Woo! They'd have me certified in a New York minute.

In fact, however, the idea of an attendant assisting in intimate relations is not as far-fetched as Meghan might think. Chigier (1981) describes a video that shows how a nurse can help two consenting adults engage in sexual relations. "This is the kind of thing that, when you think about it, is really not so wild or radical" (Chigier 1981: 137). For a number of those interviewed, the idea of two individuals with SCI having an intimate relationship was an amusing prospect. Todd laughed and said, "Well, hell, neither one of you can feel anything."

Meanwhile, Tonya opined that men with SCI are

not interested in another handicapped person. The men want an able-bodied female. They don't want a handicapped girl. I've figured that out. . . . I think females—we just want a relationship with someone we can talk to, someone that can be there for you to help you, or you can help them. That's all I want from somebody. But the guys don't look at it that way. They want a trophy. If you're in a wheelchair and you have an able-bodied person that likes you, then it's like a trophy.

Tonya added, "You would think some of these guys would be more accepting of the females that are in chairs"—but her experience suggested otherwise. In spite of Tonya's assessment, both male and female participants in the study were somewhat reluctant to get involved in relationships with other disabled individuals.

## The Ideal Partner

I asked the study participants what qualities they value in a partner, and whether their preferences had changed since their injuries. Several stated that they now place greater emphasis on finding partners who are emotionally and intellectually compatible, although some aren't certain whether this change in attitudes is related to their disabilities or simply to greater maturity. For example, Travis stated that he no longer subscribes to what is "quote normal for accepted societal physical beauty." He described how his approach toward relationships had shifted:

> My mindset used to be the ideal playboy: large breasts, nice body, that whole kind of thing. And, I think as I matured my disability had some effect on that but I think my maturity also had some effect on looking at the value of a mate as far as an intimate relationship differently. . . . I see so many people that are extremely good looking as far as physical beauty, but they couldn't carry on a conversation about anything.

At the same time, most of the participants have a clear message to convey: "Just because I have a disability doesn't mean I've compromised my standards." They still want physically attractive partners, and if their values have changed at all, it is primarily due to their own personal growth and the need to find someone who is emotionally compatible as well. For example, Stacy stated:

> I'm like six feet tall. I still like tall men, and you'd think I would prefer shorter men or I really wouldn't care. . . . I mean my physical attraction kind of changed. I mean, I think now I look for more depth and more maturity.

Stacy felt her accident had prompted her to mature more quickly, and she said that most of the college men she met were not compatible. Similarly, Edward emphasized the importance of both emotional and physical chemistry:

> I would be looking more for a lasting relationship. It's changed in that way but my preferences—I don't like fat girls, that's not changed. People say, "You're too picky in which you want your women to look like." That's the way I've always been and that's not

going to change. If they're overweight, if they don't do anything for me physically or emotionally, so I wouldn't date somebody that's not gonna turn me on.

Edward told me that he hadn't been involved in a relationship for several years. He seemed especially irritated with the effect that his injury had on his social life.

Several of Derrick's friends had arranged dates for him, but he found that he seldom liked the women they set him up with: "They're like, 'You can't be picky. You're a quad now.' And I'm going, 'Bullshit.'" During our interview, Derrick gave me his dating card—the size of a regular business card, but pink, and with a small heart in each corner. It read:

BEST BOYFRIEND YOU'VE EVER HAD IN YOUR LIFE!!!
1.) I can't run around on you! (legs don't work)
2.) I can't grab or abuse you! (hands don't work)
3.) I'm submissive in the bed (I like the bottom)
4.) I have a script for VIAGRA (never too tired!)
5.) I'll treat you like a *QUEEN* if I'm your King!
[Derrick's phone number]
SATISFACTION GUARANTEED! YOU WON'T BE SORRY!

He told me he was looking for "a nice Christian lady"—someone who would be honest, caring, and loving. He added that it wouldn't hurt if she were also rich and attractive. Only one participant, Jeremy, said that he had lowered his standards:

Your standards is a little bit lower than what they were [*laughter*] when you was up running around. But then again, they're a little bit fine-tuned.

EIW: How have your standards changed?

Man, that's double-edged right there, because I still like beautiful women.

Upon further probing, he told me that he still wanted someone attractive and that he had a special penchant for petite women. He also said, "When I was standing I really didn't care, didn't have to have a brain, now I'm more or less looking" for someone intelligent. In the end, it almost seemed as if Jeremy's standards had risen in the aftermath of his injury.

## Relationships with Service Providers

Relationships between service providers and individuals with SCI are not uncommon. Sixteen percent of women with SCI have engaged in sexual activity with health care personnel (Sipski and Alexander 1993), and approximately 50% of women dating men with SCI have had considerable prior experience with disabled individuals. Many have worked as nurses or as occupational therapists. For these women, prior contact has presumably eased their reservations about dating individuals with disabilities (Milligan and Neufeldt 1988). At the same time, marriages between disabled individuals and nurses/providers often do not succeed. This may stem from difficulties in role transition, or from the fact that some providers marry patients in the hope of achieving financial security (DeLoach and Greer 1981).

Of the 31 individuals I interviewed, eight—mostly men—said that they had dated or been involved in a relationship with a personal care attendant, occupational therapist, or rehabilitation counselor.[3] In several cases, these relationships began while the individual was still a client of the service provider. While the Code of Ethics of the Commission on Rehabilitation Counseling states that "a personal relationship compromises the effectiveness of the counselor-client relationship" (Wright and Martin 1987: 343), many study participants seemed genuinely unaware of the potential for harm inherent in such relationships. Instead, they focused on the advantages of dating a care provider—the comfort, understanding, and prior knowledge that make it unnecessary to explain everything. As Al said,

> It's easier to meet a therapist than somebody out on the street. . . . two sisters, if one's a therapist and one knows nothing about it. It would be easier to go out with a therapist just 'cause they know all about it.

Harry described how he had become involved in a relationship with a therapist he met during rehabilitation. He was frustrated because one of the female nurses—ostensibly out of jealousy—was trying to discourage his relationship as well as those of some of the other men:

> There was a couple of us guys in the rehabilitation center that was having relationships with people, and this overweight nurse who was married and tied down was pissed off because these other people in wheelchairs—of all things—having fun! "Bullshit! That's not

supposed to happen." So she was trying to break us up the whole time—trying to get her [girlfriend] to go on dates with all these big cowboy boyfriends of her husband and all this stuff. It was a losing battle.

Meanwhile, Travis was living with a woman who had been his therapist. He described her initial hesitancy to get involved with him:

> Even when we first started becoming friends and stuff, she couldn't deal with it. . . . But then we got to talking and stuff, and she would come see me when I was in the hospital. [It] gradually turned into something where we both knew that there was something there. And for the longest time she wouldn't admit to it because if I was her patient, it would be unethical in her opinion. So she couldn't get over the idea that I had been her patient. But everybody I've talked to—and I've known numerous people who've ended up marrying their therapists and stuff—it's not unethical; I was no longer her patient [when we became involved].

At the time of the interview, Travis and Mary were living together and considering marriage.

Derrick had been involved in one intimate relationship since sustaining his injury—with Ellen, a nurse's aide he met during rehabilitation. Near the end of their relationship, when things were going poorly, Ellen had encouraged Derrick's son to disobey him:

> [She] told him that he didn't have to listen to me because I couldn't do anything about it anyway, and that he had to listen to her. He was wanting to get up from the dinner table at a restaurant one night and I told him he had finish his plate. She said, "Just go ahead." And I said, "No. He's gonna sit here and finish his meal before he goes and plays video games." And she said, "Just go ahead, Ron, you don't need to listen to him. He can't do nothing anyway." And when she said that it was like a stake through my heart.

Derrick told me that he also questioned whether Ellen had been faithful to him.

Stacy had dated a personal caregiver, although not her own:

> I dated a guy this summer. Actually, I met him at that conference.
> He was the personal assistant to a guy that was there. But he lives
> in Arizona so it's not working out. He came here to visit and
> everything, but other than that I really haven't dated this year at all
> and I'm okay with that right now.

Along with those who had dated service providers, a number of participants
reported having met their intimate partners through businesses or organizations that provide disability-related services such as wheelchair repair or
vocational rehabilitation training.

## Unhealthy Relationships

Individuals with disabilities are more like to find themselves in abusive relationships than their nondisabled counterparts (Ducharme and Gill 1997;
Hwang 1997; Sobsey 1994). In particular, many women with disabilities
feel that their disabilities make them more vulnerable in relationships with
men (Tighe 2001). Moreover, certain nondisabled individuals are especially
likely to have a "prurient interest" in wheelchair users (Marks 1999: 92).
DeLoach and Greer (1981) classify individuals especially attracted to disabled persons into four groups: (1) *the walking wounded* (people who have
been deeply hurt in a previous relationship with an able-bodied person); (2)
*the would-be dictators* (those who are insecure and feel the need to dominate
others); (3) *the unsolicited missionaries* (those who try to "save" individuals with disabilities); and (4) *the gallant gesturers* (those who discount the
sexuality of disabled individuals and thereby view any liaison with them as
a basis for self-congratulation).

A few reported having been involved with partners who fit the profile
of the "would-be dictator." For example, Harry described a woman with
whom he had been involved:

> That girl I was telling you about—the one I was getting ready to get
> married to again—she didn't want me doing any rehabilitation. . . . I
> always had the dream to walk again and I'd work out and work out,
> and we'd get into these horrible fights and she'd say, "I don't know
> why the fuck you ever work out." . . . I was trying to get strong and
> she's like, "Why in the hell you even work out?" And I knew we were
> getting ready to break up, I mean you can just tell. And I'm like, "I'm
> gonna walk again if it f'n kills me."

After the relationship dissolved, Harry returned to a rehabilitation center and learned to walk using leg braces. Shannon told me about her relationship with a truck driver whom she had met a few years after her injury. She had married him just a few months after they met:

> It's all a bad experience. I've really tried to erase it. [*laughter*] He was very verbally abusive and somewhat physically abusive. . . . A very abusive personality and a very controlling person. And I don't sit well being controlled. He wanted someone he could really push around and take care of, and I didn't need to be taken care of that much.

Shannon went on to marry another man who treated her well.

As Rosa noted, individuals with SCI can themselves be abusive. She described how her former boyfriend, who also had a spinal cord injury, had victimized her:

> I was set on fire, doused with rubbing alcohol and then he set his lighter in my hair 'cause I used to process my hair and so my hair caught right on fire. And I was burned 37 percent of my body. Of course, it had to hit the upper top part, the lower half is already shot and then being set on fire messed up my top part. So I felt like that took my looks. I lost my legs in '85 and then I lost my looks in '89.

Rosa didn't know why her boyfriend had been so abusive, but she thought his attitude seemed to be, "If I can't have you, then nobody can."

## Union Formation and Dissolution

Previous studies have shown that individuals with SCI are more likely than others to be single (Berkowitz et al. 1992, 1998) and that individuals may be selected (or deselected) for marriage on the basis of their health or disability status (Brown and Giesy 1986; Donohue and Gebhard 1995). Individuals with SCI—women and minorities, in particular—are especially prone to divorce (Berkowitz et al. 1992, 1998; Bonwich 1985; Brown and Giesy 1986; Crewe, Athelstan, and Krumberger 1979; DeVivo and Fine 1985; Dijkers et al. 1995; Donohue and Gebhard 1995; Kasprzyk 1983; Richards, Tepper, et al. 1997). Most changes in marital status occur in the early years following injury (Dijkers et al. 1995). Although SCI doesn't necessarily *cause* a relationship to dissolve, it may provide the impetus to end a relationship which is "teetering on the brink of collapse" (Strawn 1966: 33). Unstable marriages are especially likely to collapse under the stress of SCI (Trieschmann 1980, 1988, 1989).

Several aspects of SCI—altered sexual performance, restricted mobility, bowel and bladder problems, reduced fertility, and attitudinal barriers—have been shown to cause stress in intimate relationships (see, for example, Brown and Giesy 1986; Crewe 1993; David, Gur, and Rozin 1977–78; Drew-Cates 1989; Dijkers et al. 1995). When one partner acquires an SCI, individual differences are frequently accentuated. This is especially true regarding pace of life, temperature preferences, income allocation, and social activities (DeLoach and Greer 1981). Those with severe injuries are more likely to divorce, as are those without children (El Ghatit and Hanson 1976). The risk of divorce is also directly linked to the number of role changes that occur—the number of roles (provider, household worker, etc.) that must be abandoned or transferred in response to disability (Killen 1987).

Intimate relationships can be especially difficult when the roles of caregiver and lover are combined (Crewe 1993; Crewe, Athelstan, and Krumberger 1979; Dodd 1991; Ducharme et al. 1988).[4] In such cases, spouses frequently experience role conflict as their marital relationships become more similar to those of parent and child or nurse and patient (Kester 1986). Among women whose husbands have SCI, life satisfaction declines as the perceived burden of care increases (Santora 1996). Men often find it difficult to assume what may be a necessary caregiving role (Morris 1989), and many women report feeling trapped by family and societal expectations into caring for their disabled husbands (Chan 2000; Oliver et al. 1988). Chronic anxiety is a common problem among the spouses of individuals with SCI (Kester 1986), and able-bodied partners who care for their disabled spouses exhibit especially high levels of vulnerability (dependency and fear of separation) (Feigin 1994).

In contrast, other studies find that SCI has only a minimal impact on the likelihood of marriage dissolution (Crewe, Athelstan, and Krumberger 1979; Deyoe 1972; El Ghatit and Hanson 1976; Guttmann 1964; Hudson 1990; Neilson 1990; Oliver et al. 1988; Teal and Athelstan 1975). In some cases, spinal cord injury may even strengthen marriages by providing greater emotional depth (Oliver et al. 1988; Quintiliani 2000). Despite the burdens and emotional upheavals that accompany disability, some wives of men with SCI view the adjustment period as a time of emotional growth and positive change in which the couple grew closer (Vargo 1984).

Of the study participants, half were single, 25% were engaged or married, and another 25% were divorced or separated. Younger individuals were especially likely to be single, as were those with more severe impairments. While many participants with high-level spinal cord injuries expressed a desire to be married, none had entered into marriage since becoming disabled (one such female was engaged, however). Among the thirty-two participants in my study, seven had been married, one had been engaged, and seven had had steady boyfriends/girlfriends (or had been in committed relationships) when they first became disabled. However, only three (all married) had remained with the individuals who had been their partners at the time of their injuries. The others' relationships dissolved soon after they became disabled. For example, Cody described how his relationship with his girlfriend ended shortly after he was shot at the age of 28:

> I guess she just couldn't take me being a paraplegic. We just sort
> of spread apart. . . . There were a lot of issues. I don't think she
> was strong enough to handle the things that had come with being
> injured.

The difficulty of having a partner with SCI was a common theme among those whose relationships had fallen apart. Walter told me that his was ex-wife could not handle the injury, and Rosa reported that her fiancé "didn't want to be strapped to the responsibility."

Several described how impaired mobility and extensive caregiving needs compromised their ability to have enduring and successful intimate relationships. For example, Fred recalled his frustration during the time he was dating Eileen, a home health care aide:

> We went to Funland [an amusement park] just for a date. I couldn't
> win her anything. A teddy bear or y'know, I couldn't. . . . And I just
> said, "Fuck it, let's go home." . . . It's hard to love a person in my
> condition. Who wants to love a person in a wheelchair that you have
> to do 99.9 percent of their daily management?

Similarly, Todd told me that his relationship with his girlfriend (whom he had begun dating prior to his injury) had become more tenuous as she assumed an increasing range of caregiving responsibilities:

> Things just didn't work out. She really never could accept my injury so I ended up breaking up with her. . . . It became to where she was like my caregiver and we didn't have any intimacy anymore or anything like that. I couldn't live that way anymore.

Todd attributed the lack of intimacy to his girlfriend's discomfort. "Ever since I had my injury, she wouldn't have anything to do with me in that respect," he said.

Several indicated that it was they—not their partners—who had broken off long-standing relationships. For example, Travis felt that things had changed so dramatically in the aftermath of his injury that it was unrealistic to expect the relationship to continue:

> When I first got hurt in high school my girlfriend—the girl I was dating—could never say it, but I think we both knew that we weren't together anymore. And finally, it's one of the moments that I'm most proud of myself because I was able to be an adult about it and basically tell her that, "Hey, we both know it's over, let's just admit to that."

At the time of his injury, Travis was a high school football player and he had been dating one of the cheerleaders. Likewise, Stan encouraged his girlfriend to date others after he was injured in a swimming accident at the age of 17. He felt it was unfair of him to expect her to continue the relationship while he was in the hospital. He explained:

> Between [where I lived] and [the hospital] was some sixty-five miles. Plus I was in therapy. And I was going to focus all my energies on getting better.

Meanwhile, Adam told me that his relationship with his girlfriend had fallen apart largely because of how he had responded to his injury:

> I was really nervous about going out into social situations because I wasn't really sure how to handle it at the time.
>
> EIW: What were you nervous about?

Accessibility. I was afraid I might get out and have some sort of accident with maybe my bowel program or my bladder program. I was just really nervous about everything at the time because it was all so new, so I just thought it was safer just to stay home, and that put a lot of strain on us.

Urey, Viar, and Henggeler (1987) stress the importance of participating in recreational and social activities outside the family, especially since the absence of these activities has been associated with problems in marital adjustment.

## Current Relationships and Post-Injury Unions

Marriages established post-injury tend to have greater stability than those established before the onset of disability (Crewe, Athelstan, and Krumberger 1979; Crewe and Krause 1988; Dodd 1991; Deyoe 1972; Simmons 1981; Simmons and Ball 1984).[5] This may be related to higher levels of self-actualization and inner-directedness among those who opt to marry individuals with SCI (Simmons and Ball 1984). Moreover, couples who marry post-injury do not have to contend with the redefinition of relationships that accompanies the trauma of SCI (Crewe and Krause 1988). Psychological assessments reveal that post-injury marriage partners are significantly more satisfied with their living arrangements, sex lives, social lives, general health, emotional adjustment, and sense of control over their lives (Crewe, Athelstan, and Krumberger 1979; Crewe and Krause 1988). Although Kreuter and associates (1994b) found no significant difference in overall satisfaction between individuals in pre- and post-injury relationships, they did note that partners from pre-injury marriages are more likely to report a decline in the frequency of sexual activity and a deterioration in their sex lives.

Of the thirty-two individuals in the sample, twelve were involved in intimate relationships at the time of the study (including nine in post-injury relationships). Six had entered into marriage after the onset of their disabilities. Of the six, four had subsequently divorced, although one had remarried a second time. A similar divorce/separation rate (four of seven) can be seen among those participants who were married at the time of their injuries. Although my sample is small, these findings suggest high levels of marital instability for both types of marriages.

While some evidence suggests that married and single people with SCI have comparable physical and mental health (Putzke, Elliott, and Richards 2001), those who are married report greater life satisfaction, possibly because they have a larger support system, are more effective communicators, or encounter fewer challenges than unmarried persons (Chase 1998; Putzke, Elliott, and Richards 2001). Among those in my sample who were involved in intimate relationships, the majority reported meaningful relationships with their partners. At the same time, however, several—both those who were involved and those who were not—mentioned that their disabilities had put them in a vulnerable position. For example, Leonard reflected:

> It seems like when you're married it can be held over your head how you need me. "You're disabled and you won't find somebody else." This, that, and the other. That's always come up. Everybody I know that's in a chair, be it male or female, that's pretty much come up in one way or another.

The individuals with the most satisfying intimate relationships are often those who can most successfully renegotiate relational roles and expectations. This frequently requires that partners redefine traditional gender roles, and it may also involve new attitudes toward sexual intimacy (Nemeth 2000). The ability to "see past the disability" is also important, especially among individuals who are getting to know one another. Walter described how he met his current girlfriend, Mandy:

> When somebody looks at me, the first thing they see is the chair, they don't see a person, they see the chair. You didn't. [*gestures to Mandy*]

Walter and Mandy were living together at the time of the interview. They were contemplating marriage, but they also reported that there were issues they needed to resolve.

While relationship instability was widespread, several participants described secure, loving marriages. For instance, Shannon stated that her current husband, whom she married in the aftermath of her injury, "is a sweetie; he's a sweetie." While Andrew and his wife had been separated for at least a year and a half at the time of his injury, they had subsequently reconciled. "It bonded us back together," he said (although they later separated again). Chris has a very close relationship with his wife, whom he married before he became disabled. "Oh yeah, we're buddies. We do about everything together. Of course, I don't try to dictate what she can do, what she can't." Meanwhile, Roger reported that his wife had been an important source of support in the period immediately following his injury:

> Everybody was real supportive through the whole thing. They understood where I was at and especially my wife, she supported me. She took over managing the business and she just said, "Okay, you just deal with this problem and I'm gonna take care of the home life." And she took care of me for three years basically. And we never really sat down and discussed how she felt about the situation. There was never really any time for that.

Roger felt that he was currently paying the price for this lack of communication. He and his wife were in counseling at the time of the interview. They were also experiencing sexual problems, and it was evident that they had many obstacles to overcome in order to make their marriage work.

## Marital Intentions

Of the 24 single (not engaged or married) participants in the study, a majority (54%) expressed an intention to marry some day. Thirty-three percent were uncertain about their future marital plans, and 13% did not plan to get married. Unmarried men were considerably more likely than their female counterparts to indicate definite plans to marry (63% versus 20%). In comparison with disabled men, disabled women are often regarded as less attractive potential marriage partners (Kutner 1987), and women are less likely than men to marry following SCI (Dijkers et al. 1995; Trieschmann 1980, 1989). While women with SCI do encounter major difficulties in the marriage market, the sex difference in marriage plans may also reflect a genuine lack of interest in marriage among some disabled women.

Men were somewhat more likely than women to indicate that their disabilities had influenced their attitudes toward marriage. The degree of impairment had no clear impact on attitudes, however. While I anticipated that those who had become divorced and/or separated in the aftermath of their injuries would be more likely to have experienced a change in attitudes toward marriage, only two of the five individuals who had experienced such a separation/divorce felt that their disabilities had affected such attitudes.

Meanwhile, however, a substantial number reported that their disabilities had prompted them to question whether they would ever find a suitable mate. For example, Travis described how his views had changed in the immediate aftermath of his injury:

> As a result of my disability I basically had realized that I probably would never get married. And I had resigned myself to that and was dealing with the ramifications of that. I was very involved in school activities and that kind of thing. . . . And then I met Mary and I've gotten very uninvolved in school activities because I'm very committed to this relationship and making this relationship work.

Like Travis, Jennifer felt destined for a life of spinsterhood following her injury: "At first, I thought that there wouldn't be a man that would want to marry a woman in a wheelchair. And I think I had that perception for a long time, until I met my fiancé."

While Stacy reported that her attitudes toward marriage were unaffected by her disability, she did admit that "it may take a little bit more time to find someone that I'll be perfect with. But other than that, I plan on getting married some day." In contrast, Tonya told me that she had voluntarily removed herself from the dating scene because of all her physical problems (in addition to her spinal cord injury, Tonya has pancreatitis):

> I assume—I may be wrong and I could be—I assume that most men do not want the problems that I have, medically or physically. This is a lot to handle. So I don't even put myself in the position to be involved with anything. I have friends that are male and they all understand. This is my problem. It's unfortunately my kids' problems, but I don't feel like I should dump it on somebody else.

While research has shown that women with SCI sometimes reject potential partners because of a perceived sense of pity, a decreased libido, or fear that sexual intimacy will hurt (Donohue and Gebhard 1995), Tonya's withdrawal seemed specific to her physical complications.

A few, primarily high-level quadriplegics with very limited arm and hand control, felt that their disabilities reduced their marital appeal because of the extensive care they required. For example, Kevin agreed strongly that his disability affected his attitude toward marriage. "I feel like a pain in the ass to somebody," he said. "Somebody always has to take care of me and that's not exactly my idea of marriage." When I asked Kevin if he thought some day he'd get married, he replied, "I have no idea."

While Ryan definitely wanted to get married someday, he was somewhat fearful of it on account of his SCI:

> I think that kind of goes back to the whole sexual and having babies thing. That's my main problem with marriage. I would love it if I didn't have to worry about that and could just find a wife and get married. I don't necessarily have any fears about getting married, but it's just finding a wife who can accept me and then the whole whether or not I can have children thing.

Vibha worried that she might eventually be abandoned if she were to marry an able-bodied spouse:

> I'm just scared that if I marry somebody who is nondisabled, later there'll be a situation where the person will probably prefer a person who's not disabled than a person who is disabled.

At the time of the interview, Vibha was involved in a long-distance relationship with an able-bodied man.

## Spinal Cord Injury and Fertility

Spinal cord injury is a barrier to male fertility. Up to 95% of men with SCI experience ejaculatory problems (Seager and Halstead 1993), and many others suffer from retrograde ejaculation whereby semen travels into the bladder rather than out through the urethra (Bielunis 1995; Hammond et al. 1992; Linsenmeyer 1997). Semen quality, particularly sperm motility, is frequently impaired in men with SCI due to a number of factors including sperm contact with urine (due to retrograde ejaculation), prolonged sitting in a wheelchair, long-term use of medications, and alterations in the testicular reflex mechanism responsible for maintaining a temperature appropriate for spermatogenesis (Becker 1978; Drench 1992; Freehafer 1997; Linsenmeyer 1997). In the absence of interventions, the successful pregnancy rate for sex partners of men with SCI is less than 5% (Griffith, Tomko, and Timms 1973; Sidman 1977).[6] Many men with SCI do produce sperm capable of impregnating a woman, however, and interventions such as electroejaculation (ejaculation resulting from an electric current placed into the rectum) offer great promise for enhancing men's fertility potential (DeForge et al. 2004; Halstead and Seager 1993; Seager and Halstead 1993; Sipski 1997c).[7] Recent research suggests that advanced fertility techniques can increase fertility rates for men with SCI to above 50% (DeForge et al. 2004).

In contrast, SCI has only a minor impact of the fecundity of women. Although women with SCI frequently experience a short break in the menstrual cycle immediately following injury, the resumption of normal menses usually occurs within four to six months of injury (Axel 1982; Ducharme et al. 1988; Ducharme and Gill 1997; Fitting et al. 1978; Garden 1991; Senelick 1998; Trieschmann 1980, 1989; Palmer, Kriegsman, and Palmer 2000; Willmuth 1987).[8] As long as they are menstruating regularly, women with SCI are unimpaired in their ability to conceive—regardless of the level or severity of their injuries (Axel 1982; Bielunis 1995; Davis 1995; Freehafer 1997; McDonald et al. 1993; Mooney, Cole, and Chilgren 1975; Senelick 1998; Sipski 1997a; Webster 1983). Since reproductive organs are protected internally, pregnancy and full term deliveries are possible (Comarr 1973; Drench 1992; Farrow 1990; Robbins 1985). Some have even argued that childbirth is easier for women with flaccid paralysis, since their abdominal muscles are naturally relaxed (DeLoach and Greer 1981). At the same time, women with SCI report that it is a challenge to find obstetricians or midwives who are willing to help them through what are perceived to be high-risk pregnancies (Fine and Asch 1988b).

Although the ability to get pregnant is not affected by SCI, little is known about the pregnancy failure rate or the incidence of birth deformities (DeForge et al. 2004). Women with SCI who carry their pregnancies to term are at increased risk of complications such as anemia, premature labor, osteoporosis, rapid delivery, urinary tract infections, pressure sores, and autonomic dysreflexia (Baker and Cardenas 1996; Becker 1978; Bérard 1989; Bielunis 1995; Davis 1995; Freehafer 1997; Garden 1991; Mackelprang and Hepworth 1990; McDonald et al. 1993; Morris 1989; Senelick 1998; Singh and Sharma 2005; Sipski 1997a; Sipski and Alexander 1992; Verduyn 1993; Willmuth 1987). Moreover, women with complete lesions above the T-10 level may not experience sensations of contraction or fetal movement (Garden 1991; Grundy and Russell 1986; Zasler 1991). For these reasons, pregnant women with SCI often need to take special care to ensure the safe delivery of their infants.

SCI also interferes with a woman's ability to use certain contraceptive methods. For example, oral contraceptives and Depo-Provera may cause an increased risk of thromboembolic disorders and are therefore contraindicated. The intrauterine device (IUD) poses the risk of asymptomatic pelvis inflammatory disease (PID) or uterine perforation, which may in turn result in infertility and/or sepsis. Barrier methods of contraception also present challenges. For example, a woman's catheter may cause a condom to tear, and the weakening of the pelvic muscles may cause a diaphragm to dislodge. Among women with SCI, spermicides have been associated with vaginal irritation and urinary tract infections (see Nunchuck 1991 for details).

## Parenting Intentions

Individuals with SCI are less likely than their nondisabled counterparts to report that their need for having and raising children is well met (Whiteneck 1993), and "taking care of children" is indicated as a key area of concern for many with SCI (Elliott and Shewchuck 2002). Although evidence suggests that mothers with SCI provide well for their children (Alexander, Hwang, and Sipski 2001; Westgren and Levi 1994), many individuals with SCI feel that their disability makes them unable to serve as parents.[9] For example, some women either relinquish custody of their children or give up their plans to have children because of the physical and financial limitations related to SCI (Bonwich 1985). A delay in childbearing is also common (Cross et al. 1991).

Of the thirty-two study participants, eight (25%) indicated a desire for children (or additional children), fifteen (47%) said they wanted no children (or no additional children), and nine (28%) were undecided. Men were more likely to express a desire for (additional) children, but there was little variation in response by severity of impairment. Although participants without children were more likely to indicate a desire for (additional) children, it is noteworthy that only seven of them (35%) planned to have any. This finding reinforces the notion that SCI alters fertility intentions.

While most of the participants in the study indicated that their disabilities had no bearing on their childbearing intentions, several quadriplegics questioned their ability to adequately care for a child. For example, Chris said, "See, I can't take care of a kid. . . . If it's a baby, it falls and crashes, I can't pick it up. I can't change dirty diapers. I can't do nothing." Kevin expressed similar concerns:

I like my little nephews and stuff, but I don't know if I'd feel comfortable having a little baby because I wouldn't be able to hold it or when it started crying and wouldn't be able to play with it a whole lot and stuff like that. So I wouldn't feel comfortable. I wouldn't feel like it was fair to that little baby having a father stuck in a wheelchair that can't do anything for them.

Several others felt that they might be able to care for a child but were concerned about their ability to fulfill traditional parental roles. For example, when I asked Todd if he wanted children, he replied:

It's kind of an iffy thing. Ultimately, I think I would, but one of my things that I have kind of in my head is I wouldn't be able to maybe do as many things with [the child]. Like if I had a son, I wouldn't be able to go out and play ball with him like a normal dad would. . . . And being able to take care of 'em and everything and stuff being in this situation. But I think I could handle it.

When I asked Todd how many children he wanted, he laughed and replied, "Twenty!" Fred also wanted a large family, but expressed reservations due to his disability:

Maybe not, because if I had my boys, I couldn't teach them how to hunt and fish, drop the meter, and they might not accept me being like this.

Fred had helped raise two twin boys while in a previous relationship, however, and he thought he had done "very well."

Some of the women remain ambivalent about the impact of their disability on their childbearing intentions. Stacy stated that her many health problems had caused her to question whether she would ever want to bear children:

I was so young when I got injured, I don't really know what I was thinking. I always thought, yeah, a husband, kids. I don't know if . . . now without the disability if I would have changed that. I don't know if I want kids. . . . If I do want kids, I don't know if I would want to have them myself or if I want to adopt or something like that. With all the internal problems I've had and just all the complications that come with it, it's scary. It's hard on your body, but I would love to adopt, or I don't know if I really want kids, either. [*chuckle*]

Stacy had sustained a number of internal injuries in the accident that left her paralyzed, and she feared the potential complications that might result were she to become pregnant. Meanwhile, Vibha expressed fears that her children might be born with her disability, spina bifida, which has a hereditary component. She also questioned her ability to care for a child.

Although one participant in the study had adopted a child, none had physically conceived children after becoming injured. Among those who stated they were uncertain or definitely wanted (additional) children, approximately half planned to have their own biological children. Men were less likely than women to indicate this intention, and several of them indicated that fertility concerns were a source of considerable stress in their lives. For example, Ryan stated,

Had I not had my injury, I don't know if I would necessarily be worrying about [children] right now. I think that I would just be worrying about who was gonna be my wife and thinking, "later down the road when we have kids." But now it's "later down the road *if* we have kids." And so I believe it definitely has changed my attitude toward that. I cherish kids. I like being around kids and some guys aren't like that, and so it definitely hurts me to know that there's a possibility that I can't have kids.

Andrew described the disappointment he felt when he was informed by the doctor that he was incapable of fathering a child:

Before my ex-wife and I split up, I went to the doctor and told him, "Look, I want to have a test done; I want to see if they can swim." . . . He said, "No." He said that from my accident and the way that I sat and the way that my testicles were so close to my body all the time, that if I did produce sperm it probably wouldn't have the capability to impregnate a lady.

Andrew told me that he was uncertain whether he trusted the doctor's prognosis, but he didn't have health insurance and could not afford expensive fertility tests. Many men with SCI express great resentment that there had been no sperm testing or routine banking as part of their rehabilitation (Oliver et al. 1988).[10] Meanwhile, impaired fertility among men with SCI may be an issue for spouses, too, since many wives of men with SCI report that their inability to get pregnant and bear children is a "major source of dissatisfaction" (David, Gur, and Rozin 1977–1978: 200).

## Summary

The physical, economic, and psychological consequences of spinal cord injury in conjunction with the social stigma of disability make it difficult for individuals with SCI to enter into relationships and sustain them. For many individuals with SCI, reduced mobility, impaired fertility, and actual or perceived losses of sexual functioning are significant barriers to the establishment of both intimate relationships and parental roles. Many study participants experienced considerable rejection in their attempts at dating, and several felt that they were likely to be passed over in favor of nondisabled men and women. At the same time, over 25% admitted that they themselves preferred an able-bodied partner. Among those who voiced this preference, most felt that dating another disabled person would only compound the frustrations and challenges associated with SCI.

For many study participants, SCI was associated with considerable instability in intimate relationships. A sizable proportion indicated that their disabilities had a bearing on their attitudes toward marriage, and many reported that their chance of finding an appropriate marriage partner was substantially reduced. Moreover, many participants—particularly those with high-level quadriplegia—felt that SCI threatened their prospects for parenthood. Many of the men expressed justifiable concerns about their physical ability to father children, and several felt as though their physical limitations would make it difficult for them to care for and raise a child. A more enabling environment that includes financial support for fertility treatment, adoption counseling, and in-home assistance would help many individuals with spinal cord injury to fulfill their parenting objectives.

# 8
# Friends and Strangers

Jennifer is a 21-year-old quadriplegic woman with a slender build and long, wavy black hair. She is friendly but soft-spoken, and she tends to avoid eye contact. Although she uses a manual wheelchair, she has limited manual dexterity and is paralyzed from the chest down. She was injured while driving at age 14: "There were some really big ruts in the road and I just didn't see 'em, and I lost control and hit a telephone pole."

Jennifer is a student at City University, where she is studying political science and criminal justice. (She plans to go to law school after college.) She lives in a two-bedroom apartment in a working-class section of the city with Wayne, her 26-year-old fiancé, and Lorraine, her personal attendant. Lorraine is in her 50s and assists Jennifer with a variety of tasks when Wayne is out working as an auditor. For example, Lorraine helps get Jennifer to school in the morning and assists with her bowel and bladder regimens. When I asked Jennifer how she felt about having Lorraine living with her, she replied, "It doesn't really bother me" but added that her fiancé "doesn't really like it. [*chuckle*] 'Cause we don't have a lot of time by ourselves."

Jennifer was in eighth grade at the time of her car accident, and she missed the entire spring semester due to her injury. When I asked what it was like returning to school the following year, she replied,

> You definitely find out who your friends are and aren't, 'cause I know a lot of people who I thought were my friends, just all of a sudden didn't have time for me because I couldn't run around and do everything that they did. . . . It made me realize that it wasn't just the popular people that were important 'cause I know before I was injured I treated a lot of people really bad.

EIW: Were you one of the popular people?

Yeah, I was. And I know that after that, I got to be really good friends with I guess you would call them "the unpopular people."

## Social Relationships

The hostile sociopolitical context in which disability occurs is one of the most significant barriers to positive identity transformation in the aftermath of spinal cord injury (Waldinger 1999). Denigration and exclusion are two common forms of "psychic oppression" experienced by individuals with disabilities (Marks 1999: 25). Individuals with normative values frequently avoid establishing friendships with disabled individuals, and many use segregation as a means of keeping social and territorial distance (Safilios-Rothschild 1970). Of course, personality, behavioral, and cognitive factors tend to mediate whatever effect disability has on social relations (Chwalisz and Vaux 2000). For example, individuals with disabilities who are depressed are more likely to elicit negative reactions from others (Corcoran 1985; Elliott 1987).

Social anxiety and social phobia have been observed among some individuals with SCI (Richards, Kewman, and Pierce 2000), and a number of studies have documented an increased tendency toward introversion (Alfano, Neilson, and Fink 1993; Tayal et al. 1997; Trieschmann 1980, 1988). Social isolation not only limits educational, vocational, and social opportunities, but it may also have an adverse impact on emotional growth (Marks 1999). Individuals with SCI who are less socially integrated exhibit lower levels of life satisfaction (Fuhrer et al. 1992), and social discomfort among individuals with SCI has been inversely linked to overall adjustment (Dunn 1977). Although individuals with SCI report that a large share of their relationships with others are characterized by reciprocity (equal give and take), they are also especially likely to report relationships with others who give more than they do (Rintala et al. 1994). Because individuals with disabilities often lack power in their relationships with others, many suffer low levels of self-esteem and may even come to expect mistreatment (Neath 1997).

## Social Support and General Well-Being

Social ties provide individuals with both instrumental assistance (practical help, financial assistance, advice, and guidance) and psychosocial support (comfort, happiness, sense of worth, a sense of belonging, affection, and love) (Chwalisz and Vaux 2000; Elliott and Shewchuk 1995; Elliott et al. 1992a, 1992b; Thoits 1995). The measurement of social support is complex, however, and encompasses the individual's perceived social support as well as the composition and structure of one's supportive network—friends versus family, for example (Pollets 1975).

Psychosocial support is one of the most important predictors of successful adjustment among individuals with SCI (Pollets 1975; White 1983). Numerous studies have shown that social networks and social support are key factors related to the acceptance, social and medical adjustment, coping, life satisfaction, and well-being of individuals with spinal cord injury.[1] Although social support does not necessarily protect individuals with SCI from stressful life events (Mills 1989), those who lack support and companionship find it harder to integrate into their communities (Dattilo et al. 1998). Likewise, measures of social integration are directly and positively related to mental and physical health (Thoits 1995). A satisfactory support network can help reduce the likelihood of depression, Post-Traumatic Stress Disorder (PTSD), and secondary physical complications such as pressure sores (Elliott and Frank 1996; Elliott et al. 1992a, 1992b; Hundley 1985; Kishi, Robinson, and Forrester 1994; Krause et al. 1999; Lyons 1985; Nielsen 2003; Rintala et al. 1992). Unfortunately, many individuals with SCI perceive decreasing support from friends and family over time (Povolny 1993). Moreover, behaviors that are intended to be supportive can occasionally have harmful effects (Silver and Wortman 1980).

Different kinds of social relationships can have different effects on psychosocial well-being. Emotion-oriented support from family members promotes greater satisfaction with relationships, although the same cannot be said of support from friends and acquaintances (Post, Ros, and Schrijvers 1999). The presence of a live-in partner is associated with increased mobility and economic self-sufficiency (Sherman, DeVinney, and Sperling 2004), and support related to social interaction seems to enhance career opportunities (Krause et al. 1999). Meanwhile, relationships in which individuals with SCI are held responsible for the nurturance of others may generate psychological and social distress (Elliott et al. 1992a, 1992b).

An individual with a disability who feels threatened by his or her condition may find comfort in meeting other disabled individuals whom he or she admires and holds in high esteem (Safilios-Rothschild 1970; Waldinger 1999). Exposure to peers or people with similar injuries may promote better adjustment through modeling and emotional support (Richards, Kewman, and Pierce 2000; Wright 1976), and the most effective support givers are likely to be individuals who have successfully faced the same stressful situations as the support recipient (Thoits 1995). In particular, friends who also have SCI may help to reduce the uncertainty associated with the onset of disability (Parrott, Stuart, and Cairns 2000).

## Friendship Networks

While the majority of individuals with SCI are either satisfied with their social lives or express only minor dissatisfaction (Oliver et al. 1988),[2] SCI undoubtedly influences social relationships and may even interfere with relationships with pets (Kleiber et al. 1995). Individuals with high levels of impairment tend to have lower levels of social contact outside the household (Morgan et al. 1984), and quadriplegic women are less socially active than their paraplegic counterparts (Inniss 1994).

While some evidence suggests that women with SCI are more active socializers than men (Gold 1983), the men in my sample were more likely than the women to report close friendships (64% of the men and 43% of the women agreed either *somewhat* or *strongly* that they had many close friends). This can perhaps be attributed to the supportive networks that many had established through various disability-related organizations. (For example, 60% of the males but only 29% of the females in the sample are members of the local SCI organization.)[3] This explanation is supported by the fact that those with less involvement in social groups are also less likely to report close friendships. Also, those with greater degrees of impairment are less likely to report strong friendship networks. This may be related to the magnitude of the obstacles confronted by those whose mobility is most impaired.

Several participants in the study stated bluntly that their disabilities were responsible for their lack of close friends. For example, Meghan said that "isolation" went hand in hand with high-level quadriplegia. Roger reported,

> I have friends, they're not close friends. They're friends that like I said, I see at the spinal cord meeting. We [my wife and I] don't have

friends like we used to: "Hey let's go out, let's go here, let's go do this. Wanna go have a drink after work?" Don't have those kinds of friends anymore.

Of the 28 participants who had sustained spinal cord injuries after the age of ten, 86% indicated that their friendship networks had changed in the aftermath of their injuries. Among those who indicated that their friendship networks had changed, 33% had lost most of their previous friends and 50% had lost a few of their previous friends; 38% had gained a few new friends and 46% had gained many new friends. Half of those whose friendship networks had changed reported both losses and gains.

The overwhelming majority of the study participants (71%) indicated that their disabilities had affected their social lives. Among those who had acquired their disabilities after the age of 10, 39% had become less social and 14% had become more social as a direct result of their spinal cord injuries. Those with greater impairments and those who do not drive—two circumstances that frequently overlap—were considerably more likely to report having become less social.[4] While men were somewhat more likely than women to indicate that their friendship networks had changed as a direct result of their injuries, they were less likely to report that their levels of social activity had changed.

## Divergent Interests and More Meaningful Friendships

Several of the research participants—particularly those who had considered themselves popular and athletic, and who had been injured in high school—found that their friendship networks changed dramatically following their injuries. Many came to realize that people they'd thought were their friends were not really there for them when push came to shove. Their disabilities therefore provided the impetus to establish new and more meaningful friendships. For example, Harry, who had been a football player on his high school team, described how his friendship network had changed:

> The juniors and the seniors I ran around with didn't hang around with me anymore. But the people I used to shun and treat like shit were there for me. Many people in my sophomore class were my friends now. And it really made me feel really real bad for a long

time; it really changed my attitude. I was really a cocky bastard there for a long time. But then when I came back and I realized that the people that used to be my friends really wasn't my friends and the people that I used to treat like shit were now my friends and it really changed my attitude on things that way. . . . I don't think I'm better than anybody else today and I don't think anybody else is better than me; I don't care who they are.

A few participants described how their injuries had taught them to distinguish between fair-weather friends and true friends. For example, Leonard said,

I don't know if I lost them because of the disability or because of the lifestyle change that I had and just kind of lost contact with them. . . . After about six months I knew my friends from my acquaintances real quick.

Likewise, Stacy reported that "after a while, you just find out who your true friends are." When I asked her why her friendship networks had changed following her injury, she replied,

I think it's just the whole patience thing and you've got to take time; you've got to go special ways, you've got to carry me up stairs. I think that kind of gets old maybe and that may have been part of it, but I would say I matured a lot and the things I might have done previously didn't appeal to me anymore, and I don't know if they thought that I just didn't want to hang out with them or whatever. It was just, "Grow up," you know?

Several individuals felt that their friends had gone by the wayside due to the inconvenience of socializing with a wheelchair user. While Ben reported that one old friend had stuck by him,

with everybody else it was almost like, "What have you done for me lately?" And since I was in a wheelchair; I was gonna be a big problem and a big pain. It seemed like people just found it easier just to drop and let it go. . . . And I didn't have a car and things like that, so I didn't pursue it.

Ben also felt that his own attitudes had changed:

I sort of tend to look at it with a jaundiced eye now. I used to be pretty outgoing, pretty nice towards people and pretty social and stuff. When I got injured, I had a more jaundiced eye towards people. . . . We tend to fool ourselves, "Oh yeah, people are really nice and basically they're okay" and that sort of thing. And then when this happens to you, then you're kinda like, "Face facts—they are louses." [*laughter*]

Ben told me that since acquiring his injury, he looked for more "real" and "down-to-earth" relationships. "I used to be able to sit there and BS with the best of them," he said. "I don't have time for that sort of relationship anymore." Indeed, several of the individuals I surveyed stated that they no longer share common ground with their former friends. For example, Paul said,

I slowed down. They didn't. They had other things going on, so they went and did their thing and I stayed in school.

Likewise, Brad reported that only a few people came to visit him at the hospital or his parents' house: "I suppose they preferred to continue to go out drinking, smoking [*laughter*], stuff like that."

## Lack of Transportation and Accessibility Concerns

For individuals with SCI, "often the use of a car [can] mean the difference between an independent, active social life and restricted mobility, or even social isolation" (Oliver et al. 1988: 66). Transportation difficulties can even limit participation in rehabilitation activities (Inniss 1994). It is therefore not surprising that a number of study participants mentioned inadequate transportation, inaccessible buildings, and wheelchair-maneuvering problems as factors that constrain their social lives. Women were more likely than men to mention transportation difficulties, a finding that is probably related to the lower percentage of female (43%) than male (68%) study participants who drove vehicles. Tonya described the difficulties she faces:

I don't like to bother people, even my disabled friends, because right now I don't have a handicapped van . . . so that's a burden upon my kids or whoever's gonna take me some place.

Several individuals who lacked convenient transportation described how they had become reclusive as a result. For example, Rosa described herself as a "homebody": "I don't go out too much, hardly at all," she said. Likewise, Ben reported that there are fewer "opportunities to be social. You don't have a car, you rely on bus system, you can't get out and around as you once used to." While Fred's dependence on others for transportation discouraged him from being more social, he was also somewhat hesitant to take up driving:

> I'm supposed to go . . . to see whether I still can handle the road, but I'm a little afraid of hurting somebody or hurting myself worse or killing myself out there. . . . I get these spasms, I don't know when they're coming on.

He was also reluctant to put hand controls into his van because that would prevent other people from driving it. "I didn't want them to convert that, mutilate it that bad for nobody else to drive it but myself," he said. Meghan also felt that transportation barriers interfered with her social life, such that she didn't really have a friendship network:

> I have acquaintances. . . . I don't have the transportation. I think if I had Mercedes Benz, and y'know [*laughter*] of course there'd be people around to drive it. But nobody wants to drive a 21-year old jalopy Dodge van. . . . It's nothing you want to be around in.

While Cody reported that he had become somewhat less social since his injury, he attributed the problem to accessibility concerns rather than transportation-related difficulties:

> Getting the wheelchair in and out [of the car] is all right, but I don't like having to worry about, well, "Is this place wheelchair accessible? Will I be able to move around in it? [Is] the ramp gonna be there?"

Similarly, Leonard mentioned how the inaccessibility of other people's homes sometimes kept him from visiting friends and family members:

> Getting in and out of people's houses can be a chore. . . . Going out to people's homes who don't have accessible homes. . . . Or if they've got steps. I've never been to my brother's house in six years. He's got

seven steps going up to his house. . . . So I tell Ken, "Hey, when you lower your house down I'll come see you."

Leonard was reluctant to ask for assistance getting up the stairs at his brother's house: "Ken's going on fifty years old and he's had three back surgeries. I don't want somebody to blow out their back for me."

Stacy felt that maneuvering in a wheelchair was a particular challenge in crowded environments:

> When you go to like a cramped bar, and "Excuse me, excuse me," and you have to tell people to move, I feel like I'm making a scene and everyone's staring at me . . . That's kind of a hassle and then stairs and things like that. It's usually not too bad because I just find some guys to help me and they don't mind it but then like everyone's looking. But other than that, everything's the same I think.

Al, a self-described daredevil, chose to ride his wheelchair in the street:

> If I'm driving down the road I've had people yell shit at me. . . . Kids, they'll yell, "Get the hell out of the road!" and "Get on the sidewalk!" 'cause I drive in the street.

If someone calls him a name, he said, "I'll curse 'em out. And if they stop, it's their ass." He added, "I'm a real bastard." At the same time, he noted that many people were helpful and friendly when they saw him—waving and nodding their heads, for example.

## Leisure and Recreational Activities

Sports and exercise are especially important among individuals with SCI since they promote social connectivity, provide opportunities for peer support, and enhance both physical and psychological well-being (see, for example, Glaser et al. 1996; Green 1996; Jackson 1987; Lee and McCormick 2004; Loy, Dattilo, and Kleiber, 2003; Rogers 1996; Slater and Meade 2004). Individuals who maintain active leisure lives are more satisfied, less depressed, and more likely to maintain confiding relationships (Coyle et al. 1993; Coyle, Lesnik-Emas, and Kinney 1994; Daniel and Manigandan 2005). Sports and recreational activities may also reduce social stereotyping by promoting the acceptance of individuals with disabilities (Glaser et al.

1996; Rogers 1996). Unfortunately, however, many individuals with SCI avoid sports due to a lack of access to facilities or a dislike of traditional sports for wheelchair users (Tasiemski et al. 2004).

While most individuals with SCI express a desire for continued participation in the recreational activities they enjoyed prior to their injuries (Lee et al. 1996), SCI has a significant disruptive effect on recreational and social activities (Glaser et al. 1996; Kirkby, Cull, and Foreman 1996; Kleiber et al. 1995; Lee et al. 1993; Mulcahey 1992; Noreau and Fougeyrollas 2000; Oliver et al. 1988; Price 1983; Targett et al. 1998; Wu and Williams 2001). Many activities, ranging from church attendance to running errands to visiting friends, have been shown to decline in frequency after the onset of SCI (Targett et al. 1998). The decrease in outdoor recreation is offset to some extent, however, by increased participation in entertainment, arts, and cultural activities. Involvement in hobbies and crafts is least likely to be affected by SCI (Price 1983). Not surprisingly, pre-injury lifestyles that centered on "embodied activity" (active participation in sports, a professional trade, or outdoor pursuits) are often associated with particularly intense adjustment problems (Lee et al. 1993). Many individuals with SCI—particularly quadriplegics—report high levels of dissatisfaction with their leisure activities (Oliver et al. 1988).

Most individuals with SCI cite environmental and physical problems as the key factors that limit their ability to engage in sports and recreation (Oliver et al. 1988). Individuals with SCI who participate in athletic activities must be attentive to potential complications including heat stress (due to impaired thermoregulation), soft-tissue injuries (resulting from overuse of the upper extremities), elbow pain, and entrapment neuropathies (Slater and Meade 2004). Overuse injuries to the upper limbs of athletes who use wheelchairs are common but not easily treated (Apple, Cody, and Allen 1996). As might be expected, independence in self-care and a lower level of injury are positively associated with involvement in social sports (Anderson 1982). While one study found no significant association between pre-injury athletic involvement and post-injury wheelchair sports participation (Kirkby, Cull, and Foreman 1996), other evidence suggests that individuals who were active in sports before their injuries are more likely to maintain long-term participation afterward as well (Wu and Williams 2001).

For many individuals, especially men, the need to discontinue participation in sports can seriously disrupt pre-injury friendship networks. Chris explained:

All your sports stop. . . . Quads are pretty well limited. You can't grab anything. They try to get you to do racing in a wheelchair. Man, that is tough on the elbows and shoulders. I've already got tendonitis in my elbows, and these things have got to last me the rest of my life so I'm not going to go out and push. You talk to some of those guys that race—they're usually young, they've got plenty of energy, but after a while that's no fun with your head pushing with all of your might every stroke. . . . I used to play racquetball every week. . . . These guys that I played racquetball and sports with were just sports friends. After I got hurt, they just kind of disappeared. But I can understand that; that's no big deal.

While Chris considered his sports buddies "good friends," he also acknowledged that they weren't "real, real close friends." Adam characterized the friends he had lost in a similar way:

They were more the superficial friends that I'd go play football with or we'd go hang out and stuff. I guess since things had changed to the point to where we couldn't do that anymore, they really didn't know how to relate to me.

Meanwhile, Todd felt that his injury had intensified his reclusive tendencies:

I've turned into a loner. I think my injury did that to me. I was always kind of a loner anyway but I would probably say more so now. . . . For one, I'm not participating in motocross which that was a big part of my social life. I'd race every weekend and be there. I like being at home now; I'm just more of a homebody. The weather affects me a lot and I just don't get out as much as I used to. I never really went to the bar scene or anything like that even when I was able-bodied and so I just never was a big social person.

Todd still enjoyed watching motocross, but he said he'd prefer to be racing. Fred, who had moved after his injury, attributed his loss of friends to the change in residence. However, his comments suggested that other factors might also have been at work: "I don't blame them if they don't want to be around me; I'm no more fun no more." Some of Fred's family members had encouraged him to move to a reservation in Montana, but he was reluctant to do so because of his mobility restrictions:

They will ask me to move up there. I would like to, the place is so pretty and we've got three uncles that have ranches; I just can't participate in the round-ups or go around and do the elk hunting scene or fishing and I hate to be the one to sit there and watch.

Meanwhile, several of the people I interviewed had found new ways to maintain active recreational and social lives following their injuries. After his injury, Jonathan learned how to swim again. He became involved in a wide variety of sports ranging from softball (with a pinch runner) to ping-pong to pool. At the time of the interview, he was preparing for a vacation in the Cayman Islands with his family where he planned to scuba dive. "I was always pretty athletic and I still am." Others participated in wheelchair athletics. For example, Walter had joined a wheelchair basketball team, and Ryan was in the process of trying to get together a wheelchair sports program on campus. The local spinal cord injury association also sponsored an annual "I-can-ski" program that gave participants the opportunity to water-ski.

## Social Stigmatization and Lack of Understanding

As Joseph Shapiro (1993: 3) notes, "Nondisabled Americans do not understand disabled ones." For many people, disability is frightening since "it taps into our fears of ostracism, illness, and death" (Fisher and Galler 1988: 176). Most Americans have only a limited knowledge of permanent disability, and nondisabled people frequently hold unfavorable or ambivalent attitudes toward individuals with disabilities. In other cases, both favorable and unfavorable perceptions coexist (Schwartz 1988; Wright 1960). Either way, a sense of awkwardness is often present. In face-to-face interactions with disabled individuals, those without disabilities tend to maintain a physical distance and to terminate interaction sooner than they otherwise would (Albrecht 1976).

The absence of clearly defined norms often contributes to strain in social interactions (Safilios-Rothschild 1970). Many nondisabled individuals experience anxiety and discomfort when interacting with disabled individuals.[5] Stigmatized individuals are frequently unsure how others will receive them (Goffman 1963), and individuals with disabilities tend to be keenly aware of others' discomfort in relating to them (Fichten et al. 1989). In social relations, there is a tendency for nondisabled persons to focus undue attention on the disability itself (Davis 1961; Goffman 1963).[6] In so doing, they may be overly gracious, overly sympathetic, patronizing, or insensitive, or they may ignore the disabled individual altogether (Bogdan and Biklen 1993; Gove 1976; Morris 1993b; Safilios-Rothschild 1970; Trieschmann 1980). This latter tendency often reflects the fear of saying something wrong (Dunn 2000; Kleck 1966) or the awkward competition between curiosity and inhibition (Makas 1993). Efforts at tension reduction may sometimes take an extreme form, including "behavioral instability, in which extremely positive or negative responses may occur" (Katz, Hass, and Bailey 1988: 48).

Individuals with SCI often report a dislike of the pity and patronizing attitudes shown by nondisabled people (Ray and West 1983; Shapiro 1993). These negative attitudes may make it difficult to develop new relationships or to reestablish old ones (Quigley 1994). Altogether, approximately two-thirds of the participants in the study (66%) agreed either *somewhat* or *strongly* that "individuals with disabilities are stigmatized in society"; 22% neither agreed nor disagreed, and 13% disagreed either *somewhat* or *strongly*.[7] Women were more likely than men to agree with the statement.

Many of the people I interviewed described how others treated them as if they had mental disabilities, were social outcasts, or were unworthy of social engagement. Harry said, "everybody's stigmatized, but I guarantee you the more different you are, the more you're stigmatized." Roger reflected,

> A lot of times I think people don't see me, they just look through me, because they really don't want to see the person in the chair. . . . People don't take me for what I am or what I can do. They're more interested in, "Let me get that for you, I'll hold the door. Look at Roger, he's in a wheelchair." People don't look at me. They look at my chair.

Jonathan agreed strongly that individuals with disabilities are stigmatized in society, primarily because people tend to equate physical disability with mental disability. While he felt that attitudes had improved in recent years, in the past this had been a very serious problem:

> They would say, "How are youuuu toodaaaayyyy." [*accentuates the slowness of the words*] "I'm doing fine, how about you?" I mean, they seemed a little retarded to me. That's just lack of exposure and ignorance on their part.

Similarly, Edward said,

> They think if your hands are like this [*gestures to his hands*] then
> you're retarded. They're not gonna think they can carry on a
> conversation with you. . . . This girl at work, she's got some kind of
> muscular dystrophy and it's affecting everything—her speech and
> she's hard to understand—and sometimes I feel sorry for her because
> people avoid her more than they avoid me.

Individuals who use wheelchairs may confront special obstacles when
they interact with people who are standing. Unless the upright person is
especially short, she or he will have to either "talk down" or bend down in
order to engage in a conversation with the wheelchair user.[8] Ben, a walking quadriplegic, described how conversations changed when he made the
transition from sitting in a wheelchair to standing upright:

> Once I got standing and I could finally stand up and look people
> eye-to-eye when they talked, then it seemed like they were talking
> to me again because I could stand and look 'em eye-to-eye, whereas
> before I was in a wheelchair and they were looking down there. It
> just kind of seemed like they were just talking over me more than to
> me.

Roger felt that his status as a wheelchair user reduced the likelihood that
people would engage with him in meaningful conversation. He described
what happened when he attended parties with his wife:

> I don't threaten people so I think people will approach me more than
> before. The only way people approach me is they just would, "Can
> I help you?" There is no more, "Hi, I'm John, glad to meet you.". . .
> People come up to me and they shake my hand and they say, "Hello.
> How's things going, Roger?" And then they fade away. . . . When
> people see me coming they move: "Oh, let me get out of your way."
> And I'm like, "I don't want you to get out of my way." [*laughter*] "I'm
> coming to talk to you."

Roger's explanation for this treatment was that individuals with SCI are
intimidating: "I feel we scare people because it's very easy for you to be in

this chair also. It doesn't take much at all." Indeed, previous research has indicated that a negative reaction to individuals with disabilities may involve a physiological component (anxiety) stemming from a perceived threat to the self-image (Vander Kolk 1976).

Several authors have explored methods of reducing the social strain between disabled and nondisabled individuals. While many studies have found that social interaction reduces aversive reactions and discomfort, others report contradictory effects (see, for example, Makas 1993; Trieschmann 1980, 1988; Yuker 1988). Many factors are likely to moderate the relationship between frequency of contact and attitude, including the characteristics of the disabled person, the characteristics of the nondisabled person, and the nature of the interaction (Yuker 1988). Meanwhile, information that clarifies the physical aspects of disability tends to bring positive attitudinal changes (Haney 1982). Individuals who are open about discussing their disabilities generate a more positive response from others (Aiello 1988; Evans 1976; Yuker 1988), and social strain may be reduced if individuals with stigmatized identities make a conscious effort to reduce tensions (Evans 1976; Goffman 1963; Meyerson and Scruggs 1980).

Several of the study participants felt that ignorance and a lack of exposure were to blame for people's tendency to stigmatize individuals with disabilities. For example, Shannon reflected,

> They don't think [individuals with disabilities] can think. And I just think it's the product of not being around and I would probably be the same way. If it's something you're unfamiliar with, you're a little unsure, a little scared. And if you don't have to deal with it, you better not. And I can't say that I wouldn't be the same way. Because I didn't know anybody in a wheelchair and probably would be fearful of approaching someone or being around them.

Shannon suggested, "I think we need to be more visible and outspoken and show 'em that we have brains." Ryan felt similarly and saw the tendency to equate physical disability with mental disability as a "big problem in society." Kevin expressed a similar view:

> I think mostly that people are ignorant. They never been around somebody in a wheelchair or somebody blind or whatever. They just don't know.

A few of the people I interviewed described how children were socialized to fear individuals with disabilities. For example, Derrick described his own experience growing up:

> My mom and dad used to tell us when we were kids, "Don't look at 'em. Don't look at 'em." You know, they're in a wheelchair. Or they're on a cane or they're blind or whatever. And I know that when I was a kid, I was kind of scared of somebody in a wheelchair. And I take time now to stop and turn my lights or honk my horn and my turn signal's on for kids and you know, try to make them where they're not scared of it.

Meghan was bothered by the fact that parents would often discourage their children's curiosity:

> Children will look at you—y'know, just stare. And I go, "Hey, what's your name?" And if you act normal, children will act normal. But their parents don't. They yank on their arms and I go, "Please don't yank their arms." Because if you do that, all they're gonna remember is that they were looking at a person in a wheelchair and you made them feel that it was inappropriate because you yanked their arm. . . . If they wanna talk to me, let 'em talk. But don't yank on their arm and drag them away. And that's what parents do because the parent is uncomfortable . . . and they're projecting off onto this child. And that pisses me off more than anything, probably. [*pause*] Oooooh. [*whistling sound*]

Meghan said she wished that parents would just say, "Johnny, if you want to talk to the lady, talk to her, but do not stare at her." At the same time, however, Meghan was sometimes bothered by staring:

> If we'd gone over to Red Lobster or something and ordered dinner, we would have gotten stares. . . . And most days you blow it off, but on a bad day you're just going, "Like, what the hell you looking at?"

She sometimes directly confronted those who stared at her:

> "What the hell's wrong? Do you want me to drool?" And they'll sit there like they're waiting for something. And I'm going, "What?"

Jennifer felt that it was mostly children who stared. She said that she had been "overly sensitive" to it in high school, but less so now.

A few individuals described how other people's unwillingness to welcome them into social activities affected their social lives. For example, Travis said,

> You're not gonna go out dancing as much, you're not gonna be as likely to be invited to people's houses because if they think, "Oh, I have two steps, how's he gonna do that? We'll just not invite him." And so you get into these situations where you don't get invited to things that you might have got invited to otherwise.

Ben had a similar view:

> It just seems like once somebody becomes physically disabled, people tend to leave them off to the sidelines a little more. They don't seem to engage them like they would a normal able-bodied person.

Some individuals with SCI report that people do not know how to interact with someone in a wheelchair (Povolny et al. 1993). Travis agreed with that assessment:

> One day I saw some friends of mine out here throwing a baseball around on the South Oval [a part of campus]. And I was like, "Come on, give me the glove." And they don't know what to do. I'm like, "My arms aren't affected. I can throw a baseball, I can still play catch, I may not be able to run after the ball real well so try to get it close to me at least." They couldn't get it—this idea that I could still play catch with them.

Ultimately, Travis's friends gave him a glove and he played catch with them for a while, but it was still awkward: "You could tell in their mind, it was like, 'What the hell do I do?'" he said. "They didn't know what to do."

Many individuals with SCI express fears regarding a lack of social acceptance (Roessler 1978), and the uncomfortable gazes and questions of strangers may sometimes lead disabled individuals to withdraw into familiar terrain (Bury 1982).[9] Ryan reflected,

> I'm not as outgoing as I would be if I were not in a wheelchair. . . . There are times when I see myself not reaching out to people because

> . . . I'm afraid of what they're gonna think or how they're gonna react.

Several of the people I interviewed described how some of their previous friends had difficulty relating to them because of their disabilities. For example, Edward lamented that his former friends

> all just kind of avoid me—like . . . walking by and they turn their head the other way. They act like you got some kind of disease that they're gonna catch if they talk to you. And this Indian friend of mine—we was best friends all through school—he won't even hardly talk to me now. It's probably because he don't know what to say. And a lot of people are like that. . . . At parties [I've] actually had to say, "Hey man, I'm the same guy." I said, "I just can't walk like I used to but I'm still the same asshole you ever knew!" And that would loosen them up and they'd go ahead and be normal to me.

## Birds of a Feather Flock Together

Goldstein (1996) maintains that humans have an innate, instinctive tendency to seek out social bonds of likeness. Individuals with SCI tend to self-segregate following discharge from hospitals and rehabilitation programs (Haney 1982). Moreover, leisure groups and social activities specifically geared for people with disabilities are integral to networking and friendship formation (Knox and Parmenter 1993; Oliver et al. 1988). These groups promote social adjustment and a sense of empowerment among individuals with SCI (Chesler and Chesney 1988; Coyle et al. 1993; Coyle, Lesnik-Emas, and Kinney 1994; Goldstein 1996; Henderson, Bedini, and Hecht 1994; Moeller and Hartman 1985; Riggin 1976; Waldinger 1999). Of course, the tendency for individuals with disabilities to form their own clubs and recreational groups may be due to external factors, such as social and psychological isolation (Safilios-Rothschild 1970).

Altogether, 75% of the participants in my study—80% of the men and 57% of the women—reported that they were members of a social group or organization. Ninety-two percent of those who reported an affiliation were members of one or more disability-related groups. The relationship between impairment and organizational involvement is curvilinear; 63% of paraplegics, 89% of quadriplegics who use manual wheelchairs, and 43% of quadriplegics who use motorized wheelchairs indicated that they were *actively* involved in a social organization. Moreover, the overwhelming majority of research participants—including those who were not members of the spinal cord injury association—described how they had gained new friends in the disabled community following their injuries. For example, Tonya reported,

> I met a para one day I was coming in at the doctor's office and I wasn't gonna say anything to him just because he was male for the main reason, I don't generally go up to men and say anything to them. So, he came over and spoke to me and I started going to church with him and his family and from there he introduced me to the spinal cord injury association and from there I met lots of people with spinal cord injuries and I really enjoy it.

Roger also reported having met "a lot of people" and having made "some good friends" through the local SCI association. SCI is "our common denominator," he remarked. Todd traced many of his new friendships to his involvement with the disabled community. He had joined the local SCI association, worked at a company that sold wheelchairs, and served as a volunteer speaker for newly injured persons. He said,

> And I meet 'em [new friends] when I'd go . . . speak to freshly injured people to help 'em out. . . . I don't get to do it anymore now that I'm working so much. . . . But I loved doing that. I wish I could figure out how to get paid for doing that.

Todd's experience is consistent with research showing that many individuals with SCI derive considerable gratification from providing help, both physical and emotional, to other disabled individuals (Goldstein 1996).

Ben described how living in a handicapped apartment complex served as a conduit for meeting other people with disabilities. There were approximately 3 or 4 such complexes in his city, and individuals living in them were connected through extensive networks: "Somebody here knows somebody there that will know somebody there."

Meanwhile, Adam maintained friendships with some of the guys he had met in rehab:

> I have a lot of friends who are in chairs now. Like Eitan, for instance. He's a friend of mine now and I probably would have never met him if I hadn't been in a chair. And then I have friends that I met when I

was in rehab that I still stay in contact with. . . . And I'm still pretty close friends with them.

Adam described how he had become much closer to one of his childhood friends who also had a disability:

> We've actually become closer friends since I've been disabled. I don't know if the disability had anything to do with that or if it's just the fact that we both live in [the same city] now, so we hang out more so we got to know each other better. . . . He's also disabled. He had both legs amputated when he was born; he's got one above the knee, one below the knee. And he's got some deformities in his hands. I never thought any different of him growing up. Now that I'm disabled I have a lot more respect for him for what he went through. . . . I think that common bond might have made us a little closer.

Unlike Ben, Al was not comfortable living in an apartment complex that served individuals with disabilities. In fact, he was eager to relocate:

> I've lived here for eight years, and there's been like eight or nine people die. . . . Two were because they had AIDS—just different things. Two OD'ed. And that's something I don't want to be around. . . . I don't like this place.

Although Al has one close friend who resides in the complex, most of his friends live elsewhere. Unfortunately, the trend for public housing is to make all units in a given area fully accessible. This results in the segregation of individuals with disabilities, since few nondisabled individuals are attracted to these units (Henderson and Bryan 1984). One possible remedy to this problem would be an adherence to universal design in the construction of public housing units.

Although Stan is a member of the local SCI association, he connects more with others on the basis of shared interests (social and political advocacy) rather than disability status

> because we're working in the same political arena. I can talk about activities, the politics. . . . The people that are in the spinal cord injury association are younger by and large and they're leaders in their own right and we come together to act as a group. . . . What is

causing us to come together is the mission of the spinal cord injury [group].

Stan considers most of the people he knows in the SCI association to be acquaintances rather than close friends.

Nathan, a member of the SCI association, said that he is friendly with people from church and work but that he doesn't have any friends "as far as going out and doing things." Nathan's lack of a friendship network may be related to factors other than his disability, however, since he often appeared to be lost in his own world. He remarked that things could be better

> if I was up and around and I was a multimillionaire, all that stuff. If I knew how to socialize better. All that stuff. I'm just a mystery and always have been, even before I got in a wheelchair.

## Friends with Disabilities

Men and quadriplegics were especially likely to report that at least a few of their friends have disabilities. More specifically, all of the men I polled reported that at least a few of their friends have disabilities (and 32% reported that half or more have disabilities), compared to 71% of the women (43% indicated that half or more have disabilities). This may reflect the men's relatively high rates of involvement with the local SCI association and the disproportionate number of men who incur spinal cord injuries. Moreover, all the quadriplegics reported that at least a few of their friends have disabilities (compared to 87% of paraplegics).

Meanwhile, those who had been injured for shorter periods of time were more likely to report that the *majority* of their friends have disabilities. Several factors may account for this: (1) individuals who were more recently injured may be more likely to maintain friendships and connections with people from their rehabilitation programs; (2) in the initial adjustment period, individuals with SCI may find it easier to connect with others who also have SCI; (3) individuals who have been injured for longer periods of time have had more opportunities to meet and cultivate friendships with individuals from a variety of different backgrounds; they are also an older population, on average.

The individuals I surveyed were also asked whether they (a) avoid friendships with others who have physical disabilities, (b) actively seek friendships with others who have physical disabilities, or (c) don't care either way. Only one, Stacy, indicated a desire to avoid friendships with other disabled individuals. The remaining 31 study participants (97%) indicated that their approach to friendships was disability-blind.

While Stacy had enjoyed meeting other disabled individuals at a conference in Washington, DC, she was finding it difficult to establish similar bonds at the university she attends:

> This summer was the first time I had been around that many people my age in wheelchairs ever, and it freaked me out when I got there. I didn't know how to react and then I started talking and I met people that were exactly like me—like the same things, like athletic, and all these things. . . . I hope people see me like that. Like there's some people that I see around here and the way they carry themselves and their social skills—I hope people don't just see me like that. . . . Like when I go out, like party, you never run into any of these people in wheelchairs. . . . Just the way people present themselves on campus. I'm kind of scared of half of 'em. . . . They just seem like they're in their own world.

Stacy did seem more outgoing and socially adept than some of the other study participants.

## Socialization and the Internet

The use of the Internet promotes social connectivity, provides easy access to information, and has been linked to improved emotional well-being among individuals with SCI (Drainoni et al. 2004; Houlihan et al. 2003). Individuals with SCI report that they most often use the Internet for e-mail, disability and health information, shopping, playing games, employment or vocational information, and chat rooms (Drainoni et al. 2004). While earlier research suggested that individuals with SCI are especially unlikely to own computers due to their relatively low rates of employment (Kruse, Krueger, and Drastal 1996), a more recent study found especially *high* rates of Internet use among individuals with SCI (Drainoni et al. 2004).[10]

Altogether, 71% of the individuals I surveyed indicated that they use the Internet to socialize with friends and family members. Females and those with more severe impairments are most likely to use the Internet for this purpose. Among the 20 respondents who were uninvolved at the time of the study, four (20%) reported using the Internet (chat rooms, etc.) to meet new people *sometimes.* Three (15%) said they do this *seldom,* and 13 (65%) said *never.* Of those who use the Internet, most use it to correspond with friends and family members.

It is noteworthy that many study participants who had not been computer literate before their injuries cultivated an interest in computer technology afterward (see Chapter 10). For many, this was a strategy to break free of the isolation—and the boredom—that sometimes accompanies SCI. For example, Adam had started learning "computer stuff" only after his injury, although he had since become "a computer nerd." Several described how they use the Internet for recreation and socialization. For example, Jay regularly uses the Internet to chat with friends and family members. Harry corresponds via the Internet with people who share his passion for Neil Young music, and Tonya uses her computer to play games and to keep in contact with friends and family.

Some individuals have been reluctant to use the Internet, however. When I asked Roger if he ever used the Internet to interact with people, he responded,

> I'm not an Internet person. I hate the Internet. . . . And I know that will have to change. I use it a lot at work.

While I initially thought that Roger might have a fear of computer technology, he said that wasn't the case. When I asked him why he disliked the Internet so much, he said,

> Um, too personal. . . . But I know a lot of bad things about the Internet. A lot of bad things.

I suspected Roger might be alluding to the widespread use of the Internet for pornography, so I said, "I guess it's sort of like anything; it's what you make of it." He responded, "Exactly. It can either create or destroy."

While a few study participants had used the Internet to find potential dating partners, several suggested that this use of the Internet was ridiculous or embarrassing. For this reason, some individuals may have been reluctant to mention their use of the Internet for this purpose. However, when I asked Jennifer how she had met her fiancé, she said, "Actually we met on the Internet, if you can believe that." [*laughter*] When I assured her that I knew several people who had met their partners over the Internet, she responded, "Everybody I talk to finds it amazing." Jennifer's fiancé had relocated from out of state to live with her. Meghan also said that she sometimes uses the

Internet to socialize and to meet new people. At the same time, however, she had met only one man in real life following an Internet correspondence and had felt uncomfortable with the experience:

> It was some weird [*laughter*]; like this is sick.

> EIW: Why was it sick?

> I don't know. I was not comfortable with that. . . . I guess because I don't believe anything anyone was telling me over the Internet.

When I asked Meghan if she ever talked about her disability when she met new people online, she responded,

> I don't really go into a lot of detail about me. . . . Like, I'd never say, "I'm disabled." Like one guy said, "Why are you typing so slowly?" And I just never told him.

Several months after our interview, I learned from Meghan that she was dating a man she had met over the Internet.

Kevin had used the Internet's chat rooms, but he had become bored with them after they lost their initial appeal:

> I've had my computer now and Internet access for about four years. When I first got it, I was in those chat rooms all the time. Did make up all kinds of lies to other people, and I made a lot of good friends in there. I talked to them just about every day or every other day or so. That lasted for a year or two and then I kind of got tired of it. So I don't use it that much anymore. But every once in a while I still go in a chat room.

Kevin told me he had never met any of his Internet correspondents in person, since all the people he connected with lived far away and he thought it would be a "waste of money" to travel across the country to meet them. However, given the isolation of many individuals with SCI, Internet technology seems to have unrealized potential as a mechanism for establishing new relationships.

## Summary

Spinal cord injury has a significant bearing on psychosocial well-being and personal relationships. The study participants identified a number of ways in which their disabilities had disrupted their friendship networks and social relations. Many complained about the tendency of others to sideline them, treat them as if they had mental disabilities, give them undue attention, or more commonly, ignore them altogether. The latter issue was a source of considerable pain for a number of them who expressed a strong desire to be included in social activities. At the same time, many individuals with SCI also forged new friendships in the aftermath of their injuries, which often arose out of involvement in various disability-related organizations. Although most report a disability-blind approach to new friendships, the shared experience of living with SCI provides a pre-existing bond that fosters closeness and comfort among many with spinal cord injury.

Although studies indicate that attitudes toward individuals with disabilities are becoming less negative in developed countries (Westbrook, Legge, and Pennay 1993), the stigmatization of individuals with SCI is widespread. A more disability-friendly physical and social environment (e.g., removal of transportation barriers) would facilitate a higher level of social participation among many individuals with SCI. Moreover, education and disability awareness may help to eliminate negative biases against disabled people (Roberts 1996) and to reduce the social strain that frequently characterizes social interaction between disabled and nondisabled individuals. Anxiety about social interactions is a two-way street, however, and individuals with disabilities may need to develop social techniques and psychological mechanisms to respond to the behavior of nondisabled individuals (including that which is unhelpful but well-intentioned) (DeLoach and Greer 1981; Drew-Cates 1989; Makas 1988; Meyerson and Scruggs 1980). In particular, psychosocial rehabilitation should confront the issue of stigma (Gove 1976) and emphasize effective communication skills (e.g., self-advocacy and self-management) to help facilitate the kinds of social interactions that can aid understanding, overcome loneliness, and encourage integration (Quinn 1985).

# 9
# Economic Conditions and Family Responses

Roger is a handsome 43-year-old man with straight dark hair, a moustache, and a deep voice. He was paralyzed four years previously by a malignant tumor on his spinal cord. While the physicians were able to treat the tumor effectively using radiation (he was in remission at the time of the interview), the tumor "strangled" a nerve and resulted in paraplegia at the T-10 level of his spinal column. Roger currently lives in a modest, middle-class home with his wife and three daughters (ages three, seven, and eight).

Roger is both angry and saddened by how his disability has affected his life. "I don't like being in the chair," he said. As a direct result of his injury, Roger went from owning his own construction company to selling doors for commercial buildings. He reported a family income between $35,000 and $49,999, and when I asked him how his injury had affected his financial situation, he replied:

> Oh, man! Ohhh. [*laughter*] Let's just put it this way: financially and credit-wise right now it's so bad that I had to beg a bank to give me a checking account. 'Cause of what this has done, the credit history that I have accumulated after not working for two and a half years, not having an income. But even though you don't have an income the bills are still coming in.

Although Roger had health insurance at the time of his injury, his policy was woefully inadequate. The health insurance

> was nothing. That got ate up in the first seven months. And everybody thinks, "Well, you have health insurance," but there are

certain things you got to look at in health insurance. The health insurance that I had—I took out as an umbrella. The men that worked for me wanted insurance, so I took it out as an umbrella. I had to have it to be able to cover my men. . . . And so I just took out a policy, I think it only covered up to thirty-five thousand dollars. After thirty-five thousand it's like, "They ain't paying for it."

Roger told me that he and his wife were about $65,000 to $70,000 in debt.

During the course of our interview, Roger's wife, who was also home at the time, maintained her distance. Roger told me that his relationship with his wife was seriously strained as a result of the challenges—financial, physical, sexual, and emotional—that resulted from his disability. In describing how his disability affected his life on a daily basis, Roger reflected on his relationship with his children. He was in

a depressed mode not being able to do the things I want to do. I can play with my children, but not the way I want to play with my children.

At the same time, Roger felt his children provided the inspiration for him to go on living:

I look at them and they're the reason why I carry on. They're the reason that I learn to do the things that I do now, why I wake up every morning and go to work. When they accomplish something, it brings a twinkle to my eye.

Roger expressed sadness over what he perceived as abandonment by his extended family:

How can I put this? My family's been a real jerk. [*laughter*] . . . When we needed their help, they kind of stepped back. . . . When I first became paralyzed, . . . there were lots of things that in my eyes I feel my mother and my brother should have done for my wife that didn't get done. Here's my wife running a business, trying to keep her head above water and when she gets off of work she runs, picks the kids up from daycare. She's pregnant at the time, comes home, feeds the kids and then right after that she gathers them up and comes and drives to the hospital and sits with me at the hospital. In my opinion, my mother and my brother should have said, "Give us the kids, we'll make sure they're fed, go see Roger." But there wasn't any of that.

Roger felt this had "put a wedge" between him and his mother and brother. "I love my mother, I love my brother, but it made me cold," he said. Unfortunately, family conflict can disrupt the process of rehabilitation and has been linked to depression and distress in the aftermath of SCI (see, for example, Boekamp 1998; Boekamp, Overholser, and Schubert 1996; Drew 1997).

## The Economic Consequences of Spinal Cord Injury

Spinal cord injury is an expensive disability. The average first-year health care and living expenses for someone with high quadriplegia, low quadriplegia, and paraplegia are $710,275, $458,666, and $259,531, respectively. Expenses in each subsequent year average $127,227, $52,114, and $26,410 (National Spinal Cord Injury Statistical Center 2005). Overall, spinal cord injury costs the nation over $12 billion each year (Berkowitz et al. 1998).[1] Although SCI is considerably less common than most major diseases, the aggregate cost of spinal cord injury is one-tenth that of cancer and one-third that of stroke (DeVivo, Whiteneck, and Charles 1995).

Spinal cord injury has both direct and indirect costs. Average annual expenses are estimated at $14,215 for personal assistance, $11,169 for SCI-related medical care, $3,086 for medication and supplies (catheters, disposable gloves, powders, etc.), $1,612 for wheelchairs and repair, and $708 for vehicular modifications (Berkowitz et al. 1998). Home modifications included as first-year expenses average $26,040, and annual recurring costs average $466 (Berkowitz et al. 1998). The primary indirect cost of SCI is the economic output that is lost as a result of the inability to work. Estimates of this amount have ranged from $16,821 (Berkowitz et al. 1998) to $57,613 annually (National Spinal Cord Injury Statistical Association 2005). The economic impact of SCI varies considerably according to the individual's resources and work status, education, severity of injury, the disability benefits received, and the possibility of legal compensation (National Spinal Cord Injury Statistical Center 2004, 2005; Oliver et al. 1988).

Spinal cord injury creates financial stress that often extends to family members. Many individuals with SCI turn to family members for economic, instrumental, and social support, particularly in the immediate post-injury period. In response, family members also must respond and adjust to the disability of a loved one. For this reason, spinal cord injury has come to be viewed as a "family disability."

## Economic Status and Life Satisfaction

SCI generally brings a dramatic drop in earnings as well as an increase in various forms of government assistance (Berkowitz et al. 1998). In fact, the median income of individuals with spinal cord injury is less than two-thirds that of the general population (Berkowitz et al. 1998). The median personal income among study participants was $12,500, a figure that reflects, in part, the high concentration of students in my sample.[2] The 13 persons currently working (median personal income = $36,500) earned far more than the 11 students (median personal income = $6,786) and the 8 individuals not working (median personal income = $4,375). Moreover, men reported substantially higher incomes than women, paraplegics had higher incomes than quadriplegics, and those with the most severe impairments reported the lowest incomes of all.

The economic status of many of the participants in the study was related to the circumstances of their injuries. Specifically, individuals who had been injured as a result of someone else's recklessness and who had been awarded financial settlements were generally better off than those who had incurred their injuries as a result of their own negligence or bad luck. Meghan, who had been injured when she lost control of her car on an icy road, was acutely aware of these disparities. She felt that people who received generous financial settlements could never really understand the struggles she confronted:

> People that have got lawsuits because of their injury have more resources and they have more money. It's like anyone who's able-bodied.

While none of those who had received settlements indicated that their lives were as simple as Meghan suggested, many did report that the financial compensation provided a certain level of economic security and peace of mind. For example, Stacy told me she was financially "set for life." She had been injured as a result of a car accident in which her seatbelt malfunctioned. A subsequent lawsuit against the car manufacturer resulted in a generous award:

> I don't have to worry about [money] in the future, I don't have to worry about paying all these medical bills and finding insurance that will cover me and all those type of things. But [*sniffle*] it's not made it any easier like emotionally but it helps. I mean that's a big stress in your life. If I had to get a job right now to pay for tuition and stuff like that, that would probably be hard.

Meanwhile, Chris had received a workers' compensation settlement that provided some financial security (he had been hit by a vehicle while walking near work). He said he had invested his share of the money and that all things considered, he and his wife were "doing fine." He noted, "We live within our means, plus Social Security."

In general, individuals with SCI who have lower incomes report more psychological distress (Brenner 1990) and lower subjective well-being and life satisfaction (Decker and Schulz 1985; Lee and McCormick 2004). There is a positive association between satisfaction with income and length of time since injury, since over time people become more likely to obtain work or compensation, or to adjust to living on a reduced income (Oliver et al. 1988). The possibility of legal compensation is also important. Oliver and associates (1988) found that 84% of those who had settled compensation claims were satisfied with their financial circumstances. In contrast, 56% of those with no possibility of compensation and only 9% of those with outstanding compensation claims were satisfied.

My study confirmed that income has a considerable influence on emotional well-being. For example, while 88% of the study participants with personal incomes over $35,000 agreed with the statement, "I am a happy person," only 50% of those with personal incomes of less than $15,000 did. The receipt of a legal settlement was closely tied to reported happiness, as none of those who had received a settlement reported that they were unhappy. Moreover, those with jobs were more likely to report that they were happy (77%) than those not working (63%). Interestingly, all eleven students in the sample agreed that they are happy people.

## From Riches to Rags

Many of the individuals I interviewed described how their injuries had caused economic devastation in their lives. Derrick, who had fallen asleep while driving, reported,

I lost my house, and my three businesses had to be auctioned off to completely get rid of everything. And then the money for that had to be applied to all my medical bills before the state would do anything. That's after 20 years of paying taxes.

Derrick was getting $749 each month from Social Security and lived in a garage apartment behind his mother's house. He complained that he was having difficulty paying for attendant care and car insurance:

And now the state's not paying for my personal care so I'm having to pay for that out-of-pocket and every dime I get from Social Security Disability goes to pay for personal care, and then Mom and Tom [my stepfather] have to add money on top of that.

Although another driver was responsible for the auto accident that had left Fred paralyzed, that driver had had no insurance. As a result, Fred received only $7,000—money he used to buy his first wheelchair. He described how he had subsequently gone into debt:

I'll just show you the bills they sent me every month. There's no way I could pay 'em back. I told 'em I could pay maybe five bucks here and there, but a hundred thousand dollars, I mean that's *nuh-uh*.

Fred had moved in with his aunt due to the financial problems that had resulted from his accident.

## Ongoing Financial Challenges

Several of the people I interviewed noted how the high costs of their disabilities presented ongoing challenges for themselves and their families. Jay described how his disability had affected his family when he was growing up:

My father being an electrical draftsman, he wasn't making tons of money. And having six kids and my mother didn't really ever work so it was hard and he provided for a family of six and he was a very great dad and stuff like that. But things like the deductible for a pair of braces took away maybe my brother's baseball uniform or something like that or my sister getting a piano. I mean, I was a priority as far as my medical stuff.

Meanwhile, Vibha had experienced considerable difficulty getting insurance because she was considered a "high risk" case. She could only afford a nominal health insurance program through her university. To illustrate the inadequacies of this policy, she described how she had recently been hospitalized at a rate of almost $700 while her insurance had paid only $250. When she needed surgery for complications from bedsores, she had to return to India to get the operation:

> If I was to get operated here, the operation would have been thirty thousand and I would have got a thousand from my insurance. . . . I went in the spring semester midway. I had to get incompletes in that semester.

In India, Vibha explained, the operation cost about $3,000. When I pointed out the irony—that she had been forced to travel from an industrialized country to a developing country in order to get a necessary operation—Vibha replied, "It's sad."

Derrick described how he was in a struggle with Social Services to get a new wheelchair:

> I've been arguing and battling with the Department of Rehabilitation Services for over two years now because that chair has been so defective.

> EIW: Which chair?

> The other chair—the old chair. And now this chair I got in January and the next month I informed my counselor that it was so uncomfortable and nothing happened. So I wrote a letter the next month after talking to him again, told him that I still wasn't doing better after seeing numerous doctors here . . . I called him and he informed me that I needed to get a refund for this chair before they'd consider getting another one like the old one which was what I'd requested to begin with. And instead of doing that, he never helped me pursue that. And it's left me in this chair since January and now it's August and I've been in that bed more than I've been in this chair by far.

Unfortunately, wheelchairs are costly and often do not last through the interval after which insurance companies will pay for a replacement.[3] Many other essential supplies are also expensive. While the use of old, deteriorated wheelchair cushions has been linked to the development of pressure sores (Donovan et al. 1988), a new wheelchair cushion can cost several hundred dollars (the *AirFlo* Wheelchair Cushion retailed for $434 in 2005). Specialized equipment for individuals with disabilities is often notoriously overpriced, and individuals with disabilities are seldom in a position to negotiate these expenses (DeLoach and Greer 1981).

## Government Support

Two federal programs administered by the Social Security Administration provide entitlement benefits for individuals with disabilities: Social Security Disability Insurance (DI; Title II of the Social Security Act) and Supplemental Security Income (SSI; Title XVI). For both DI and SSI, disability is defined as the inability to engage in any substantial gainful activity by reason of a physical or mental impairment that is expected to end in death or to last at least twelve months. The eligibility criteria for DI and SSI differ, however. DI is a social insurance program that was founded in 1956 for disabled workers, and eligibility is contingent on prior employment in jobs covered by Social Security. SSI, established in 1974, is means-tested, requiring beneficiaries (those who are 65 or older, blind, or who have a disability) to satisfy income and asset criteria. The SSI disability program has recently expanded more quickly than DI (Rupp and Stapleton 1998).

Altogether, 38% of the participants in the study received DI and 28% received SSI (three of them—9%—received both DI and SSI). The average person with a severe physical disability has to expend considerable energy to deal with multiple bureaucracies, and our social welfare system has set unreasonably low income limits that often result in the loss of financial assistance, attendant care, and medical treatment benefits (Trieschmann 1988). The tax benefits to individuals and families who care for persons with disabilities have also been described as woefully inadequate (Perlman 1983).

Perhaps unsurprisingly, one of the most frequently voiced complaints among individuals with high-level quadriplegia was their inability to afford payment for adequate in-home care. Since most insurance policies make no provisions for attendant care, many families cannot afford even a part-time unskilled attendant (DeLoach and Greer 1981). Although Medicaid and Social Services provide some support for custodial care, the underlying premise of these programs is that individuals must be destitute in order to receive tax-supported assistance. As a consequence, individuals with chronic disabilities requiring attendant care frequently must make a choice between essential assistance and work, a choice that is undesirable from the perspective of both the consumer and the government (Adams and Beatty 1998).

The availability of and satisfaction with personal assistance services is one of the most important external factors influencing the rehabilitation outcomes of individuals with SCI (Chase 1998; Nosek et al. 1993). Unfortunately, complaints about personal attendant care are also pervasive (Neath 1997). Meghan told me that she sometimes spends the entire day in her wheelchair because her personal care attendant doesn't show up:

> I was in and out of the hospital, staying in bed two days, staying in my chair two days, and that's all I was doing. I had water and crackers in bed with me and my medication most days. And I was on the phone to different people. That was all I could do. . . . One lady told me once, 'cause I was saying "This is not right" and I was going through my little spiel which she's probably heard before. She said, "Oh, stop whining." And I said, "It's not whining when you can't get out of bed, when you haven't eaten in two days, or if you have eaten it's been carry-out or carry-in or whatever." . . . We really need help. We are dying. We are going to nursing homes and there's no reason.

Meghan said that she received less than $1,000 each month from the government and had been paying out-of-pocket for her personal care:

> I think that my government should pay people [i.e., assistants] if it's seven dollars a hour, ten dollars an hour, or whatever it is. I think they should pay that money to allow me to get up at five o'clock in the morning. And people say that that's a little bit much, but I don't think so because the reason it's not asking a bit much is because if you allow me to get up at five o'clock in the morning or whatever and go to bed when I want to go to bed, I'm going to do something that is gonna be productive and then I won't need the government's help.

Because she was having so much difficulty meeting basic needs, Meghan felt that her other concerns often seemed trivial:

> It doesn't matter if a place is handicapped accessible if you can't get out of bed. If you can't get out of bed and go to a shower and get

your hair washed and go to a movie theatre, what difference does it make if the movie theatre is accessible?

Kevin was in a similar predicament since he was paralyzed at the level of the neck. Although he had a regular personal care attendant who visited every day, much of his custodial care was performed by his parents (especially his mother). He had very real concerns about who would take care of him in the future:

Someday Mom and Dad's gonna croak.

EIW: Is that something you're scared of?

When I stop to think about it, yeah. But I think it will be a while. Hopefully, I'll be busy doing other things by then.

Several of the people I interviewed reported that the money they received from Social Security (between $500 and $600 per month) was barely enough to cover their basic living expenses. For example, Jennifer said she was dependent on her fiancé for transportation because she could not afford a wheelchair accessible vehicle.

In contrast, a handful of participants in the study—particularly those in public housing—reported that they were living comfortably with the government assistance they received.[4] For example, Ben, who got $616 each month from DI, seemed to be making very good use of the assistance he received. He lived in handicapped housing and paid $170 per month in rent, $10 for bank services, and $35 for the phone, which left him with approximately $400 to meet other living expenses. Al also lived in public housing and received "around 530-something" each month. "I live comfortably," he quipped.

Vocational Rehabilitation (VR) helps individuals with SCI (among others) secure employment commensurate with their abilities. VR assists with local job searches and promotes awareness of self-employment and telecommuting opportunities.[5] Nearly 16% of the individuals I interviewed receive VR benefits. Adam was very grateful for the VR assistance he received:

They pay for tuition, give you vouchers for books. It's a pretty good system. They do a real good job of trying to get people back into the workforce after you've been injured. . . . It makes you to where you can become self-sufficient, and I'm a big supporter of that.

## The Cliff Effect

Disabled workers risk losing their income support and health benefits if their earnings rise above the allowable maximum. The system of economic support for individuals with severe disabilities "can be described as an all-or-nothing system: earn a little and lose a lot" (Roberts 1989: 240). Supplemental Security Income benefits decline as earnings rise, and the Social Security Disability Insurance program cuts off assistance to those who earn more than $830 per month ($1,380 for blind individuals) (U. S. Social Security Administration 2005). This sudden loss of economic support has been described as the "cliff effect" (Arnold 1998: 1361).

For a low- or middle-income worker, the loss of government benefits can make employment financially disadvantageous (Daniels and West 1998). Because full-time workers are no longer regarded as disabled under many government programs, they are unlikely to receive financial assistance to help meet expenses. Unless they have good-paying jobs, they may actually find themselves in a worse financial situation than their nonworking counterparts (Ernst and Day 1998). Moreover, going to work often means the loss of Medicaid benefits, and private insurance is prohibitively expensive for many disabled individuals (Trieschmann 1980, 1988). As a result, many low-income individuals with SCI avoid work altogether and subsist entirely on government welfare programs (Krause and Anson 1996a; Quintiliani 2000). This becomes a Catch-22. While most rehabilitation efforts are intended to promote full-time employment, many people with disabilities cannot afford to take a job (Trieschmann 1980).

Recent years have seen expanded efforts to promote the employment of people with disabilities, including the Ticket to Work and Work Incentives Improvement Act of 1999. As a result of this act, most SSI and SSDI beneficiaries receive a "ticket" they may (voluntarily) use to obtain vocational rehabilitation, employment, or other support services from an approved provider of their choice (U. S. Social Security Administration 2002). Once accepted, these tickets become a contract between the Social Security Administration and the providers. The SSA agrees to pay the employment networks for helping disabled individuals find jobs. Moreover, Medicaid and Medicare programs were expanded in 2000 to provide benefits for a greater number of working people. For example, Medicare's Part A premium-free hospital insurance coverage is now available to most Social Security Disability beneficiaries who work.

Meanwhile, the study participants are keenly aware of the tensions between receiving disability benefits and working. For example, Adam commented,

> There are people who aren't able to do things on their own and they do need someone there to help them out. And they're not able to go out and get a job and pay for it themselves because they're afraid if they go out and get a job then they're gonna lose their benefits. So it's kind of a tricky situation.

Likewise, Travis described his struggles:

> Every time I've worked, I've always had difficulty with Social Security. They're supposed to allow you to work a certain amount without automatically cutting off your benefits. . . . But because of the bureaucracy that they are, they don't do very well with managing people who are on Social Security trying to work. It makes it really hard because of the fact that by the time they figure out what the hell is going on they're saying, "Well, you owe us money."

## Shelter but Not Serenity

The independent living movement in the United States has actively promoted the self-determination of individuals with disabilities: the right to live independently outside their parents' homes, nursing homes, and other institutions (DeJong 1979; Frieden and Cole 1985; Morris 1993c; Roberts 1989; Staas et al. 1988; Starkloff 1997). Although independent living has been a major objective of the disability rights movement, this goal may ignore or undervalue long-standing relationships and harm the self-esteem of people who cannot live without a great deal of help from others (Wendell 1996). While autonomy and dependence are recurrent themes in Euro-American conceptualizations of disability, many minority-group cultures value sociality (family and community membership) more than individual ability (Ingstad and Whyte 1995).

The opportunity to make residential decisions is a key factor in the life satisfaction of individuals with SCI (Boschen 1996; Oliver et al. 1988). The majority of individuals with SCI live with relatives following their discharge from rehabilitation (Bamford, Grundy, and Russell 1986), and most individuals with SCI living in the community identify family support as their most important source of help (Melendez 1992).[6] It is estimated that 70% to 75% of caregiving is provided by relatives (Berkowitz et al. 1992, 1998; Shapiro 1993). In most cases, women—especially wives and mothers—are the primary caregivers for individuals with severely disabling conditions (Elliott and Shewchuk 1998; Elliott, Shewchuk, and Richards 2001; Nosek et al. 1993; Shewchuk and Elliott 2000; Traustadottir 1993). While living with family members has been linked to greater satisfaction in the performance of daily tasks (Boschen, Tonack, and Gargaro 2003), reliance on family members for caregiving can add stress to relationships (Morris 1989). It may also lead to poor outcomes if family members deny or avoid the realities of disability, such as postponing independent living and thereby prolonging dependency on family members (Zirpolo 1986).

Quite a few of the people I interviewed complained about insufficient housing for wheelchair users, and several quadriplegics reported that there were no nearby independent living facilities for those requiring extensive personal assistance. A number of those I spoke with had moved in with their parents or siblings immediately following their injuries because they either lacked financial resources or required instrumental help in order to accomplish daily activities. Kevin, who had moved in with his parents after his injury, described how his need for attendant care had rendered him an appendage of his mother and father:

> They want to go down to the lake this weekend. They've got a cabin down there. . . . They want to go down there this weekend and take a bunch of new stuff and do a bit of work. And I don't wanna go, but I'm coming—stuck along with them.

Derrick described how he had moved into a garage apartment next to his mother's residence after returning home following rehabilitation:

> I was single and living alone. I had no nowhere to go unless I came here. And the doctors tried to get me to be put in a nursing home. And my mom and [her] husband thankfully made this and added the bathroom so that I could have a shower out here and everything.

Leonard and his wife divorced during his rehabilitation, and he subsequently moved into an apartment his parents had built alongside their home. Meanwhile, Andrew, his ex-wife (who got back together with him after his injury), and their two children moved in with his mother, since they had no other way to support themselves. He felt that living at home was "rough" because he was not in a position to help his mother financially:

> Luckily for me I had a good family support team system behind me
> and after six months I finally got a lump check [from Social Security]
> and that was over two thousand. So with that I gave my mom quite a
> bit of money and then we got our own place.

Nathan also went from living on his own to living with his mother after
being discharged from rehabilitation:

> I went home, and my momma took care of [me] 'til I got well. And
> then I started school. . . . And when I got out of there I went back
> to [my hometown] for a while and then I come up here and went to
> work.

At the time of the interview, Nathan had moved out and was living with
his brother (see Chapter 6).

## Spinal Cord Injury as a Family Disability

Many of the problems that affect individuals with SCI—financial hardship
and prejudice, in particular—also affect their families (Barnes, Mercer, and
Shakespeare 1999; Kester 1986). Of course, the individual's role within the
family is important, and the disability of a major breadwinner is likely to have
a more disruptive effect than the disability of another family member (De-
Loach and Greer 1981; Killen 1987). Some authors have argued that family
adjustment to SCI is similar to patient adaptation—that it is characterized
by a variety of responses such as anxiety, accommodation, and assimilation
(Bray 1978). During the days immediately following injury, families may
experience an even greater sense of helplessness than the disabled individual
(Weller and Miller 1977b). For example, the parents (especially mothers)
of patients with pediatric SCI show greater post-traumatic stress than do
the patients (Boyer et al. 2000). Of course, there is considerable variation
in family members' responses, making stage theories of adjustment overly
deterministic (Oliver et al. 1988). At the same time, family members often
experience feelings of frustration, isolation, guilt, and resentment following
the permanent impairment of a loved one (Alfano, Neilson, and Fink 1994;
Weller and Miller 1977b).

   Among the family members of individuals with SCI, social support tends
to reduce stress, promote psychological health, and increase life satisfaction
(Ell 1996; Kester 1986; Pelletier, Alfano, and Fink 1994; Santora 1996;
Ziolko 1993). Counseling may also help family members reduce the stress

associated with SCI (Ziolko 1993). Most family members express a desire to have their questions answered honestly, to have complete information on the disabled individual's physical impairment, to be assured that the patient is getting the best medical care, and to have a professional to turn to for advice or services (Meade et al. 2004). Close relatives also express a desire to feel helpful to the individual with SCI, to be able to cope with home and family responsibilities, to receive adequate emotional and social support, and to deal with major future effects of the injury (Hart 1981). Family members' emotional and social needs are often overlooked as families become preoccupied with short-term needs rather than long-term family growth (Hart 1981; Meade et al. 2004; Steinglass et al. 1982).

Many of the people I interviewed described how their family members initially reacted to their injuries with shock and disbelief. Harry, whose injury occurred during a high school football game, reported,

> My mom freaked. . . . My mom didn't care what the extent was or what the problem was, she just wanted it fixed. And they had to sedate her and . . . they had to have my step-dad calm her down.

Similarly, Al said that his injury was "heartbreaking" for his family, but because of his positive spirit he felt they were more effectively adjusting to the injury. "Right now, they see my attitude and I know that it's still hard for them but it's not as hard," he said. As Al's experience demonstrates, the perception of the disabled individual's overall psychosocial functioning strongly influences the extent of long-term stress on family members (Neilson 1990).

In some instances, family members—especially parents—may become riddled with guilt as a result of their relative's injuries. For example, Brad told me that his mother "thinks it's her fault that this happened 'cause she let my sister and I go on this boat trip" where his accident happened. Likewise, Jennifer said that her dad "kind of feels guilty because he was the one that let me drive that day, so he kind of blames himself." Meanwhile, both Jennifer and Brad reported that their parents were strong sources of support.

## Caregiving and Conflict

Disability often causes strain in family relationships (Cleveland 1980; Killen 1987), and there are many opportunities for stressful exchanges among the family members of disabled individuals (Ell 1996).[7] This most often occurs as family members assume new roles as caregivers and financial providers. Caregiving is inherently stressful, and family caregivers are at risk for depression, anxiety, and a variety of other health complications (Elliott and Shewchuk 1998; Elliott, Shewchuk, and Richards 2001; Kester 1986; Perlman 1983; Shewchuk and Elliott 2000; Steinglass et al. 1982). Caregivers often experience financial stress, and they sometimes must withdraw from school, quit their jobs, increase their working hours, reenter the labor market to replace lost income, or take jobs that provide less stressful conditions and greater flexibility (Berkowitz et al. 1992).

Harry's experience living at home with his mother and stepfather illustrates some of the tensions inherent in these kinds of caregiving arrangements:

> [My mother] was under all this stress. I was a lot weaker. She had to get up at night and help me go to the bathroom; they had to take care of me and I was in those modes to where I was letting people take care of me. . . . The doctor told my mom, "If you don't get him out of the house, you're gonna die, it's gonna kill you. You need somebody to help him." You know, they didn't have the money to hire somebody to help me personally. So when I was 18 years old they put me a nursing home.

At the nursing home, Harry felt he had hit bottom:

> I went from high school to a nursing home. . . . And I've got this guy named Alex that comes up to my door that's on Thorazine going, "Well, well, well, well." And he'd look down, his slobber would hit the floor and I'm like, "What the hell am I doing in here with all these old people?"

After experiencing considerable humiliation and mistreatment in the nursing home, Harry lost weight and gained the strength to do transfers on his own so that he could enter a rehabilitation program. In retrospect, Harry seemed to feel as though his experience in the nursing home motivated him to become self-sufficient. "I'm thankful for my parents that put me in the nursing home," he said.

As Harry's case illustrates, the mothers of children with disabilities may experience severe role strain as their desire to care for their dependent off-spring conflicts with the maternal role prescription to foster independence (Cleveland 1980). While family members frequently serve as primary sources of emotional, therapeutic, and financial support, tension frequently ensues as children (including adult children) with SCI try to reconcile their need for help with their desire for independence. In turn, SCI can complicate the process of becoming independent from one's parents (Davies 1982; Morris 1989). As Stan noted, he and his parents had

> had a good relationship prior to my disability. And there were times that were strained afterwards because I was in that growing up stage of trying to become independent. And it was far more difficult for me to become independent than someone who is able-bodied. So there were those growing pains.

Although injured as an adult, Chris experienced similar tensions in his relationship with his father. At the time of his injury, Chris's mother was in the hospital being operated on for a cancerous cyst. She later died while he was in the hospital recovering from his injury. Chris's father, who was torn up "from both ends," subsequently

> switched all his attention from Mom to me. So he was at the hospital a lot. But when I went to rehab, they wouldn't let him come in that much so he was recuperating in his own world. . . . And of course after I got home now he wanted to come up here all the time. And he was lonesome and he overprotected.

After his injury, Chris felt it was "really tough" to go out in public, and his father tried to protect him from having to face other people by telling them not to visit him. In retrospect, Chris felt that his father's approach had been counterproductive: "I know better now that you want to expose yourself to this as quick as possible to get over that hump," he said. Interestingly, individuals with disabilities who are unmarried seem to achieve greater functional independence than those who are married, possibly owing to anxiety-ridden or overprotective families who make it more difficult for them to recover fully (Safilios-Rothschild 1970).

Some evidence suggests that unmarried young men are less likely than unmarried women to be welcomed back home after disabling injuries (Safilios-Rothschild 1970), and a few men described how they had been turned away in the aftermath of their injuries. For example, Fred reported that when his accident occurred, "friends and family just kind of turned their back and tiptoed away real fast." While he had received support from his brother, an aunt, and a cousin, his mother was unavailable:

> My mother, she was not very, you know – what's the word?
>
> EIW: She wasn't there for you?
>
> No, she wasn't there [from] day one. There was just no feeling there at all.

After he was discharged from rehabilitation, Fred moved in with his aunt, with whom he still lives: "I'm very lucky that my aunt took me in because I'd be probably dead [if she hadn't]," he said. "I'm not a nursing home type of Indian."

## Sibling Stress

The brothers and sisters of children with SCI are often acutely sensitive to the ramifications of having a sibling with a chronic disability. In some instances, the attention given by parents to the child with a disability results in neglect or jealousy (Davies 1982). Parental preoccupation with the immediate crisis of the injury, months of rehabilitation, and years of caregiving may cause siblings to feel that they are missing out on parental involvement (Palmer, Kriegsman, and Palmer 2000). Brad described his case:

> It screwed up our lives for quite a while. . . . My sister probably didn't get the attention she needed in her final year of school because my parents were at the hospital a lot the first three or four months, just a fair amount of the school year.

Kevin felt that his disability may have contributed to family problems:

> My oldest brother started going out to bars and getting in fights. And my youngest brother started smoking a lot of pot and getting in trouble at school and stuff.

He felt that his brothers had nonetheless been very supportive of him. Meanwhile, Jennifer asserted that her brother was never fully able to come to terms with her disability:

> At first I think it was just disbelief. . . They wanted to believe that it wasn't gonna be permanent. And my brother, he never really has dealt with it; he still has problems. He says that he doesn't like seeing me like this 'cause I was so active before and he doesn't like to see me just sit there.

In general, male family members—especially brothers and fathers—have a more difficult time accepting individuals with SCI (Drew-Cates 1989).

## Parents with Disabilities

Fifteen percent of American parents have a disability (Through the Looking Glass 2005) and they remain a stigmatized group whose suitability for child-rearing is sometimes questioned. For example, many rehabilitation professionals have expressed concerns about the effects of socioeconomic changes associated with physical disability (including SCI) and the presumed reversal in parental roles (Buck and Hohmann 1984). At the same time, children's adjustment does not appear to be adversely related to either the financial security or the employment status of fathers with SCI (Buck and Hohmann 1984), and maternal SCI does not negatively affect children's individual adjustment, attitudes toward their parents, self-esteem, gender roles, or family functioning (Alexander, Hwang, and Sipski 2002). Moreover, adult children whose fathers had SCI show no evidence of adverse psychosocial development (Buck and Hohmann 1981). While some evidence suggests that children experience distress in the period immediately following a parent's SCI, this may be resolved through regular parental contact, family support, reassurance, and explanation (Webster and Hindson 2004).

Most evidence suggests that the children of disabled parents tend to develop a greater sense of responsibility and personal involvement with their parents (Trieschmann 1989). In particular, the children of parents with SCI often have an increased sense of independence and tend to be self-sufficient, empathetic, sensitive, and helpful (Buck and Hohmann 1981; Reinelt and Fried 1993; Shaul, Dowling, and Laden 1981; Trieschmann 1989). At the same time, some parents worry that their need for assistance places too many demands on their children (Trieschmann 1980), and many try diligently to avoid being seen as dependent (Shaul, Dowling, and Laden 1981; Quigley 1994). Roger described how his disability affected his three young girls:

It has opened their eyes and has given them a chance to see a completely different side of a different life. They want to do things for you and that basically drives me nuts 'cause I want to be independent.

Tonya felt that her disability was a constructive force in her children's lives:

I don't think my kids see it right now, but I think it's going to make them better people. . . . More sensitive to others. More sensitive to any kind of people. More open and accepting to people.

At the same time, she felt that her eldest son sometimes acted out in response to her SCI:

I have one child that's twelve, and he accepted it because he was fairly young when this happened. He didn't have the problem with it. Now, I have a son that's fifteen and he's had a problem with it since the day I was injured [eight years before]. He's been angry and bitter about it. And he still is resentful about it, he's never accepted it and I just assume that with age he will come to terms with it and there's nothing I can do about it.

A few respondents complained that their disabilities keep them from full involvement in their children's activities. For example, when I asked Cody how he thought his disability had affected his children, he responded:

I don't participate in their life as much as they probably would want me to. . . [My daughter] was a student queen and I just didn't feel like going through the hassle of making sure that they had places for me to sit and all that stuff.

## Closeness and Comfort

The majority of individuals with chronic disabilities report high levels of emotional closeness with their families (Kutner 1987), and increased family closeness and compassion following the onset of disability—particularly between parents and children—have been documented in previous research (Cleveland 1980; McMillen and Cook 2003). Stacy, who had been injured in an accident in which her maternal grandmother was killed, described her family's response:

> My dad's parents—it changed them a lot because they were the type that you didn't give hugs goodbye to; you were just like, "Bye, see you later," y'know, you never said "I love you" and everything. I think my dad said the only time his father ever said he loved him was like when he told him he was getting married. That's the only time. But now we're always giving hugs . . . and I say, "I love you."

Stacy also felt that her parents had grown closer in the aftermath of the accident. "I just really admire their relationship," she said. "It could have been just total hell, it could have ripped our family apart, but it didn't." In describing how his injury affected his relationship with his parents, Adam reported:

> It did bring me closer, especially my dad. But it did create some tension because it frustrated me that I wanted to do more but he was really, really overprotective. And he was afraid to let me do more so that did cause some tension. But other than that, I think it probably brought us more closer.

Travis described how his family—especially his father—was a source of considerable strength and comfort in the aftermath of his injury:

> I think that I was really lucky. My father was a disabled veteran.[8] . . . And so even though I hadn't been immersed per se in the disability culture, I knew what it was to try to overcome a disability and so I had somebody that could help me with that in some ways.

Travis reported that his father was the closest person in his life for many years.

## Summary

Economic distress frequently accompanies physical disability, and many individuals with SCI have difficulty maintaining or finding employment, securing adequate health insurance, making ends meet, or living solely on the income provided by government assistance. Trieschmann (1988: 293) contends that "the primary consequence of SCI for most people is sustained financial destitution and insecurity in order to quality for financial aid from the state." While money can never fully compensate for disability, "it can add choice and meaning and significantly improve the quality of life" (Oliver et al. 1988: 126). Indeed, "the old adage 'money can't buy happiness' may need to be rephrased as 'money may not insure happiness, but it damn sure helps'" (Clayton 1992: 112). The comments of several of the people I spoke with reinforce these sentiments.

Economic well-being and employment are two areas in which individuals with SCI report especially low levels of satisfaction (Fuhrer et al. 1992; Krause 1992b). This seems to be particularly true among individuals with high-level quadriplegia, many of whom are preoccupied with meeting basic living expenses and avoiding institutionalization. Personal assistance services are the "new, top-of-the-agenda issue" among disability activists (Shapiro 1993: 251), and many individuals with high-level quadriplegia voiced major concerns related to the costs of independent living and attendant care. On the other hand, the financially secure study participants—particularly those who had received large cash settlements as compensation for their injuries—seemed considerably more comfortable with their living conditions.

Spinal cord injury often has a dramatic impact on the friends and families of disabled individuals. Not only do family members need a supportive environment in which to express their emotions, but those who are caring for individuals with high-level quadriplegia often require ongoing financial and social support as well as respite care. Since family members have a major impact on the rehabilitation process (Boekamp 1998; Rosenthal 1989), rehabilitation therapists need to pay special attention to the social and family roles of individuals with SCI. Rehabilitation efforts that involve family members may be instrumental in reducing feelings of anxiety, helplessness, and frustration among the families of disabled individuals (Rohrer et al. 1980). While the majority of people I interviewed reported that their disabilities interfered with family roles and relationships, several also pointed to a renewed sense of family closeness and caring that emerged in the aftermath of their injuries.

# 10

# Education and Employment

Stacy is an attractive 20-year-old paraplegic college student with braces on her teeth and shoulder-length jet black hair. She has a slender build and is six feet tall. She works as a residential assistant (RA) in the dormitories and has her own room on the second floor of a high-rise dormitory. In her room is a queen-sized bed and a couch. A stuffed moose sits on her bed, and several more are lined up on a shelf.

Stacy's spinal cord was severed in a car accident on Father's Day in 1996 when she was 15 years old. She was in a car with her family (father, mother, grandmother, and sister) when they came upon an oil truck stalled on top of a hill. The truck had no lights or flashers on, and their car rammed into it. Stacy was in the back seat, and her seatbelt malfunctioned—"It kind of held me there and pretty much just cut me in half." Her 52-year-old grandmother was killed in the accident, and several family members sustained severe injuries. Although Stacy initially went through periods of anger and depression, she now characterizes herself as a happy person. She neither agrees nor disagrees that her disability is a positive force in her life.

At the time of the accident, Stacy had been very involved in school athletics (e.g., basketball and cheerleading). As a result of her injury, however, her activities shifted away from sports and toward academic achievement:

> I couldn't really do a lot of the things I used to do. In [my hometown] there's not any wheelchair athletics, so that kind of shifted my whole focus. I kind of turned to the academic part: I was in student council, on the constitution team, which is kind of like a

debate team. And we went to nationals with that, and that took a lot of my time so I just shifted gears and went into that mode.

She also started taking honors classes and graduated with honors. She remarked that "I probably would have never done that" before the injury.

Stacy is studying advertising and would someday like to do advertising for a large corporation. "I would love to work for Budweiser or something like that," she said. Although she did not feel that her disability had any bearing on her career aspirations, Stacy expected to encounter problems related to disability discrimination when she began applying for jobs:

> I think once I enter the workforce, like when I start interviewing for jobs, that will be when I kind of face things 'cause I don't know what they're gonna think of me or how to present myself. That's something I'm gonna have to figure out.

## Educational and Vocational Achievement

Educational achievement and participation in the workforce are central to quality of life among individuals with SCI. Highly educated individuals adjust more effectively to their disabilities (Alfano, Neilson, and Fink 1993; Bulman and Wortman 1977; Katz and Kravetz 1987; Livneh and Antonak 1997; Shnek 1995; Shnek et al. 1995). They tend to have a more positive self-concept (Green, Pratt, and Grigsby 1984) and are less prone to depression and anxiety (Scivoletto et al. 1997; Shnek 1995; Shnek et al. 1995). Individuals with SCI who have high levels of education also tend to have better social functioning and higher life satisfaction (Post, de Witte, et al. 1998). They lead more intellectualized lives, have a greater capacity for fantasy, and are better able to avoid the frustrations associated with immobility (Nickerson 1971). Because physical disabilities often limit the kinds of manual labor that individuals can perform, highly educated individuals are also less likely to be disadvantaged in the labor market.

Like education, employment plays a key role in quality of life for individuals with SCI (Brenner 1990; Chase 1998; Clayton and Chubon 1994; Crewe 2000; Decker and Schulz 1985; Dowler, Batiste, and Whidden 1998; Krause 1990, 1992a, 1992b, 1996; Krause and Anson 1997a; Krause and Crewe 1987; Lundqvist et al. 1991; Oliver et al. 1988). Society attributes a high value to gainful employment, and the unemployed are often perceived to be dependent on others (Dowler, Batiste, and Whidden 1998). Among individuals with SCI, employment encourages social integration (Mackelprang 1986) and promotes self-efficacy (Shnek 1995; Shnek et al. 1995). Moreover, those who are working report fewer problems, more satisfaction with their lives, and better overall adjustment (Krause 1990; Krause and Anson 1997a; Krause and Dawis 1992).

Of course, work is valued not only for its instrumental properties (i.e., sustenance or financial prosperity) but also for its role in identity formation, self-esteem, and physical and mental well-being (Safilios-Rothschild 1970). The transition to employment appears to enhance many areas of life adjustment, whereas the loss of employment has the reverse effect (Krause 1996). The need for productive work appears to be ongoing, since the beneficial effects of employment appear to subside once employment is terminated (Krause 1992a). Psychosocial and vocational adjustment have even been linked to survival rates among individuals with SCI, possibly because individuals with less active lifestyles are less likely to seek medical treatment (Krause and Crewe 1987).

## Educational Rights and Accommodations in the Schools

Since the 1970s, federal law has guaranteed the educational rights of disabled individuals. Section 504 of the Rehabilitation Act of 1973 specifies that "no otherwise qualified handicapped individual" can be excluded from participation in any program or activity receiving federal financial assistance. In 1975, Congress passed the Education for All Handicapped Children Act (Public Law 94–142) to guarantee "a free appropriate public education" for all disabled children. In recent years, the Education for All Handicapped Children Act (now referred to as the Individuals with Disabilities Education Act) has undergone various amendments to extend the scope of its coverage and to change the procedural aspects of planning and evaluation. Further support for nondiscrimination in the schools has come from the 1990 Americans with Disabilities Act (ADA), which extends disability rights to the private and nonfederal public sectors.

Several study participants described the challenges they had confronted prior to the implementation of legislation guaranteeing equal access to education. Two older men, Stan (age 50) and Jonathan (age 49), recounted how they had broken new ground when they had been mainstreamed into schools and colleges many decades earlier. Jonathan said,

I was injured when I was seven. . . . This was my first and second grade years and then I . . . went just to regular school which [was] unheard of—especially back then. No one ever did it. . . . So that was late 50s, early 60s. You didn't see people in wheelchairs even out.

Jonathan described how his parents, and especially his father, went to great lengths to ensure that the school was accessible for him:

My mom and dad were pretty good about raising me just like you would just raise a child, only this child happens to be in a wheelchair. . . . And as we went through school, the schools weren't accessible. So my dad was pretty active in the community and . . . pretty well-known and he would make sure that as I went from grade to junior high school, and junior high school to high school that we set it up to where it was accessible enough for me to get around and go to class and so forth.

Even so, Jonathan felt his disability had prevented him from being as active in extracurricular activities as he might otherwise have been:

The chair kind of makes you different. I mean, even as a child you see that and you kind of have a little bit of a negative frame of mind sometimes no matter [what] people say to you or try to encourage you. Sometimes you just don't wanna go to the trouble or it's too much hassle.

When Stan was injured at the age of 17, he wrote a letter to U. S. Speaker of the House Carl Albert requesting accommodations so that he could attend college. Nearly two weeks prior to his injury, Stan had watched Albert give a speech during which he had said, "If ever I can do anything for you, please give me that opportunity."

Little did he know and little did I know that eleven days later I broke my neck. . . . I knew that I had to go to college and . . . so I wrote him a letter and I said, "Where can I go to college? I need help." . . . And within six weeks he wrote me back a letter and said, "I have given [a state university] a grant of so many hundred thousand dollars over a six-year period to become a demonstration site for the removal of architectural barriers and that you can go to school there." And this was in 1969 before any law that mandated the fair treatment or the civil rights of individuals with disabilities.

Like Jonathan, Stan recalled that individuals with disabilities were rarely seen in public during this era. Perhaps as a result of this, the stigmatization of individuals with SCI was often quite blatant. Stan recalled a particularly upsetting episode that had occurred while he was in college:

> I was in a TGNY store . . . and I was buying some peanuts and M&Ms and a lady just hit me over the head with her purse. Bam! . . . I looked up at the lady and I said, "Why did you hit me over the head with your purse? That hurt!" And she said, "You shouldn't be out in public." And I said, "What? I'm going to college here. . . . I'm a student." She says, "You're horrible to look at. . . . You should be in a nursing home or at home, or finding someone to take care of yourself." And that hurt me, but it hurt me enough to make me mad. And I always remembered it.

On the other hand, Jay (age 37) who was injured as an infant, attended a special "disabled school" up until third grade because "they didn't know anything about mainstreaming." Jay described how accessibility barriers had precluded him from attending the Catholic school where many of his siblings were enrolled:

> The reason I didn't go was 'cause the Catholic school wasn't accessible to get around.
>
> EIW: But you were walking on crutches, right?
>
> Yeah, but it's still four flights of stairs, upstairs with no elevator or anything like that. I might be superhuman in trying to do things [*laughter*] but I wasn't that stupid.

The main problem, according to Jay, was going up the stairs. Going down the stairs was less of an issue: "You can pretty much fly down if you got the handrail, if you've got the handrails close enough to each other," he said, chuckling. Although Jay never enrolled in the Catholic school, he did attend public schools. When I asked him if he had experienced any negativity because of his disability, Jay responded,

I don't think it was different than much. High school kids are cruel a lot of times anyway. I do remember being called "Crutch" and it bothering me at first, but then I understood psychology enough: I told everybody to call me "Crutch" and when they saw it didn't bother me, it wasn't fun for them to do anymore. [*laughter*]

Meanwhile, Travis felt that far from being unaccommodating, the teachers in his high school had let him get away with too much:

When I first got hurt, I had teachers that cut me too much slack and I took advantage of them. And that's my fault for taking advantage of it, but maybe if they'd been a little bit harder on me it would have probably been better for me.

Among the study participants currently enrolled in college, nearly three-quarters (73%) agreed either *somewhat* or *strongly* that their colleges and universities provided them with necessary accommodations. It is interesting to note that the individuals attending Flagship University reported higher levels of satisfaction than those attending smaller colleges in the region. It is likely that the larger universities have more resources to accommodate students with disabilities.

Stacy, described as the beginning of this chapter, reported that disability discrimination was not something she'd experienced at Flagship University:

I've had no problems. I'm very independent, though. . . . [I've] talked to people that use electric chairs and they have a little more problem. If you have a problem you tell the Center for Student Life and they get it fixed.

Stacy also seemed to have a more carefree attitude toward accommodations than many of her compatriots at the university:

When we [the disabled students] were out having our meeting, they were talking about how someone had to pick him up and put him on the van for something and they were all bitching about it. And I just thought, "That doesn't bother me at all."

EIW: What do you mean "pick him up and put him"?

There wasn't a lift, so he had to pick him up and just put him on the seat. And that could be embarrassing, but I don't have a problem with that at all, and I guess some people just get offended more easily.

Meanwhile, a handful of the students in my sample indicated some degree of dissatisfaction with college/university services and accommodations. Ryan, who was president of the Disabled Students' Association, reported serious problems with accessibility at Flagship University, including inaccessible doors and buildings lacking elevators. He felt he had a clear mandate:

> I believe there are certain things on campus at Flagship University that I would like to get changed, that I believe are blatant discrimination on the parts of disabled students that I would like to get changed. . . . They say, "Oh, but we don't have the money." Well that's bullshit. And pardon my language, but that's discrimination. You have to change it.

Previous research has shown that problems with accessibility in the schools (e.g., small doorways, steps without ramps, and small bathrooms) may discourage reintegration, promote isolation, and emphasize disabled identities (Low 1996; Mulcahey 1992).

## Educational Attainment and Aspirations

Overall, 16% of the participants in the study had a high school education or less, 44% had completed some college, 9% had an associate's/technical degree, and 31% had a bachelor's degree or higher (the educational attainment of each individual is specified in Appendix). Compared with the U. S. population overall (ages 18–54), the study participants were somewhat more likely to have graduated from high school and to have attended some college (U. S. Census Bureau 2003). Women were more likely than men to have attended college, and there was no consistent relationship between degree of impairment and educational attainment. While the relatively high level of education among the study participants is undoubtedly linked to the selectivity of the sample, it is also the case that physical limitation often brings a reorientation toward intellectual achievement (White 1983). Moreover, individuals with SCI often return to school to strengthen their occupational skills (Chase 1998; Crewe 2000; Dijkers 1996; Duggan and Dijkers 2001; Krause 1998a). While individuals with SCI have somewhat lower-than-average educational attainment at the time of their injuries (Go, DeVivo, and Richards 1995), they have higher-than-average educational attainment ten years post-injury (Dijkers et al. 1995).

Several of the people I interviewed reported that they had become more academically focused in the aftermath of their injuries. For example, Jeremy reported that his injury had motivated him to get a degree in management information systems. He described himself as more of a "roughneck" prior to his injury and felt he had become more intellectually oriented since then. Likewise, Paul, who was studying architecture, reported, "I wouldn't be here right now if I wasn't disabled." When I asked him what he thought he'd be doing instead, he responded, "Probably pumping gas somewhere. I was not a good student."

For many, educational support from Vocational Rehabilitation provided a meaningful use of time as well as an avenue to economic independence. Several of the people I interviewed had participated in a vocational computer training program sponsored by Goodwill. Andrew described the Goodwill program as his "first step to going back to work." Edward, who had worked as an electrician and welder prior to his injury, had initially been hesitant to enroll in the Goodwill program, but it turned out to be a positive experience for him. He eventually graduated at the top of his class, even though he hadn't known how to turn a computer on and off when he began. The class was a one-year offering co-funded by the state, Rehab Services, and several charities.

In some cases, the return to educational activities was motivated by a desire for intellectual and social stimulation. For example, Leonard starting taking classes in history, business, composition, and other subjects at a local college after his injury

> mainly just to get some extra education—really just to get out of the house. Just to do some things, meet some people, just to get out and do something.

Previous research has shown that men with SCI often become less judgmental and rigid about what does *not* interest them (Rohe and Athelstan 1985). Several of the people I interviewed described how they had switched or were contemplating a change in their college majors because they wanted practical job skills. For example, Ben had initially wanted to work in carpentry, but now he felt that computer science would be a more sensible career path:

> Now I'm going to school working with computers. . . . Not that I'm a big computer buff, but that seems to be where the money is and so that's what I want to do.

Meanwhile, Adam was considering switching majors from zoology to education:

> I've always enjoyed science but it just doesn't seem like a major where you can do very much if you're physically disabled. The only thing I can really see doing is . . . becoming a professor and I really did not want to go long enough to do that. So I think if I switched to education then I can keep zoology as a minor and I can teach high school zoology and I'll still be involved in what I want to do.

A few described how they had lingered in college, at least partly because vocational rehabilitation had provided such extensive support services. For example, when I asked Harry how he felt about state benefits for individuals with disabilities, he reflected

> Well, I'm gonna be totally honest with you. . . . I don't think they should have gave as much money as they did because had they tightened the reins on me, I probably would have changed my attitude and some of the things I done and had a lesser debt and been out of school already.

Brad also reported that he was in school "for a very long time" because he had spent a lot of time "goofing off."

## Employment Experience

Most individuals with SCI are able to return to work, or to use the time formerly spent on work doing other useful activities (Schönherr et al. 2005a). Nonetheless, many are unsatisfied with their vocational status (Post, Van Dijk, et al. 1998). Estimates of the post-injury employment rate of individuals with SCI have ranged from as low as 11% of persons injured in the late 1970s who resumed work in New South Wales (Selecki et al. 1986) to as high as 75% of those who had ever worked in a 1980s sample of persons injured for at least 6 years in the United States (Krause 1992c).[1] This wide variation may be attributed to inconsistent definitions of employment (*currently working* versus *ever worked,* for example), different sociocultural contexts, and variations in the composition of the sample populations (time since injury, amount of vocational training, etc.). While most early studies simply classified individuals as either *working* or *not working,* many recent researchers have broadened the concept of employment to encompass all productive activities, including meaningful activities that do not necessarily result in paid remuneration (volunteer work, homemaking, etc.) (DeVivo et al. 1987; Young et al. 1994).

Recent U. S. research suggests that while the majority of working-age individuals with SCI are employed prior to their injuries (59%–73%), fewer than 30% are working post-injury (Chapin and Kewman 2001; Dowler, Batiste, and Whidden 1998; Duggan and Dijkers 1999, 2001; Krause and Anson 1996a; Krause et al. 1999). Over time, employment rates tend to increase, and most studies show that 30% to 40% of those with SCI are working ten to fifteen years after their injuries (Dijkers 1996; Krause et al. 1999).[2] In fact, it usually takes approximately five years from the onset of SCI to the first post-injury job, and six years to the first full-time post-injury job (Krause 2003). Many return to work for the same employers they had previously worked for (Tomassen, Post, and van Asbeck 2000), and the likelihood of returning to employment quickly is higher for those who do (Krause 2003; Krause and Anson 1996a; Schönherr et al. 2005b).

Many demographic variables influence post-injury employment, including educational attainment, severity of injury and functional limitation, age, race, and sex. In short, young, white males with higher levels of education, less severe injuries, and fewer functional limitations are the people with SCI most likely to be working.[3] Variables that seem to influence employment *directly* include age at the time of injury, education, motivation to work, ability to drive, and social support (McShane and Karp 1993). The effects of some variables are interactive. For example, gender is more important in determining reemployment chances among blacks, for instance, while level of injury is more critical among whites (James, DeVivo, and Richards 1993).

Other factors that encourage a return to employment include (1) the ability to visualize a return to employment, (2) boredom or dissatisfaction with not working, (3) social support, (4) transportation, (5) adequate personal care, (6) a supportive work environment, and (7) adequate financial remuneration for working (Morehouse 1996). Contextual factors such as disability compensation and the structure of the labor market also moderate the relationship between disability and employment (Szymanski 2000; Tomassen, Post, and van Asbeck 2000). Individuals who complete vocational rehabilitation programs are also more likely to be employed (DeVivo et al. 1987). Psychosocial characteristics such as high motivation, optimism, positive self-esteem, an achievement orientation, and the presence of positive role models also encourage productive activity (see, for example, Chapin and Kewman 2001; DeVivo et al. 1987; Kemp and Vash 1971; Krause 1997). Employment is also more likely among those with high intelligence (DeVivo et al. 1987; Herron 1987).[4]

Altogether, 41% of the study participants were employed; 25% were enrolled in school but not working, 9% were working students, and 25% were neither working nor going to school. Women and those with more severe impairments were especially unlikely to be working. (The fact that all the participants under age 30 were enrolled in college is an artifact of the sampling method.) Among the 16 employed participants, 50% were employed in professional/technical occupations, 19% in managerial/administrative positions, 13% in service positions, 6% in sales, 6% in clerical/administrative support, and 8% in agricultural/related positions (see Appendix). The individuals I surveyed were disproportionately concentrated in the professional occupations due to the high number of computer programmers and systems analysts in the sample. Research indicates that the overwhelming majority of nonemployed individuals with disabilities want to be working (Eaton, Condon, and Mast 2001; O'Brien 2001). While a few nonworking study participants had voluntarily opted out of the labor market, most expressed a desire for paid employment. Meanwhile, the participants identified a number of barriers—both internal as well as external—that precluded employment or resulted in underemployment.

## Internal Obstacles to Employment

Among individuals with SCI, the inability to work can most often be traced to disability-related physical limitations (Berkowitz et al. 1998; Inge et al. 1998; Krause and Anson 1996b; Schönherr et al. 2004). Older individuals are especially likely to cite health-related problems as factors that preclude their ability to work (Krause and Anson 1996b). Mobility and position restrictions also interfere with the development of satisfying careers (Bozzacco 1993). High-level quadriplegia brings special challenges: severe physical disability (limited or no movement below the neck) and decreased respiratory function.[5] Individuals with the most severe impairment are likely to require special skills training in order to participate in meaningful vocational and creative activities (Lathem, Gregorio, and Garber 1985; Sargant and Braun 1986).

Both prevocational and vocational programming may help individuals with SCI overcome the work-related challenges associated with physical impairment. The former includes assistance in the development of productive work habits, the practice of personal hygiene, the refinement of writing and other motor skills, and other ancillary instruction such as driver training. The latter includes the implementation of changes in the work environment and in prescribing, fitting, and using job-specific adaptive equipment (Kanellos 1985).[6] At least some individuals with SCI are likely to need transportation, housing, financial assistance, independent living services, medical assistance, and personal assistance services (Inge et al. 1996). At the same time, telework—paid work conducted from a remote location—holds particular promise for individuals with SCI, since it minimizes the effects of many work-related hindrances such as mobility limitations, transportation needs, and the fatigue imposed by medical complications (Bricout 2004).

Many study participants identified physiological complications as factors inhibiting their success on the employment front. Several described how bowel and bladder problems, chronic pain, recurrent urinary tract infections, and pressure sores prevented them from obtaining steady employment. Kevin told me he that there were "lots of different reasons" why people with SCI didn't work, but physiological factors were key:

> My back is giving me nothing but hell. I've got one friend and he pretty much can't do anything because he has bowel problems all the time.

Likewise, Tonya described how her bowel and bladder problems contributed to her withdrawal from the labor force:

> You'd have to have an employer that was understanding. . . . I have infections all the time and with that suprapubic. . . . I thought that was gonna be the end of my problems, but it really hasn't.

Meanwhile, Fred was trying to lose weight so that he would be eligible to join an independent living center, go back to school, and eventually return to the working world. (Fred is 6'1" and weighs approximately 325 pounds.) He reported that the likelihood of achieving his goals depends on his ability to get his health under control:

> It just depends on how my health turns out. [I'm] constantly fighting urinary tract infections, that's not good for anybody. That, and other things. . . . I had a decubis [ulcer] on my bottom and it just got a bad bug, bad bacteria in there—just couldn't shake [it] off very well. . . . I've had three surgeries on my bottom and it's just pretty tender down there.

Like Fred, Jonathan felt that the physical challenges of SCI seriously constrained his employment options:

> Obviously, I had to do something [where] I could sit on my butt and use my hands and talk and those kinds of whatever tools I have.

## Not Enough Hours in the Day

Although productive employment is associated with subjective well-being, it also results in considerable stress for many individuals with SCI (Krause 1997; Morris 1989; Ville et al. 2001). In spite of the advantages of productive activity, traditional full-time employment has many hidden costs as well as negative short-term and long-term physiological effects. These include decreased strength and energy, physical pain, and wear and tear on the body (decreased ability to perform activities of daily living) (Ernst and Day 1998). Because many routine activities (dressing, bathing, etc.) take significantly longer for individuals with SCI, these regimens may sometimes become the focal point of the individual's life (Strauss and Glaser 1975).

Chris had other concerns—that full-time employment would undermine his social life. He described what it was like for one of his friends with SCI:

> Emily, she's a para, she gets up at three or five o'clock in the morning to get dressed to go to work. Doesn't get back probably 'til 5:30 at night and she's got to fix dinner, eat out, whatever. . . . I mean, it

takes all day long. . . . And so it's pitiful, but she's a trouper, though, 'cause she's been doing this for quite a few years.

Chris himself was ambivalent about employment: "I hate thinking about going to work because that'll just end all the social activities that I've [been] doing," he said. "You just don't have any time."

Stan, who worked as an educational advocate, described a similar daily routine. In order to be at work at 8:00 a.m., he had to get up at 5:00 or 5:30 a.m. He described the toll working full-time had taken on his body:

Now I'm over 50, working behind a desk, working long hours, I don't get the exercise that I should and I'm stiffer of course today than I was when I was 17. Arthritis sometimes sets in.

## External Barriers to Employment

Barriers in the social environment—employer attitudes and inadequate accommodations, for example—prevent many individuals with disabilities from obtaining appropriate jobs (Baldwin 2000; Inge et al. 1996, 1998; Marti and Blanck 2000; Scheid 2000; Shrey 1983). Workplace adaptations are often inadequate, and many individuals with SCI who don't have regular employment report that they might have returned to work if more job modifications had been made (Schönherr et al. 2004). Undercover studies have revealed that employers are less likely to hire wheelchair users than equally or less qualified people without disabilities (Inge et al. 1998). Racial minorities appear to be especially vulnerable, since the difference in employment rates between whites and blacks is larger post-injury than pre-injury even when a variety of socio-demographic variables are taken into account (Meade et al. 2004).

Employers may be reluctant to hire individuals with disabilities because they fear the possibility of discrimination lawsuits (Willborn 2000) or increases in the company's group insurance rates and/or workers' compensation claims (Muller and Wheeler 1998).[7] Many employers also hold negative attitudes and misconceptions about the costs of accommodating disabled workers (Miller 2000). Quadriplegics frequently have difficulty with fine motor skills such as typing, sorting, pushing buttons, assembling small pieces, or holding writing utensils, whereas paraplegics are more likely to express concerns about gross motor skills such as driving, lifting, walking, carrying objects, and working at a standing height (Dowler, Batiste, and Whidden 1998). If a desk must be raised to accommodate a wheelchair, furniture leg raisers can be installed for less than $25. A workstation that allows manual height adjustments can cost anywhere from around $200 to $950, while a hydraulically-operated workstation might cost anywhere from $600 to $2500 (2004 dollars) (Dowler, Batiste, and Whidden 1998). Other necessary accommodations range from mouthsticks and voice dictation systems to environmental control units that provide for the manipulation of office equipment (overhead lights, computers, etc.) (Targett, Wehman, and Young 2004).

Many individuals with SCI have substantial work-related expenses that may render employment unprofitable, especially when combined with the potential loss of social welfare benefits. Quite a few of the people I interviewed, particularly those with high-level quadriplegia, described how external barriers including discrimination, lack of accessibility, and problems with transportation precluded employment. Derrick, who uses a power wheelchair, described how he had been repeatedly rebuffed in his efforts to obtain a job:

> I applied for a job at Lowe's Building Supply after being in the building business for 20 years, owning my company for 15 years and running numerous crews, building homes and really involved in the building industry. . . . And I have far more experience than any of their managers do with materials and that kind of thing and customer relations. . . . They didn't hire me. They didn't even call me.

Derrick had applied for numerous other jobs and had grown weary from all his fruitless efforts. "It's not like I'm just a dumbass that sits in a wheelchair," he said. Meghan also described how she had lost numerous positions to less qualified workers, a pattern she attributed to her disability and to the fact that she was an opinionated woman. "If this ain't discrimination, I don't know what it is." Several others reported that employers are unwilling to give them a fair shake. When I asked Roger if there were situations in which people did not want to get involved with a disabled person, he replied:

> Work-wise, my job. I was very fortunate that the employer that I have hired me. I wasn't his first choice, but I turned out to be his best choice. [*laughter*] . . . This was my first job [since my injury].

[*laughter*] It was my first application and my first interview, and I didn't get the job 'cause he hired somebody else, but the person that he hired quit three days later and he called me.

In spite of this, Roger seemed convinced that no one would seriously consider him for a job as a building contractor—the position he had held prior to his injury. "Not because I don't think I can, but because I don't think anybody out there is gonna give me the opportunity."

Stan had similar feelings. Although he had been working for many years, he also had been passed over for at least one job because of his disability:

I remember applying for what I thought was getting my first job. And it was with a blue-chip company. And the guy who was going to sign the contract for me to work for this high-tech company—when he saw me, it was as if his facial expression went from happiness to sadness when he came to realize that I was in a chair. At that time the offer was rescinded and the offer was never made for some nefarious reason.

Likewise, Jay, a paraplegic who maneuvered around using crutches, described how he had lost a job because a potential employer didn't feel as though he had the desired presentation:

They were looking for a professional image and almost as soon as they saw me. [*laughter*] . . . My body even—walking and stuff like that—I was kind of floppy and stuff.

The effects of discrimination extend into the workplace as well, often through inadequate promotions and pay raises, reassignments, disability-related harassment, and insensitivity on the part of co-workers and employers. When I asked Edward if he felt he had experienced any discrimination at work, he responded,

Just not being asked to go places or it's more like being ignored. Just walking down the hall at work, people that don't know you, some people will say "Hi" and some people just look the other way. . . . So it's kind of an avoidance more than it is discrimination. You get a lot of that.

Others reported that employment discrimination took less subtle and more pernicious forms. For example, Andrew reported that he occasionally had bowel and bladder accidents at work, and he felt as though his employer used these incidents to humiliate him and create a hostile work environment:

> I've even seen personal handwritten notes that he's left on his desk stating, "Andrew pissed in his pants and had to leave early. He left such-and-such project undone." Put it just that bluntly.

> EIW: Notes to himself?

> No, notes that I believe were intended to go in my employee file.

Andrew told me that he routinely made copies of these notes. After he had been at the company for several years with no promotion and "measly salary raises," he went to see a lawyer:

> I told her I felt like I was being discriminated against. I told her that he didn't like me because I had long hair. He didn't like me because I was in a wheelchair and he didn't like me because I was Hispanic. . . . And nothing ever really happened. It's still somewhere in limbo right now.

Shannon described how she had been reassigned to a different position in her company after her injury simply because her (former) boss didn't want to have a wheelchair user working for him. As far as Shannon was concerned, there was no logical reason for the transfer:

> The attorney that I worked for . . . was of a mind that I couldn't do the work I was doing before although there was nothing to say I couldn't. He didn't want me back so [the company] found a different position for me in another department.

In order to make the case that the transfer was medically necessary, Shannon was sent to a company physician who said that she wasn't suited to her previous position. In the end, however, Shannon seemed to feel her reassignment was a blessing in disguise. "It probably helped my career." Tonya, who had worked as a medication technician in a retirement home, was also dismissed from her previous job:

I wanted to go back to my original job doing medication. . . . I didn't understand why I couldn't go back but they didn't want me back 'cause of my disability. They said that I couldn't do the job, but I could still do blood pressures and give medication and do the basic care so I didn't understand.

Several of the study participants who did not have extensive job experience—particularly the college students—anticipated that employment discrimination would be a factor in their future careers. Although Ryan didn't feel that employment discrimination against people with disabilities was a problem in the field he wanted to enter (sports broadcasting), he did feel that it was a pervasive problem in society:

I believe in employment there's definitely a lot of discrimination against people in wheelchairs. . . . The stereotype is that they are retarded or they can't do everything that everybody else can do and so I believe that there's some job discrimination: they're like, "Oh, well, hey we can't hire this person. He has a handicap. Well, what can he really do for us?"

On the other hand, a small handful—many of whom had never been employed in the formal sector since sustaining their injuries—felt that employment discrimination was *not* a serious problem. For example, Jonathan pointed out that individuals with disabilities were employed in a wide variety of occupations:

In the late 50s, early 60s, you didn't see people out in the workplace. And nowadays you see people. I went to a restaurant the other day and there was a gal in a wheelchair seating people. I'd never seen that before 'til a week or two ago. And you would have never seen that 20 or 30 years ago at all.

Likewise, Cody said, "You really don't hear that much, 'This person was denied a job because he was in a wheelchair.'" Cody felt that racial discrimination was more widespread.

Meanwhile, Edward—who worked as a computer programmer—praised the fact that his employer was especially sensitive to the concerns of individuals with disabilities:

Never had a job I liked this much. . . . I ask for stuff because of my disability: just two weeks ago I asked . . . if I could have parking right by the door. Only upper management's allowed to use it. They said, "Okay." So I got a parking spot right there and I just walk in the door and just sit down. . . . So they treat me pretty good. They treat all the disabled people fairly good.

## Career Changes and Career Aspirations

There is strong evidence that vocational interests remain relatively stable following SCI (Rohe and Athelstan 1985; Rohe and Krause 1999b), and a preference for jobs that are incongruent with physical abilities may contribute to the relatively high rates of unemployment (Rohe and Athelstan 1982). For this reason, vocational planning for individuals with chronic disabilities must account for the security and stability needs of clients—in particular, the desire to remain in employment that is familiar and the need for jobs that offer security as well as adequate health and retirement plans (Lassiter 1983).

Out of necessity, however, many individuals alter their feelings about work in the aftermath of SCI. In particular, they tend to give greater consideration to jobs that draw on creative talents or that emphasize administrative work rather than physical labor (Ogden 1983). Many move from manual trades and sales positions into administrative, clerical, or finance jobs (Athanasou, Brown, and Murphy 1996; Castle 1994; Yoshida 1991, 1994b). Computer-related work is especially common among individuals with spinal cord injury, and the amount of time using a computer for work tends to rise in the aftermath of SCI (Frega 1996).[8] Computer technology can lessen the impact of the mobility limitations associated with spinal cord injury (Kruse, Krueger, and Drastal 1996), and intensive computer users are especially likely to return to their previous jobs (Berghammer et al. 1997).

Altogether, approximately two-thirds of the study participants agreed either *somewhat* (13%) or *strongly* (56%) that they had adjusted their career aspirations because of their disabilities. Those injured at younger ages were less likely to report that their career aspirations had changed. For example, when I asked Jay, who had been injured as an infant, whether he thought he might have had a different occupation in the absence of his SCI, he replied,

There's no way to tell. . . . [It's] something I grew up with all my life and planned for and I remember my tenth grade math teacher said, "You should do this and you should go to the vocational school for programming."

EIW: So that's what you did?

Yep. So I don't know if I would have done it different. But I think MIS [Management Information Systems] is a good field for people with disabilities.

Meanwhile, he also emphasized that individuals with disabilities should have the right to pursue whatever career paths they choose.

Many of the people I interviewed expressed frustration, disappointment, and a sense of loss and sadness at their inability to continue with their pre-injury work. For example, Ben, who had been employed in construction prior to his injury and was in college studying computer science, lamented his inability to continue with his previous job:

I'd like to get back into carpentry but I know that's an impossibility but [*laughter*] I like to work with my hands and stuff. . . . not that it's impossible, but the dexterity not being there slows me down . . . so there's no way I could make a living at it. As a hobby I could work at woodshop probably just fine and do my little thing if I wasn't pressured for time and to make money.

A few participants described how physical complications conspired to put an end to their pre-injury career paths. Roger had been forced to give up his construction company following his injury because he was unable to manage the business effectively (he was in and out of the hospital so often that his employees started taking advantage of the situation, and his business began to falter). He described his career trajectory in the aftermath of his injury:

Before I used to estimate a building—taking a building, digging the hole, and building it from the ground up. Right now I'm estimating doors. [*laughter*] You know, the cost of, you know to figure out how many doors goes into a commercial building and I sell doors. It's a job. It's not where I want to be, it's not what I really want to do. I would much rather be working for a construction company estimating the job, but that's kind of difficult because most companies today, an estimator is also a project manager and a project manager has to be on the job site. . . . If I go into a construction office and say, "I wanna be your construction manager," they're gonna look at me and look at my chair and just say, "I just don't see you out in the field."

Roger seemed depressed and frustrated by the path his career had taken:

It's like you just get kicked in the head. I know what I can do and I'm not going to brag, but I'm very good at what I do and I'm a very excellent problem solver, and especially when it comes to building buildings. . . . And I feel like I'm wasting that because I'm not able to do that for a contractor or myself. Not because I don't think I can, but because I don't think anybody out there is gonna give me the opportunity. . . . Even my therapist says that, "You need to get out of what you're doing."

Similarly, Derrick agreed strongly that he had adjusted his career aspirations in the aftermath of his injury. Prior to his accident, he had owned both a construction company and a business called *The Skydiving Elvis Impersonators:*

I owned five suits with the flashing lights and the shiny eagles on the chest and we made skydives. . . . And I've made night jumps into [a college stadium], and lots of concerts and everything. I was team captain, owner, and spokesman for the team.

After his accident, however, everything had to be sold at auction in order for him to get Medicaid and Medicare to pay for his medical expenses.

A number of participants expressed regret that their wheelchairs constrained their ability to work outdoors. For example, Jonathan, who worked as a financial analyst, agreed strongly that he had changed his career aspirations as a result of his disability "I'd probably have done something more physical, outdoors," he said. Kevin reflected on his career options in a similar manner:

> Before I got hurt I was thinking about being a geologist or maybe a marine biologist—where you get to run around outside all the time. But after I got hurt I didn't see any way that was possible. . . . I can't see myself enjoying any kind of career or job . . . all my upbringing and values and everything was more outdoor-oriented. We were always going to the lake and camping out, stuff like that.

Unfortunately, those who participated regularly in outdoor activities may experience greater psychological problems in the aftermath of severe disability (Hardy and Cull 1983).

Numerous participants described how their career trajectories had shifted away from blue-collar, manual labor toward service work or white-collar, intellectually-oriented employment—especially computer work. For example, after his injury, Adam bought a computer and started teaching himself computer skills because he "wouldn't be able to physically do any kind of manual job." Similarly, Jay had pursued a career in computer programming because he felt it was a field that made practical sense—it was a job he could do "without anything getting in the way." Andrew seemed somewhat nostalgic for the physical work he had done prior to his disability. After his injury, he participated in the Goodwill training program and went to work for Hertz as a computer programmer:

> Well, what I used to do was write Cobol programs. . . . I didn't like it, though, and I felt like I was just getting paid for nothing because I would show up and they wouldn't give me projects, and the projects they would give me were not that hard. And so I felt like maybe I was just a tax deduction for the company or something and I was really starting to get depressed because before that I was working as a welder in construction, pretty much physical labor and I liked that. I felt like I was earning my money.

Andrew ultimately remained with Hertz and worked his way up to a position as a production management specialist. "I like my job," he said. "I stay busy now, all the time."

A few participants had planned to work in professional careers—as musicians, physicians, etc.—but had been forced to change their career aspirations. Prior to his injury, Stan had played both cornet and piano. He had planned to go to college to become a band director, but he lamented, "You can't play instruments." For instance, playing the piano takes a lot of finger dexterity and 'course you're having to use your feet to operationalize the pedals. And you have to have a little bit more balance and on a cornet—I'm breathing from my diaphragm, my chest muscles have been paralyzed so uh [*pause*], I can't finger the valves.

After his injury, Stan obtained a bachelor's degree in elementary education and special education and a master's degree in guidance and counseling.

Although most of the participants who were no longer able to work in their previous occupations had tried to improve their skills in order to obtain new positions, a few had used the presence of the disability to be excused from working altogether. Because Chris was financially secure, he didn't need to work, and he attributed his lack of employment to his physical condition. At the same time, he still felt nostalgic for his pre-injury employment as an aircraft technician:

I always worked with my hands. I liked that much better. I never did want to go to college; never did work behind a desk. . . . I like physical things. Mental things bother me. [*chuckle*]

He didn't seem very optimistic about his prospects:

I'd love to be back in aircraft but you can't get in an airplane in a wheelchair. The only options for people like me would be supervision or computer work. Can't type very fast. I can't spell, either [*chuckle*] Oh, I don't know. . . . I'd go in there and work on that computer for three or four hours and I'm just, "Ahhh! Ahhh! I gotta get outside and kill something."

Not all the study participants had negative feelings about their career changes, however. Edward had worked as an electrician and as a welder prior to his injury but had became a computer programmer after completing the Goodwill training program. When I asked him how he felt about this career change, he replied that it was

something I should have got into a long time ago anyway. I mean, the money is about ten times more than what I made.

Cody had an experience similar to Edward's. Prior to his injury, he also had been an electrician. He completed the Goodwill computer training program, obtained a job as a programmer, and reported that the career change was a "smooth transition."

Six of the participants, including two women enrolled in college, felt as though their disabilities had little or no bearing on their career goals. Jennifer, who wanted to become a lawyer, disagreed strongly that she had made any adjustments in her career goals. Travis's aspirations also seemed unrelated to his disability:

> I want to work within the university . . . within student affairs. Ultimately, dream, I would love to run a university because I think I'm delusional enough to believe that I could make a difference.

Travis plans to get a Ph.D. in student affairs, or to attend law school.

## The Disability Employment Sector

Several study participants had held or sought jobs providing services to individuals with disabilities. Those who worked in the disability employment sector reported that employers were particularly sympathetic to their needs and to the challenges they confronted. A few also expressed a desire for jobs in the disability sector because they felt that their experiences with paralysis had made them especially sensitive to the concerns of disabled individuals.

Before his injury, Todd had aspired to be a motorcycle sales representative. After his accident, however, he started to work in various organizations that provided services and equipment to individuals with disabilities—first at an independent living center and later at a durable medical supplier. At the time of our interview, Todd was working for a small, family-owned company that modified vehicles for people with disabilities:

> [My] title is *Business Services*. Now what I do there is unfortunately I answer the phone. [*chuckle*] And I also do a little bit of some proposal work for people needing equipment. . . . I do some evaluation; I do some sales—not a great deal yet. I do in-services to hospitals and organizations. I made a catalogue for the company. I'm

currently trying to redo our web site for the company. I write some letters that I hope to put in with some of the publications.

Although Todd complained about the salary and the "secretarial-type duties" he performed, he was grateful that his employer was sympathetic to the physical problems he sometimes encountered:

> They're real good about my [disability]—if I have a bad day or something. And I had to miss a few weeks because of a pressure sore. And you don't have to dress up, so it has its advantages.

Meanwhile, Jeremy said that he'd like to contribute to the employment of individuals with disabilities:

> Down the road I [want] to create a network for people with disabilities that they can work out of the home doing maybe contract work for the government and stuff like that. . . . And maybe like have a central location where you can meet maybe once [or twice] a month so they're not too isolated. . . . Have a club-like thing.

A few participants provided counseling to disabled individuals or were contemplating such a career. Vibha described how her prior experience in this area had been especially meaningful:

> I worked in a rehabilitation center for four years in India. And before that I had worked as a volunteer in the same place.
>
> EIW: How was that experience?
>
> It was very enriching, but very challenging because the idea of counseling hasn't picked up in India and I had to counsel the poorer class of people who seem to think that the counseling was all about giving advice and they were hoping to get quick solutions. So it was very difficult, too.

Vibha was majoring in psychology and planned to earn a master's degree in family or rehabilitation counseling.

## Summary

Education and employment are major influences on the quality of life of individuals with SCI. Although a few participants complained that inadequate accommodations in education were a problem, the most troublesome instances of exclusion and segregation were confined to older individuals who had attended school prior to the implementation of ADA and other antidiscrimination legislation. Most of the students currently enrolled in college reported relatively few disability-related educational barriers.

In contrast, the occupational arena is fraught with difficulty. Participants described how physiological barriers (impaired mobility, loss of bowel and bladder control, etc.) and external constraints (prejudice and discrimination) had resulted in widespread unemployment and underemployment. For this reason, it is important to assess "whether each individual client should be adapting to his surrounding or whether it is the hostile environment itself that needs to be changed" (Hammell 1994: 12). While many of those I spoke with lamented the fact that they can no longer participate in outdoor work or physical labor, many also described how they had cultivated new vocational interests. As a direct result of their injuries, many had returned to school to study computer technology, and several had established successful careers in that area. A few described how their experiences with SCI had motivated them to pursue careers in counseling or rehabilitation work. At the same time, many of those who were unemployed or underemployed seemed frustrated and depressed with their inability to obtain the jobs they desired.

For some individuals with spinal cord injury, physical complications and economic barriers render full-time employment an undesirable objective. Although independence—including employment—has long been the primary goal of rehabilitation, some may sacrifice their health in the name of independence. There are many individuals with SCI "whose bodies are abused more by overuse than disuse" (Corbet 1993: 22). Many researchers have argued in favor of a broader approach to vocational rehabilitation—one that more effectively achieves its true purpose of maximizing individuals' strengths while minimizing resource depletion (Corbet 1993; Ernst and Day 1998). This new approach must emphasize flexible work schedules, allow for sufficient financial compensation, and place value on a wider range of productive activities including volunteer work, participation in community activities, and the fulfillment of family responsibilities (Howard and Howard 1997; Kemp and Vash 1971; Trieschmann 1980, 1989).

# 11
# Conclusions

Jonathan is 49 years old. He lives with his wife Becky and their 14-year-old adopted son in a large, rustic home. The house is surrounded by scrub oaks, and the interior of the home conveys Jonathan's love of the outdoors. The spacious living room has a big fireplace and shelves full of books and family photos. Jonathan met Becky through his younger sister, Susie, the two of whom had attended grade school together.

Jonathan is upbeat, with a warm and outgoing demeanor. He has a moustache and beard, salt-and-pepper hair, and is in good physical shape. He works as a financial analyst, and his annual family income exceeds $100,000.

Jonathan was injured in a car accident and became a paraplegic at the age of seven. His mother was driving, and they had just entered an area of low visibility. (Workers had been burning grass off the railroad tracks, and smoke from the fires was blowing across the highway.) His mother slammed on the brakes as they entered the dense smoke, and they were rear-ended by an 18-wheeler:

> I remember waking up at [the local] hospital and I couldn't get up. My dad was sitting there and something wasn't right. I had a fractured skull and a broken nose and knocked two or three teeth out. They were worried about brain damage and they didn't know I had a spinal injury. It's like back in the caveman days. . . . I kept telling my dad I couldn't move my legs and I had to go to the bathroom. . . . I didn't know what I needed or what I had but I kept thinking I had something that was holding me down. . . . There was

spinal injury without anybody even knowing it. Yeah, that's hard to believe.

Three days later, Jonathan was transferred to a metropolitan hospital where he was correctly diagnosed with an SCI.

Jonathan is paralyzed from the nipple down. "If it'd been much higher, I'd be a quadriplegic," he reflected. "There's an upside there to it." In general, Jonathan seemed to have little patience for people who didn't make the most of what they had in life:

> Everyone has their limitations and sometimes it's a severe limitation like a physical disability and sometimes it's a mental limitation— you know, pessimism or paranoid or delusional or whatever the limitation happens to be. But everybody has some type of limitation and that's what life's all about, dealing with your limitations and making the best out of which, being the best person you can possibly be. And try to be a contributor and make a difference in the world in spite of whatever that limitation is.

Jonathan drew inspiration from those who struggled to improve themselves, and he especially admired Christopher Reeve:

> I think he's fantastic. I really do. . . . I'm like, "Okay, this is it, I'm in a wheelchair, I've gotta do the best I can." And he's going, "Well, we'll be walking in five years." And I'm going, "Goollly boy, that's so far out there." I don't think that will; I mean it may not happen in twenty years, much less five or ten years, but that's what keeps him going. And if that works for him, that's great.

While Jonathan seems well-equipped to accomplish his personal and professional goals despite his impairment, he still harbors hopes that he might someday be cured and walk again:

> There's always that flicker and . . . that would be fantastic, but if it didn't happen, I can deal with that. I'm where I am. I'm just gonna do the best with what I've got. . . . My dad used to say, "Even if they do come up with a cure, I don't know if Jonathan would be interested in something like that." But I think I would.

## To Walk or Not to Walk

Morris (1991: 34; 1993b: 105) argues that "one of the most oppressive features of the prejudice which disabled people experience is the assumption that we want to be other than we are." While the dominant view of disability is one of personal tragedy with disabled individuals viewed as victims or objects of pity, few disabled people view their impairments in such negative terms.[1] Indeed, one study revealed that only 49% of individuals with physical disabilities answered *yes* to the question, "If you were given one wish, would you wish that you were no longer disabled?" (Weinberg and Williams 1978). At the same time, many disabled people would welcome medical interventions that might eliminate their impairments (Finkelstein 1993).[2] Mobility issues are among the areas of greatest concerns among individuals with SCI, and decreased mobility is frequently ranked as the most problematic consequence of spinal cord injury (Estores 2003; Glickman and Kamm 1996).

Until recently, physicians offered no hope for extensive recovery of bodily functions following SCI. Today, however, researchers and clinicians are more optimistic about the potential for at least partial recovery. Some promising rehabilitation strategies include weight-supported training on a treadmill to improve walking skills for those with partial SCI and the use of functional electrical stimulation of nerves and muscles to assist in stepping movements (Fouad and Pearson 2004).[3] Increasingly, techniques such as the electrical stimulation of muscles, the use of restorative devices, improved drug therapies, and advances in nerve regeneration are being studied and used (Hingley 1993). Transplanted embryonic stem cells and endogenously born stem cells (those already present in the spinal cord) offer great promise for repairing nervous system damage (Myckatyn, Mackinnon, and McDonald 2004). Meanwhile, many of the treatments designed to enhance axon growth have shown potential when used in the first two weeks after injury. Individuals with longstanding injuries may benefit more from a combination of rehabilitation training and pharmacological modulation of neurotransmitters (Houle and Tessler 2003).

While only a few participants viewed their disabilities in exclusively negative terms, the overwhelming majority said that given the option, they'd prefer to be free of SCI. Adam distilled the sentiments of most of them when he stated, "I would like to walk, but if I don't I'm gonna make the best of what I've got." Similarly, Todd thought a cure for SCI would be nice, but it wasn't anything he lost sleep over: "If it happens, it happens; if it doesn't, it doesn't."

During the acute phase, many individuals with SCI express positive expectations about being able to walk again (Lohne and Severinsson 2003). Several study participants were initially preoccupied with the possibility of a cure. Todd said that when he was first injured, "I asked God every night, 'Please let me walk again.'" In general, however, the participants' emotional investment in a cure for SCI appeared to subside with the passage of time. Although Jeremy would someday like to walk again, it's not a major concern in his life:

> That's something that with time kind of fades. Initially, I thought I'll be walking again within two weeks and then as you get older you go, "It's cool if I do, it's cool if I don't." [*laughter*]

Some nonetheless drew comfort and inspiration from the idea that they might walk again. When I asked Andrew if he had hope that he'd be walking again, he responded, "Oh yeah, I never lost that hope. I think that's what kind of keeps me going every day." Harry, who was 33 at the time of the interview, told me that by the time he turned 40 he hoped to have graduated from law school, be walking, and be married, with at least one child. Likewise, Adam reported,

> I'm hopeful. They're doing some pretty, pretty neat stuff with medical research. . . . I'd definitely like to see more money in spinal cord injury research. I think there's a chance that they could find a cure for it.

Stacy also seemed confident that medical science would someday yield a cure:

> I think they'll have a cure sometime. I've been told five years, but I mean I've been told that since I was hurt. I heard a doctor on CNN the other day say a year. Last summer I got really excited about that. It was like, "Oh, I'm gonna go get these things that will keep my muscles in my legs going. Oh, won't it be awesome if I walk down the aisle?" But really, that was just a phase. I'm excited for it. I mean

> I'm not counting on it. . . . I don't pray every night, "Oh, find a cure,
> find a cure."

Harry insisted that a cure for SCI already existed but had not yet been made
available to the public:

> They're just fighting over who's gonna get the Nobel prize and all
> the money and the publicity over it. . . . Am always paranoid about
> the government. I don't think that they want it to come out so fast,
> the medical industry will lose millions and millions if not billions of
> dollars every year from people like me. . . . It's political! . . . And I
> can't even walk . . . because some asshole wants to get his name on a
> damn trophy and get some money out of it and live rich the rest of
> his life? That's not fair.

Others were considerably less optimistic about the prospect of a cure.
When I asked Shannon if she thought she might someday walk again, she
replied,

> Would I love to? Yeah! Do I think it's gonna happen? No. Maybe
> someday down the road, but if it does happen I don't think it's gonna
> for people that have been injured for a long period of time.

Shannon also emphasized that the physical transition from not walking to
walking would be a difficult adjustment to make:

> You'd be learning like a baby. And it would be painful. It would be
> hard. I mean, you're gonna actually stand up and walk. . . . I'm not
> sure I would be willing to go through that pain. Believe it or not.
> [*laughter*] I don't know that I would 'cause these muscles haven't
> done a lot in a lot of years.

Ryan, who had been paralyzed for 13 years, said that he thought walking
"could throw my whole body out of whack." Likewise, Stan said he didn't
really think about walking for the "simple reason that the adjustment . . .
you would have to make being disabled to having more function would be
disruptive." At the same time, both Ryan and Stan said they'd want to walk
if given the opportunity.

Stan also felt that the process of helping people to walk again would be very costly to society—that it might not make sense from a utilitarian perspective:

> Who would pay for it? Who would pay for those procedures? I mean, would you have the means individually? Are we gonna have some HMO in the sky?

Meghan was surprised to find that not all people with spinal cord injuries would want to be cured:

> There are people who don't want to walk? Why? Why?
>
> EIW: There are a variety of reasons. You would know.
>
> No, I don't know, that's why I'm asking.
>
> EIW: For example, some people find that their disabilities give them meaning and purpose in life, and some become activists because of their disabilities.
>
> Oh, bullshit. I can be an advocate, but I want to walk. I don't need to be in this wheelchair to be an activist. My God, that is the saddest thing I've heard. Were they invisible before? I want to wipe my own butt and brush and floss my own teeth and have sex all night long in different positions. I don't need this paralysis.

## Christopher Reeve

In 1995, Christopher Reeve (well-known for his role in the *Superman* films) was paralyzed in an equestrian accident and quickly became the most famous American with SCI. Initially, Reeve was paralyzed from the neck down and unable to breathe. Prompt medical attention saved his life, and delicate surgery stabilized the shattered C-1 and C-2 vertebrae where his injury occurred. Over time, Reeve gradually regained sensation in parts of his body—down the spine, in his left leg, and in areas of his left arm. In September 2000 he moved an index finger, and the news was received with surprise by scientists who had not expected to see progress so long after his injury (Martin 2004). Reeve died on October 10, 2004, as a result of complications associated with a severely infected pressure sore.

After sustaining his injury, Reeve took a leading role in the effort to find a cure for SCI. In collaboration with philanthropist Joan Irvine Smith, he helped launch the Reeve-Irvine Research Center in California. The Center was established in 1996 to study diseases of the spinal cord with the objective of finding a cure. Reeve and his wife Dana also founded the Christopher Reeve Foundation, which merged in 1999 with the American Paralysis Association. The Christopher Reeve Paralysis Foundation (CRPF) provides funding for research to treat and cure SCI and other central nervous system disorders. It also provides grants, resources, and advocacy to improve the quality of life for individuals with disabilities. While Reeve had been very optimistic about the possibility of spinal cord regeneration, many individuals with SCI do not share his sentiments about the pace of research and recovery (Cole 2004).

I asked the study participants what they thought about Christopher Reeve as a role model, and how they viewed his advocacy on behalf of individuals with SCI. Approximately half enthusiastically supported his efforts. Another 40% had mixed opinions, and approximately 10% expressed unfavorable views. Many of those who supported Reeve said that they appreciated his efforts to raise funds for SCI and to increase disability awareness. Several also admired his personal strength, and numerous individuals drew inspiration from his conviction that people with spinal cord injury would someday be walking again. For example, Stan reflected,

> I think he is a superman. . . . Anyone who can bring awareness and money and research and other resources to inclusion, I think, "Sure. Welcome." He's already a member of the disability community. He should be welcomed with open arms and respected for what he can do and the changes that he can empower others to bring about.

Likewise, Ryan praised Reeve for the hope and inspiration he gave others:

> I think he's a great role model because he has shown people with disabilities there's no reason to give up. He has taken his disability and he has just run with it. I've never seen him whining. I've never seen him complain about life on TV. I have seen him saying, "Hey, y'know, let's find some cures."

Todd even went so far as to say that Reeve's injury was one of the best things that had happened to the SCI community

> because of his being out there, visibility and everything. . . . A lot of disabled people feel like he should be fighting more for our rights than the cure.

> EIW: And do you agree?

> I think Chris should do what he wants to do. It's up to him.

Indeed, quite a few participants expressed unequivocal support for Reeve's efforts. Leonard said, "I'm all for what he's doing," and Nathan reflected, "Who wouldn't like Superman?" Harry not only admired Christopher Reeve, but he also had special respect for Dana Reeve, his wife:

> I hope he lives long enough to see the cure. . . . He's one of my idols. I tell you who I look up to more than him and that's his wife because . . . she's taking care of him in a lot of ways. I mean, I'm sure he's got money and he's got nurses and stuff that take care of him, but she don't have to stay with him. And I look up to her big time. I'm like pulling for them so bad. . . . I have a fear that if Christopher Reeve lost his wife, that he'd give up.

While nearly all the participants in the study commented that Reeve had done much to raise disability awareness and funding, several lamented the fact that it took someone famous to draw attention to SCI. Andrew reflected,

> People have been suffering spinal cord injuries since the Vietnam War. Before! And all of a sudden a light is shed on it only when somebody famous is hurt. What about everybody else? Do they mean less than Christopher Reeve?

In a similar vein, Shannon said, "Spinal cord injuries deserved [the] attention it's getting now before he was ever injured." Jeremy worried that the impact of Reeve's efforts was waning over time:

I hate that it takes someone being very popular for society to start looking at disabilities. And he's fading. And so, what are we gonna do? Pick another candidate? [*laughter*]

A few study participants felt that there were negative aspects to the publicity that Reeve had generated. For example, while Roger expressed support for all the attention that Reeve was drawing to SCI, he also felt that Reeve presented an unrealistic representation of what it's like to have a spinal cord injury:

I think our government needs to do more educating—putting people in chairs out there. Putting them into the limelight. Letting them shine. The only person right now that is shining in the limelight is Christopher Reeve.

EIW: Is that a good thing?

No, I consider it a bad thing because Christopher Reeve has the money and the resources to do the things he's doing. And people that see him look at that and say, "Well, what does he need?" . . . Or, "Look at him, he's able to do it." But there's people out there that are like him that can't because they don't have the resources that he has.

Likewise, Brad commented, "He is lucky with the resources and people that he has." Several respondents noted that Reeve might not be able to understand the everyday experiences of ordinary people with SCI. While Vibha stated that Reeve was a good spokesman for individuals with disabilities, she also felt that "he probably wouldn't be able to empathize totally with the common man who's disabled because of his money." At the same time, she acknowledged that he would "know how it feels to be disabled."

A handful felt that Reeve's efforts and activities would have no favorable impact on people with SCI. For example, Tonya suspected that Reeve himself was the main beneficiary of all the media attention he had generated:

I feel very sad that he suffered that injury but I would feel that way for anybody. In my opinion, I don't think it's been very helpful to the spinal cord injury people from an everyday regular level. I don't think it's had any effect on us, really. . . . I'm sure it's helped him, and because he's so famous and he's benefited from it. . . . I think he's brought attention to the issue, but I don't think he's brought attention to us. He brings attention to himself.

Indeed, several participants seemed to resent the fact that because of his wealth and celebrity status, Reeve didn't really experience SCI in the same way that they did. Meghan commented,

> He doesn't have a clue. . . . He has not had the barriers that most people in wheelchairs [have] because he's a celebrity. And he has money and probably has people at his beck and call so he does not know the problems that we have run into when you are in poverty. . . . He's just like Ted Kennedy. Kennedys have, whatever, promoted things to help minorities, but they're white, wealthy people. What do they know about it all? . . . They really mean well, but they don't know.

Jay echoed Meghan's sentiments, declaring that Christopher Reeve presented a false image of what life is like for most people with SCI. Likewise, Shannon remarked,

> He can get anything he wants. Any piece of equipment, you know, in multitudes for free. I'm sure they just give it to him for the publicity it will give them. Gosh, we can't do that. [*laughter*] . . . But would I trade places with him? Hell, no. Because he's got a lot more severely injured than I am. We always say, "Quads wanna be paras, paras wanna be AB [able-bodied]."

A few stated that they had nothing against Reeve but did not connect with him ideologically. As Adam said, "His whole thing is, 'I'm gonna walk, I'm gonna walk, I'm gonna walk.' My whole thing, 'I would like to walk, but if I don't I'm gonna make the best of what I've got.' " Similarly, while Stacy felt Christopher Reeve had done wonders for raising disability awareness and had been chosen "obviously for a reason," she didn't care for his attitude:

> He's not Christian; he doesn't believe in God. And his attitude seems to be like ever since he got in his chair, his goal has been to get out. It hasn't been to accomplish things. . . . It seems like he's miserable in

his wheelchair. And I can understand that, but it seems like . . . his purpose is to get out of the chair. I don't like his attitude.

Meanwhile, a few participants defended Reeve against the criticism that others had directed at him. For example, Kevin stated,

Lots of disabled people get real pissed off at him and I don't understand that. He's brought so much awareness, and he's brought in so many millions of dollars for research and everything. It's bad for him to have it happen to him, but it's good for us. I don't really know why people get all pissed off at him. They say he should just accept it and learn to live in a wheelchair and stuff. Well, I don't agree with that at all. If there's any way in hell I can get out of here, I'd like to do it.

Adam also disagreed with the people who had been "slamming him." He added, "He's just doing like the result of us—just dealing with it in his own personal way."

## Stem Cell Research

The use of embryonic stem cells to treat neurological disorders is a controversial topic. In 2001, President Bush declared that while stem cell research would be allowed on 60 genetically diverse stem cell lines currently in existence, no additional federal funds could be used for (1) the derivation or use of stem cells lines derived from newly destroyed embryos, (2) the creation of any human embryos for research purposes, or (3) the cloning of human embryos for any purpose (White House 2001).

While many disability scholars are critical of the biomedical approach, most of the study participants who discussed this topic said they hoped stem cell research might someday yield a cure for SCI. As Stan said,

I think it's wonderful. Any means by which a medical procedure can improve the condition of spinal cord injury—oh, *do it, do it.* Stem cell research is not hurting anybody. It is not promoting anything illegal, it is just human cells that are available and why not use it? . . . I think the administration's stand has been, "Federal funds cannot be used," and there's already private monies being used. We're talking about improving the lives and conditions of people who are paralyzed, the quality of life, longevity. . . . For every muscle that you get back in return, there are more day-to-day living skills that you can perform independently. I'm for that.

Andrew expressed similar sentiments:

From what I heard, it's supposed to do really good things for anyone with a spinal cord injury. I just don't understand the conflict that there is with it because what I understand is that it was taken from fetuses of unborn babies. . . . I see where it would be controversial, but I don't see a problem. I wouldn't have a problem with some stem cells being put in if it would help me out. Isn't that selfish and awful?

I told Andrew that I didn't think his attitude was selfish or awful. He continued,

It's a touchy issue with people. I think that human beings are a little selfish and on one hand, they would be really against it, but if they could secretly have the stem cells implanted to improve their health they would do it. . . . They may be outwardly against it, but if it could profit them actually to where they could walk and be independent again [pause]

EIW: You think they'd do it?

Yeah. I know I would be one of the first people to volunteer.

Adam was optimistic but also more cautious:

They're doing a lot of really good stuff with stem cell research and it's promising, but I'm not gonna hold my breath. I mean, I'm not gonna wait for it. I'm gonna go ahead and get on with my life.

Oliver (1996a: 100) contends that "the pursuit of restoring the ability to walk or nearly walk is better understood . . . as a millenarian movement rather than the logical application of modern medical knowledge" (a millenarian movement is one that promotes social change through miraculous means). Among the people I inteviewed, Shannon seemed to have similar doubts about a cure for SCI, stating that stem cell research provides "false hope for people."

A few of the study participants had mixed feelings about stem cell research. Meghan remarked,

> I don't know enough about stem cell to tell you anything. I've been surviving so I can't give you intelligent remarks about [it]. I really haven't done any reading on stem cells. I'm more concerned about the pain issue. The older I get, the worse the pain gets. But if it helps anybody, I'm for it.

When I asked her how she felt about using stem cells from aborted fetuses, she replied,

> If they're going to abort them, why not use the spare parts? What would be the ethical question? People are not going to stop getting abortions. The only problem, say that it proves to be helpful. . . . are they going to pick someone to get pregnant and intentionally abort the fetus just to get the stem cells? . . . It's kind of a slippery slope.

Roger told me he was conflicted about using stem cells from aborted fetuses and was reluctant to advocate such research aggressively:

> It's real hard for me because I've had people approach and say, "Will you get on the Internet and approach our government about what they're doing with abortion babies?" In one point, you're throwing it away, why not use it? But in my other point as a religious person, I can't because I don't believe in it. It's wrong. I mean, this coin flips constantly. It's a very hard issue.

Meanwhile, Roger suggested that the mothers of stillborn children should routinely be asked whether they want to donate their deceased infants' stem cells.

## "It Could Have Been Worse"

I asked the study participants how they viewed SCI in comparison with other disabilities, and whether they felt it would be better or worse to have other impairments. In response to this question, many said they were fortunate that their impairments weren't as bad as they could have been. For example, Jonathan reflected on the advice his father always gave him when he was growing up:

> I don't care how bad it is, Jonathan, there's always somebody worse off than you are. So you're not to feel sorry for yourself. . . . Because you can handle it, and the reason you can handle it is look out there and see all the people that are worse off than you are. You've got some problems, but it could be a whole lot worse. So, you're lucky. You're lucky you're not a quadriplegic instead of a paraplegic.

Leonard, a quadriplegic, reported,

> When I was in rehab, I looked around and I'm going, "Oh, I could be a lot worse. . . . I could have had a higher injury; I could have had a brain injury." It could have been worse. So that's the way I look at it.

Many paraplegics expressed gratitude that they didn't have quadriplegia. For example, Stacy reflected that in rehab

> I was surrounded by quadriplegics. . . . people on ventilators, using the sip-and-puff wheelchairs, where they had to use a straw to drive and things like that. And it really made me realize that I was very fortunate. . . . There was a whole joke in our whole rehab center about quads versus paras: They kinda didn't like the paras because, "Hey, y'know, look at all the things we have and they don't.". . . It was just kind of like, "Oh, quit whining," y'know? [*chuckle*]

Tonya said she could imagine herself having most disabilities, including blindness, but that it would be "difficult" to be a high-level quad:

> I have a friend that's a high quad. . . . He has an electric wheelchair. He can push around with that, but he can't be left at home for long

periods of time because if he were to drop something he couldn't get it. He can breathe on his own and that's good, but that's scary because you're helpless pretty much.

Indeed, several of those with high-level quadriplegia feel that their disabilities are especially undesirable. Kevin, a high-level quadriplegic who uses a sip-and-puff chair, told me that blindness would be "pretty bad, but I don't think it would be worse." Meghan, who also had high-level quadriplegia and required daily attendant care, felt that being blind "would be better because you could still dress yourself; you could still live on your own."

At the same time, many participants—including quite a few young paraplegic men—singled out blindness as being one of the worst disabilities. This is consistent with previous research showing that when nondisabled people are asked what disability they most dread, blindness is the most frequent response (Vash 1981). For example, Andrew reflected,

> Sometimes I think about people who can't see and it's just so sad to me. There's so many beautiful things in the world and that would not be one of the things that I would want to lose. . . . That would be just too tough.

Similarly, Roger said,

> I'd rather be in a wheelchair than be blind. [*laughter*] I don't mean to laugh, but definitely. I don't know what I would do if I was blind, I don't know how I would handle that. . . . "My God, I'm in a wheelchair, now I'm losing my sight, this is all I need." [*laughter*]

> EIW: [*laughter*]

> Do they have seeing-eye dogs for wheelchairs? [*laughter*]

Vibha disagreed, stating that blindness would not be worse than other impairments: "I say all disabilities are as debilitating as each other."

Meanwhile, many participants reported that deafness would be preferable to SCI. Andrew reflected, "I think that you can overcome [a hearing impairment]. You know, take lip reading classes." He jokingly added, "I'm kind of deaf anyway, so. [*laughter*]" Similarly, when I asked Edward whether he'd prefer to be deaf, he replied,

I don't know. That would be a close one. Ummmm. Not being able to hear. Can I try it first? [*laughter*] That would be hard to take, too, but I'm almost to say that spinal cord injury's worse than that.

Roger pointed out that an individual who is deaf "can hear through his sight."

In assessing whether one disability would be worse than another, many focused on the degree to which the disability would hamper their independence. For Meghan, the worst thing about having high-level quadriplegia was "the loss of your independence." Edward said he was thankful that his paralysis was not as bad as when he was first injured:

> I know what it's like to be worse to where you're trying to move your hands and you can't, and try to feed yourself and you end up sticking yourself in the forehead or whatever.

Edward added that whenever he got very depressed, he reflected on how "it could be worse."

Harry mentioned another disabled student when reflecting on the degree to which different disabilities affect one's quality of life:

> If I get depressed about something or I get pissed off about something, Joseph comes in my head.
>
> EIW: And Joseph is?
>
> Joseph is this guy on campus; he's got some kind of bone disease and he's all crippled up. . . . He looks micro. He's got this huge normal-sized head and he's got this little bitty body. . . . He rides in this little wheelchair with a big back on it and stuff. . . . If I ever get depressed—I mean, I've done things in my life, not only before I got hurt but since I've got hurt, that he'll never do in life.

Similarly, Roger described his friend Herb, who has multiple sclerosis:

> I wouldn't trade that for nothing. I would rather be blind than have MS. Every day something is failing on him. He first lost mobility and walking. Um, then his voice. He can still talk, but I can't talk to him on the telephone. . . . He's married, it's real hard on his family,

because here is a man that went from walking, to walking with a walker, to being in a wheelchair, to losing bodily functions, to losing his ability to talk, and a lot of people when they talk to him they think he's brain damaged and he's not. . . . And that frustrates him because he wishes to be understood and treated like a normal person. . . . He is dying a millimeter at a time and that has to be so hard. The last time I talked to him he just said, "I'm ready to die, I want to die." It took me 25 minutes to understand what he was trying to say, so that even made it worse once I finally understood.

Disabilities that hinder communication were felt to be especially unpleasant, and some respondents mentioned cerebral palsy as the disability they would most dislike. Stacy described her conversation with a woman with CP:

[She] was like, "It's so annoying that I have all these things I want to say and no one's patient enough to listen." And I thought how horrible would that be. And no one would want to listen to you.

For others, a mental disability would be even worse. Adam stated,

Mental disabilities, that seems like that would be really bad. You know, a situation to where you . . . look perfectly normal but your thought processes don't work right.

Vibha also stated that a mental disability would be worse than her current condition: "It's gonna be tougher to be mentally challenged, right?"

A few felt that they could handle their own disabilities but weren't sure if they'd be able to deal with any others. For example, Shannon said that she wouldn't trade places with either a blind or deaf person:

You think anything is [worse] that you don't have because you know how to cope with yours. And that's my perspective.

Meanwhile, Andrew told me that the hardest disability would be "to be blind, deaf, mute, and in a wheelchair. Then you'd really be in a fix." Travis quipped, "I think also being mute would be difficult because you couldn't communicate. But I think that a lot of people would be really happy if I was mute."

## Toward a Revised Conceptual Framework

Most of the study participants have a strong desire to walk again, and many hope that biomedical innovations will eventually yield a cure for SCI. All are well aware of the challenges posed by spinal cord injury, but the majority are also grateful not to have impairments they regard as more serious, such as blindness or cerebral palsy. In general, respondents most fear those disabilities that result in the greatest loss of independence.

Scholars in the field of disability studies—many of whom have disabilities themselves—have stressed the importance of viewing disability as a condition created by social barriers rather than physical limitations. Among my study participants, however, the problems associated with impairment and illness are regarded as central to the experience of disability. More generally, the views expressed by individuals with disabilities are often at odds with those voiced by scholars and activists in the field of disability studies (see, for example, Fadem et al. 2003). We might speculate, for instance, that scholars with physical impairments are systematically different from the general population of individuals with disabilities. The fact that they are able to engage in creative and scholarly pursuits suggests a degree of independence not shared by some others. For example, individuals who are actively engaged in research and writing may be less likely to be preoccupied with the physical limitations associated with impairment (e.g., chronic pain, etc.) or with the economic struggles associated with financial destitution. Scholars with spinal cord injury may also be more likely to have higher levels of education as well as pre-injury aspirations that are less incongruent with the physical limitations imposed by impairment.

This study suggests that the individuals most likely to view their disabilities in biomedical terms are those for whom *impairment* and *illness* most fully coincide. For individuals who experience all the secondary complications associated with SCI—chronic pain, spasticity, pressure sores, etc.—the physical manifestations of their impairments are central to their understanding of what it means to have a disability. No matter how accommodating his social environment may be, Kevin's primary objective is to get his pain under control. Wheelchair accessibility doesn't help Meghan on those days when she is unable to get out of bed. On the other hand, those individuals whose impairments carry fewer secondary or illness-related complications may be more likely to view their disabilities in social terms. For an individual who sees his or her disability chiefly as a mobility problem, social remedies may be an effective means of response. For someone who sees his or her disability as a complex of impairments and chronic illnesses, a biomedical response may be more appropriate.

These results further demonstrate that each individual may view his or her disability in social terms when discussing certain topics and in biomedical terms when discussing other issues. When talking about their sexual lives, for example, study participants focused largely on the physical challenges they encountered—problems such as motor impairment, spasticity, and loss of erectile functioning. When discussing how their disabilities influenced their educational experiences, most of them emphasized cultural factors and environmental barriers such as discrimination and the scarcity of accessible educational facilities. Although the participants in the study pointed to physical as well as social barriers in almost every arena of life, there was a greater tendency to emphasize biomedical challenges in those areas most closely linked to physiological functioning.

While social scientists and disability activists have stressed the importance of viewing disabilities primarily in social terms, such a perspective may minimize the physical difficulties associated with impairment. Even the emotional pain and loss experienced by many individuals with SCI often have their origins in biological rather than social conditions. For example, Ryan expressed sadness that he may never have the biological capacity to father a child. Roger voiced his frustration at being unable to get an erection or to enjoy sex the way he had prior to his injury. For at least some individuals with SCI, the most complete remedy can be found not in better adoption laws or better awareness of sexual alternatives, but in the restoration of biological functioning. Although community-residing individuals with spinal cord injury express serious concerns about a wide range of issues—physical (e.g., bowel and bladder concerns), environmental (e.g., adequate housing and parking), and social (e.g., interpersonal relationships)—many believe that their problems could be most fully addressed by finding a cure for SCI (Elliott and Shewchuk 2002).

The interaction of social and biological factors may be more important than previously believed. Many study participants told me that the worst thing about having SCI was that they could no longer participate in the activities they used to enjoy: sports, occupations involving physical labor, running around with their children, etc. Many participants were quite explicit about the ways in which social and biomedical factors interact with one another—the ways in which their problems with intimate relationships are grounded in both physiological limitations and their partners' difficulties adjusting to those limitations, for example.

Theoretical models in the sociology of disability might also be improved through a better understanding of the experiences unique to those individuals with a particular impairment. In the same way that each racial or ethnic group has unique cultural assets and distinct modes of communication, so too do particular groups of individuals with disabilities. Just as the experience of American blacks is distinct from that of Asians or Latinos, the experience of someone with a spinal cord injury is distinct from that of someone who is blind or deaf. While the idea of pan-disability, like that of pan-ethnicity, may prove to be a valuable tool for promoting minority-group consciousness and advancing the cause of civil rights (Linton 1998), there is a much-neglected need to distinguish between those ideas that are most useful politically and those that are most useful in advancing our understanding of disability.

## Toward Prevention and a Cure

Several authors have warned that the desire to eliminate, cure, or control disability should not take precedence over the need to value and accommodate disabled individuals (Hahn 1994; Linton 1998; Wendell 1996). Unfortunately, the public health profession's emphasis on the avoidance of risk and disability may have the unintended consequence of stigmatizing individuals with disabilities (Wang 1993). A curative approach may also be perceived as threatening by disability activists who attempt to portray disability in a positive light. Efforts to prevent impairment (or disability) can easily develop into plans for sterilization, euthanasia, and other practices that attempt to eliminate disabled individuals from society (Sobsey 1994).

Indeed, an important distinction must be made between the prevention of impairment and the exclusion of people with impairments (Abberley 1987). While it is certainly beneficial to warn consumers about the possible physical injuries that may result from unsafe behavior, this should be done in a way that does not devalue the lives of individuals with disabilities. Environmental and legislative campaigns have led to significant reductions in the number of spinal cord injuries, and collaborative efforts between legislators, public health officials, education providers, and consumers are undeniably important (O'Hare and Hall 1997). Individuals who have sustained spinal cord injuries are often uniquely qualified to speak to audiences on a personal level (O'Hare and Hall 1997). They may also be especially likely to do so in a way that both empowers individuals with SCI and encourages others to practice health-conscious behaviors.

More broadly, however, we need to recognize what Neath (1997: 198) refers to as "the social construction of disability through the social creation of impairment." Referring to this issue, Oliver (1990: 13–14) notes,

> Just as we know that poverty is not randomly distributed internationally or nationally, neither is impairment. . . . If poverty is not randomly distributed and there is an intrinsic link between poverty and impairment, then neither is impairment randomly distributed.

Likewise, Krause (1976: 213) states that

> if God is a minor source of disabled individuals, then two major sources are certainly poverty and the factory. The poor are beaten before they start, by second-rate medical service, bad living conditions, and absence of preventive care. They are born on welfare, develop physical, mental and social disabilities because they are on it, and they stay there.

Indeed, the disability literature presents ample evidence that various types of impairment are especially widespread among members of the lowest social stratum (Alexander 1976). For this reason, efforts to prevent SCI must extend beyond targeting individual behaviors to examining the oppressive living conditions that give rise to impairment (Sutherland 1993). In particular, violence and drug use—factors implicated in quite a few SCI cases—are concentrated within certain communities and certain subpopulations. Both are linked to socioeconomic problems such as poverty, racism, and environmental stress. The most effective model of prevention may therefore be one that challenges oppressive conditions and relationships while promoting social and economic justice.

# Notes

## Chapter 1

1.  See, for example, Abberley (1987, 1996); Barnes (1996, 1998); Barnes, Mercer, and Shakespeare (1999); Barton (1996, 1998); Brisenden (1986); Davis (1996); Deegan and Brooks (1985); Fine and Asch (1988c); Finkelstein (1980); Finkelstein and Stuart (1996); Gliedman and Roth (1980); Hahn (1994); Linton (1998); Marks (1999); Morris (1991); Neath (1997); Oliver (1996a); Shakespeare (1996, 1998); Swain et al. (1993); and Wendell (1996).

2.  Oliver (1990, 1993a, 1993c) contends that the idea of disability as an individual pathology arose in conjunction with the rise of capitalism: "Disabled people could not meet the demands of individual wage labour and so became controlled through exclusion" (Oliver 1990: 47). Similarly, Finkelstein (1980: 10) argues that "large scale industry with production-lines geared to able-bodied norms [led to] the growth of hospital-based medicine and the creation of large asylums." On the other hand, Barnes and Mercer (2003) point to the lack of evidence that disabled people were mainstreamed into the productive life of feudal societies prior to industrialization.

3.  Hahn's (1994) description of the "minority group model" includes three postulates: (1) that the major problems confronting disabled people can be attributed primarily to social attitudes; (2) that almost every facet of the environment has been shaped by public policy; and (3) that at least in a democratic society, policies are a reflection of pervasive attitudes and values (Hahn 1986, 1988a, 1988b, 1993). It is important to realize, however, that individuals with disabilities are different from other minority group members in several important respects. An emphasis on civil rights as a common feature of race, gender, and disability discrimination may downplay the unique characteristics of each minority group (Finkelstein 1993). For racial minorities, "biological difference serves only as a qualificatory condition of a wholly ideological oppression," whereas for individuals with disabilities the biological differences are themselves part of the oppression (Abberley 1987: 8). Finkelstein (1993) points out that if an operation were available that could transform black

people into white people or women into men, it would be universally rejected by these groups. The same cannot be said of most treatments for disabling conditions.

4.   For a detailed critique of the social model of disability, see Marks (1999).

5.   Charlton (1998: 167) contends that "having a disability is essentially neither a good thing nor a bad thing. It just is. . . . In the real world, some people with disabilities have a generally good life and others a generally bad life. Some of the people with disabilities living a good life do so in spite of their disabilities; others may be living a good life because of their disabilities. . . . Everyone is different."

6.   Throughout this book, I distinguish among individuals with low, medium, and high levels of impairment. The individuals in the *low impairment* category include 14 paraplegics and 2 walking quadriplegics. Those in the *medium* category (a total of nine) are quadriplegics who rely on manual wheelchairs and are able to care for themselves (although they may require assistance with a bowel program). Those in the *high impairment* category (a total of seven) use power wheelchairs and/or require daily assistance for a variety of tasks (transfers, food preparation, etc.). Because there are only two walking quadriplegics in the sample, individuals in the *low impairment* category are referred to as "paraplegics" in the discussion of results.

7.   The questionnaire was developed in consultation with an undergraduate student who himself has a spinal cord injury. Individuals were given $10 for completing the questionnaire and $15 for participating in the in-person interview. Two participants, both males, refused to accept any payment. One man who completed the questionnaire did not opt for an interview, and two women I contacted declined to participate. Another woman initially expressed interest but never followed through after several attempts to contact her.

8.   In contrast, other writers in the area of disability studies have specified particular instances where the use of the term *handicap* may be appropriate. Wendell (1996: 22–23) argues that *handicap* "may be useful to refer to specifically any loss of opportunities to participate in major aspects of the life of society that results from the interaction of disability with the physical, social or cultural environment of the person who has it."

9.   A number of concrete suggestions regarding language have been put forward (see, for example, Blaska 1993 and Kailes 1985). Hadley and Brodwin (1988: 148–49) argue that (1) a form of the verb *to have* is the preferred way to refer to an individual's association with his or her disability; (2) a disability should never be represented as causing an individual's emotional or behavioral reactions to it; (3) a disability should not be indicated as the sole cause of circumstances resulting from social reactions to it; and (4) wheelchairs, prostheses, and other assistive devices are simply tools that people use in their various activities, and language should represent this fact. These guidelines were often violated by the participants in my study, several of whom felt that their impairments *were* the primary factors behind the major life changes they experienced. Interestingly, most felt no need to disentangle their impairments from their (and others') attitudinal, behavioral, social, economic, and other responses to SCI.

## Chapter 2

1. See Go, DeVivo, and Richards (1995); Stover (1996); and Trieschmann (1988).
2. Among a sample of 78 recently-injured individuals with SCI, the main concerns included: sexual functioning (58%), bladder control (58%), weight (51%), diet (42%), bowel control (41%), skin care (35%), sleep (32%), smoking (27%), drugs (13%), caffeine (12%), and alcohol (6%) (McColl and Skinner 1996).
3. SCI cases are also frequently classified as either upper motor neuron (UMN) or lower motor neuron (LMN) injuries. Upper motor neurons carry impulses between the cerebral cortex and the spinal cord; they are essential for voluntary movement. Lower motor neurons carry impulses between the spinal cord and the musculoskeletal system; they can cause reflex activity even without cortical control as long as the reflex arc is uninterrupted. An upper motor neuron injury is one in which the UMN pathway is broken while the LMN pathway is not. UMN injuries are therefore characterized by spasticity, since the reflexes are uninhibited and hyperreflexic but outside conscious control. A lower motor neuron injury is one in which the LMN pathway is broken. LMN injuries cause a state of "flaccid paralysis," since stimuli from the nerves do not even reach the spinal cord (Hammond et al. 1992).
4. Efforts to compare the racial/ethnic composition of the SCI population to that of the national population are complicated by inconsistencies in the racial/ethnic definitions used by the U. S. Census Bureau and in the National SCI Database (Go, DeVivo, and Richards 1995).
5. One of the women who completed a questionnaire had spina bifida rather than spinal cord injury, but I included her in the sample since the two conditions are associated with similar physiological and social difficulties.
6. Meanwhile, Rohe and Krause (1999a) report that males with SCI are less determined than the general population, have lower energy levels, and are socially retiring. Their findings refer to all males with SCI, however—not just to those whose actions played a part in their injuries.
7. For a comprehensive overview of the history of spinal surgery, see McDonnell (2004).
8. While most studies indicate that higher-level injuries are associated with poorer perceived health status (Dew et al. 1985; Tucker 1980), at least one study has reported the opposite relationship (Patterson 1989).
9. Spasticity is a "neurophysiologic condition characterized by hyperactive deep tendon reflexes and increased muscle tone" (Maynard et al. 1995: 145). Many individuals with injuries to the cervical or thoracic regions have muscle spasms which may or may not be apparent to others. Maynard and associates (1995) caution against viewing spasticity as a negative complication of SCI, since it can sometimes have beneficial effects (e.g., maintaining muscle tone). Nonetheless, the involuntary movements associated with spasticity may interfere with functional activity and can be painful (Maynard et al. 1995). Males and quadriplegics are more likely to experience spasticity than females and paraplegics (Maynard et al. 1995).
10. Gerhart and associates (1997) report that paraplegics are more prone to pressure sores than quadriplegics.

11. Fuhrer, Rintala, and associates (1993) found no association between the presence of pressure ulcers and depression, however.

12. While indwelling catheterization is the most commonly used method for all individuals with SCI in the acute phase, intermittent catheterization is the most commonly used method at the time of discharge from the hospital (Cardenas et al. 1995). In an analysis of the bladder function and bladder management approaches used by individuals with SCI, McColl and Skinner (1996) reported that 22% had normal bladder function, 33% had near normal function, and 45% had a neurogenic bladder. Among those who had some type of bladder management program, the following methods were used: intermittent catheterization (31%), external collection (24%), indwelling catheters (8%), tapping/straining/crede (6%), and incontinence pads (4%). (Some individuals used multiple techniques.) The use of different management strategies varies according to type of impairment, number of years since injury, and place of residence (Cardenas et al. 1995).

    There is no acceptable external urinary collection device for women (Trieschmann 1988), and indwelling catheterization is the method of bladder management for many females (Cardenas et al. 1995; Trieschmann 1989). Others will rely on "bladder training," in which they train their bladders to respond to a particular sensation or movement (Morris 1989). Although one study found that the choice of a particular bladder management technique is unrelated to life satisfaction among individuals with SCI (Brillhart 2004), many of those who rely on bladder training have a constant fear of accidents (Morris 1989).

13. A study of bowel regimens revealed the following post-injury rates of usage: manual evaluation (68%), digital stimulation (53%), suppositories (49%), oral laxatives (29%), and high-fiber diet (23%), as well as several other techniques (see Glickman and Kamm 1996). (Some individuals relied on more than one strategy.)

14. Some of the individuals I interviewed relied on less conventional bladder/bowel regulation programs. One used adult diapers for her bladder program, and two had had colostomies.

15. The SCI Pain Task Force of the International Association for the Study of Pain has recently proposed a new pain taxonomy that may help promote comparability and precision. The taxonomy has three tiers: (1) broad-type pain resulting from damage to the nervous system itself; (2) broad system pain, which affects an entire organ system—musculoskeletal, visceral, etc.; and (3) pain concentrated in particular structures or areas (bone pain, joint pain, dysreflexic headache, etc.) (Finnerup and Jensen 2004).

16. Neurogenic bladder is the loss of normal bladder function caused by damage to part of the nervous system. Depending on the site of the injury, the damage can result in underactivity (inability to contract and expel the contents of the bladder) or overactivity (frequent or overly rapid contraction of the bladder). Upper motor neuron injuries—those above the sacral level—tend to result in reflex or spastic bladders. In these cases, the bladder holds a smaller volume of urine, and contractions result in frequent, small urinations. Among those with lower motor neuron injuries, flaccid bladder is the more common complication (Hammond et al. 1992).

17. The use of antidepressants is also controversial because of the drugs' physiological effects on the body. For example, the use of tricyclic antidepressants may be especially dangerous for quadriplegics who have tenuous control of their blood pressure, and could result in serious cardiovascular complications (Stewart 1977). Selective serotonin reuptake inhibitors and other nontricyclic antidepressants are therefore often the treatment of choice (Richards, Kewman, and Pierce 2000; Stewart 1988, 1977). Stewart (1988) suggests that electro-convulsive therapy may be a viable treatment for individuals with SCI who suffer from depression.

18. Heinemann (1983) cautions against categorizing persons with SCI as being prone to substance abuse, since this may further contribute to their stigmatization.

19. Substance abuse may also have direct, adverse effects on the health of individuals with SCI. For example, drinking large quantities of alcohol can sabotage intermittent catheterization (O'Donnell et al. 1981–1982), stress the bladder, and result in the loss of reflex control so that the patient is unable to gain control of urinary functioning (Radnitz and Tirch 1995). Vomiting with alcohol intoxication can be potentially fatal for quadriplegics who lack the trunk muscles needed to divert vomit from the trachea by rolling to the side (Stewart 1988). The use of substances may also interact with prescribed drugs and lead to deleterious health consequences. For example, warfarin compounds, given to patients as anti-clotting agents, can result in life-threatening internal bleeding when combined with alcohol.

20. Dantrolene sodium (Dantrium) and Baclofen (Lioresal) are used to treat spasticity in individuals with SCI. Soma is a skeletal muscle relaxant used to relieve the pain of muscle injuries, spasms, sprains, and strains.

## Chapter 3

1. Researchers have used several classification schemes to characterize responses to disability and SCI. For example, Weinberg (1988) identifies three distinctive groups of disabled individuals: those who embrace the disability, those who are resigned and adaptive, and those who are forever bitter and unhappy. Meanwhile, Anspach (1979) outlines a four-dimensional model called Stratagems of Disability Management, which refers to *normalization, disassociation, retreatism,* and *political activism.* With regard to SCI in particular, Nagler (1950) describes seven psychological reactions, including anxiety and reactive depression, psychotic reaction, the indifferent group, the psychopathic reaction/aggression pattern, dependency reaction, reaction of the quadriplegic patients (those who, because of physical limitations, find it difficult to channel their aggressive drives into productive accomplishment), and the so-called normal reaction (those who make the best of their disabilities). Heinrich and Tate (1996) identify seven different factors that characterize individuals' psychological responses: anxiety, depression, mental block, interpersonal sensitivity (feeling uneasy with others), spinal cord injury (feeling weakness or numbness in the body), hostile suspiciousness, and general somatization (poor appetite or nausea).

2. Stone (1984) describes four basic ways to approach the phenomenon of disability: psychological, economic, sociological, and political. Marks (1999) also describes four frameworks for examining disability: (1) *the social model of disability*, which

focuses on the social and environmental barriers that oppress disabled individuals; (2) *phenomenology*, which addresses the interpersonal and experiential aspects of disability; (3) *post-structuralism*, which focuses on the discourses that constitute disability; and (4) *psychoanalysis*, which addresses the intrapsychic experiences of and defenses against disability.

3. For an early review of stage theories of adjustment, see Woodbury (1978). Dunn (1975b) argues that the emotional response to spinal cord injury consists of four key stages: shock, mourning, denial, and depression. Similarly, Weller and Miller (1977a) have identified the most common reactions as shock, denial, anger, and depression. Singleton (1985) outlines five developmental phases: shock, realization (recognition that the injury is a threat to self-preservation), defensive retreat (a desire to return to a pre-injury state, both emotionally and physically), acknowledgment, and adaptation.

4. Estimates of depression among individuals with SCI are complicated by the use of different definitions and assessments of depression (Elliott and Frank 1996; Skinner, Armstrong, and Rich 2003). For example, some studies evaluate a wide range of depressive disorders, while others include only the most serious manifestations of clinical depression (Boekamp, Overholser, and Schubert 1996). Many studies do not differentiate between clinical depression and the depression associated with grief or mourning (Howell et al. 1981). Moreover, some authors measure depression by assessing the extent to which patients exhibit clinical symptoms of depression (e.g., fatigue, insomnia, weight loss, disruptions in appetite, and mobility problems). These symptoms may be complications associated with SCI or the side effects of drug treatments, and therefore misleading as indicators of clinical depression (Boekamp, Overholser, and Schubert 1996; Elliott and Frank 1996; Overholser et al. 1993).

5. The relationship between the physiological changes and the emotional responses associated with SCI has been a topic of considerable debate. Some researchers have argued that the physiological changes that accompany SCI result in a lower frequency and intensity of emotional response. For example, Overholser and Schubert (1993) report that there is much indirect evidence to support the somatic suppression hypothesis—the notion that patients have difficulty experiencing any intense emotion because of the suppression of physiological arousal. Hohmann (1966) contends that spinal cord transection disrupts affectual arousal and substantially reduces feelings such as anger, fear, and sexual excitement. Hahnstadt (1985) reports that individuals with SCI show a significant reduction in autonomic responsiveness to emotional stimuli. On the other hand, SCI results in alterations of the hypothalamic pituitary-adrenal axis and alters rhythms of catecholamine excretion (Boekamp, Overholser, and Schubert 1996; Frank et al. 1985). These alterations may interact with daily stress to "create a fertile environment for depressive episodes" (Frank et al. 1985: 253). Other research has found no evidence of a decline in affective response following spinal cord injury (Chwalisz, Diener, and Gallagher 1988; Cobos et al. 2004; Lowe and Carroll 1985), and Cobos and associates (2004) suggest that emotional reactions may even be intensified among individuals with SCI.

6. For example, Coping Effectiveness Training (CET) significantly reduces depression and anxiety in individuals with SCI (Kennedy et al. 2003; Kennedy, Taylor, and Duff 2004; King and Kennedy 1999). Through lectures, practical exercises, and group discussions, CET fosters the development of participants' perceived control and confidence in dealing with the consequences of SCI (Kennedy, Evans, and Beedie 2003). The effectiveness of these programs is maximized when they are introduced relatively soon after the onset of SCI (Kennedy, Taylor, and Duff 2005).

7. By bringing together many individuals with SCI, rehabilitation programs have the potential to promote community and encourage the formation of friendships and supportive networks. Participants in a group psychological intervention program at a hospital-based spinal cord injury program in Britain stressed that their interaction with other participants was one of the most helpful aspects of the program (King and Kennedy 1999). At the same time, patients spent only a small proportion of their time interacting with other patients (Kennedy, Fisher, and Pearson 1988).

## Chapter 4

1. While vaginal lubrication and penile erection are thought to be homologous functions, females with SCI retain this ability far more often than males with SCI (Donohue and Gebhard 1995).

2. The use of Vaseline is discouraged since petroleum jelly is non-soluble in water and can become a breeding ground for bacteria. Vegetable oils may be used, but not with latex condoms (Perduta-Fulginiti 1992).

3. While a large number of men and women with SCI report that they can achieve fantasized orgasms similar to those experienced by neurologically unimpaired individuals (Keller and Buchanan 1993), these orgasms may be different and less intense than those experienced by nondisabled individuals (Comarr 1970; Fitting et al. 1978; Money 1993; Phelps et al. 1983). Money (1993: 191) contends that among paraplegics, the orgasm "becomes a memory and a penumbra of its former self," although Bregman and Hadley (1976) report that most women with SCI describe orgasm in terms similar to those used by able-bodied women. Whipple and colleagues (Whipple, Gerdes, et al. 1996; Whipple, Richards, et al. 1996) describe the physiological orgasmic responses (i.e., changes in blood pressure and heart rate) among women diagnosed with complete SCI in response to vaginal and cervical stimulation.

4. The decline in sexual activity is less pronounced among women. In a study by Mackelprang and Hepworth (1990), 62% of men but only 41% of women reported reduced sexual activity. Donohue and Gebhard (1995) found that while some females had sex less often after SCI, an equal or greater number experienced coitus at least as often as their nondisabled counterparts.

5. As Heslinga and associates (1974: 76) note, "Handicapped people whose arms are powerless are not able to masturbate or achieve a state of relaxation: This can give rise to . . . 'Bräutigamschmerzen' ('bridegroom pains'), that is to say a painful sensation in the groin and abdomen, radiating to the testes and glans penis."

6. Ellen Stohl (1987: 70), a woman with quadriplegia who appeared as a *Playboy*

centerfold, remarked that "after the accident, the first thing I asked my mom was, 'Will I live?' and the second was, 'Can I have sex?'" Meanwhile, Stohl's appearance in *Playboy* was criticized by disability activists because many of the pictures disguised her disability and did not realistically represent the sexuality of disabled individuals (Zola 1987). Cole and associates (1973), referring to interviews with injured veterans, report that many patients mourned the loss of sexual abilities more than any other functional loss. Glickman and Kamm (1996) report that loss of sexual satisfaction is ranked third behind mobility and sensory losses, while Ray and West (1984) conclude that sexual difficulties are not an especially important issue among individuals with SCI.

7.   Sexual intercourse in the sitting position or with the head of the bed elevated may reduce the likelihood of autonomic dysreflexia (Comarr and Vigue 1978b).

8.   In their study of disabled male veterans, Berkman and associates (1978) reported that 79% felt they were a desirable partner. Kettl and associates (1991) found that for women, the effect of SCI on body image is more pronounced than any change in the frequency or quality of sex. Meanwhile, Bonwich (1985) found that women with SCI considered themselves just as attractive post-injury as pre-injury.

9.   For a candid discussion of the advantages and disadvantages of the various techniques used to treat erectile dysfunction, see Ducharme and Gill (1997) or Palmer and associates (2000). For a more technical review, see Rivas and Chancellor (1997) or Stein and associates (1993).

10.  Priapism, a condition where an erection will not subside, can cause the blood in the penis to congeal and fail to drain. As a consequence, tissue damage and cell death results. If untreated, priapism can lead to the loss of any natural erectile ability (McCarren 1990; Stein et al. 1993). Papaverine has also been associated with fibrosis (the development of scar tissue) in the penis, which may result in difficulty maintaining erections. Widespread fibrosis may also cause pain and curvature of the penis during erection (McCarren 1990).

11.  Seventy to eighty percent of paraplegic and quadriplegic men practice oral-genital sex (Cole, Chilgren, and Rosenberg 1973; Phelps et al. 1983). The percentage of females who performed oral sex "often" on their male partners increased from 0% pre-injury to 42% post-injury for quadriplegics and from 16% to 32% post-injury for paraplegics (Donohue and Gebhard 1995). For males, the respective increases were from 29% to 52% and from 26% to 50%. The majority of individuals with SCI report that oral sex is appealing (Cole, Chilgren, and Rosenberg 1973).

12.  Hwang (1997) argues that sexual rehabilitation should focus less on the negative aspects of sexuality and more on reassuring newly disabled individuals that they will be able to have satisfying sex lives. Some authors recommend peer or group counseling as a forum which allows individuals with SCI to voice their concerns in an empathetic environment and to learn from the experiences of others (Mayers 1978; Miller 1988; Steger and Brockway 1980; Tepper 1992). At the same time, many individuals with SCI express a preference or desire for individual sexual counseling (Miller 1988; Zwerner 1982).

13.  The husbands of women with SCI are less sensitive to their wives' preferences in sexual activities than the husbands of nondisabled women. The husbands of

women with SCI also report less pleasure from sexual activity (Urey 1986; Urey and Henggeler 1987).

14. Men with SCI are more likely than nondisabled men to use feminine adjectives when describing themselves (Romeo 1992; Romeo, Wanlass, and Arenas 1993). Loughead (1983) found that men rated themselves lower on masculine characteristics (assertiveness, aggressiveness, independence) after experiencing a disabling injury. Disability had no impact, however, on men's self-ratings for feminine traits (yielding, loyal, sympathetic, sensitive, and dependent).

## Chapter 5

1. Fitchett and associates (1999) report contrary results—that religion does not promote adjustment and recovery among disabled individuals. Their study includes individuals with many different disabling conditions, including stroke, joint replacement, amputation, etc.

2. *Religion* is usually taken to include any formally organized structure for expression of one's supernatural beliefs, whereas *spirituality* represents a personal belief in a supernatural or divine power. These two categories are not mutually exclusive, since many individuals who have strong spiritual beliefs participate regularly in organized religious activities.

3. India is a predominantly Hindu society, and the concept of *dharma* is central to Hindu theological teachings. *Dharma* is a theological doctrine which justifies each individual's current status as the inevitable result of past behavior (Hanks and Hanks 1948).

4. Given the strength of the religious community in the American Heartland, it is perhaps not surprising that so many study participants found refuge in spiritual and religious belief systems. While the current study has focused on the spiritual attitudes and experiences of individuals, it may be helpful to consider the role of the broader religious environment (e.g., the cohesiveness and religious nature of the community at large) when examining how individuals respond to disability.

## Chapter 6

1. Countries where legislation has supported euthanasia (e.g., Nazi Germany, The Netherlands) are cited as examples where state-sponsored euthanasia has had adverse consequences for individuals with disabilities (Bristo and Burgdorf 1998). In Nazi Germany, the concept of "life unworthy of life" was developed to justify the killing of individuals with disabilities (Coulter 1988). Some evidence suggests that the majority of Dutch euthanasia deaths are involuntary (i.e., decisions are made without the patient's knowledge or consent) (Russell 1998) and public opinion in the Netherlands supports the notion that "defective" children should not be allowed to live (Miller 1993).

2. There have been several high-profile cases involving individuals with SCI who have wanted to die.

[1] In a 1989 case that right-to-die advocates see as a successful precedent, David

Rivlin died in a Michigan nursing home. Rivlin had been paralyzed as a result of a surfing accident he sustained eighteen years before he committed suicide with the aid of medical support. He relied on a ventilator and lived in a nursing home in Michigan against his will due to an inability to pay for in-home support services. After several years in nursing homes, Rivlin concluded that he would rather be dead. Mr. Rivlin was given his "right to die" and obtained a court order authorizing a doctor to sedate him and disconnect his ventilator. Days before Rivlin died, a reporter asked him what he thought about society's view of disabled people. "It sucks," said Rivlin. "Transportation, attitudes, financial help, it's all bad" (Longmore 1996).

[2] Kenneth Bergstedt, a 31-year-old man who had been a quadriplegic since the age of 10, expressed a desire to be extricated from a life of paralysis sustained by a respirator (Coleman and Drake 2005). Bergstedt was dependent on his father, who supported his son's decision to die as his own death from lung cancer was imminent. Bergstedt believed that he would be forced to live in a nursing home after his father's death and saw no options for independent living. He had his ventilator discontinued and subsequently died. The Nevada Supreme Court, ruling after Bergstedt's death, concluded that Bergstedt's suffering "resulted more from his fear of the unknown than any source of physical pain. . . . It is equally clear that if Kenneth had enjoyed sound physical health, but had viewed life as unbearably miserable because of his mental state, his liberty interest would provide no basis for asserting a right to terminate his own life with or without the assistance of others" [McKay v. Bergstedt, 801 P. 2d 617, 637 (Nev. 1990)]. Ruling after his death, the Nevada Supreme Court—which had supported Mr. Bergstedt's request for physician-assisted suicide—recognized that he had not been properly informed and had not made a free and intelligent life-or-death decision (Not Dead Yet n.d.).

[3] Larry McAfee, a Georgia man, became a quadriplegic as a result of a motorcycle accident. After exhausting his finances, McAfee was transferred to various institutions including an Ohio nursing home and the intensive care unit of an Atlanta hospital (Russell 1998). Feeling that he had lost control of his life, McAfee went to court to establish his right to discontinue his ventilator. Publicity about the case led to interaction with disability advocates and an outpouring of community support. For example, UCP (United Cerebral Palsy) offered him assistance to regain control of his life and to work in computer engineering (Longmore 1997). Encouraged by this public support, McAfee decided against exercising his court-recognized "right to die," fought to avoid placement in a nursing home (he transferred to a group home), and obtained a job. In the years that followed, interviews with McAfee made it clear that the reason he had wanted to die was because the state of Georgia had not provided him with alternative living arrangements outside of a hospital or nursing home.

3.  According to Batavia (1998: 329), many disability programs are "based on an outdated premise equating disability with unemployability." Believing that most benefit programs promote an entitlement mentality, Batavia recommends a new system with four types of benefits: (1) a permanent disability pension for individuals with no capacity to work; (2) a temporary disability benefit for the vast majority of

beneficiaries; (3) an early retirement benefit; and (4) provision benefits, including personal assistance services, assistive technology and training to enhance the employability of temporary disability recipients. Goldman (1998), on the other hand, is critical of time-limited benefits and recommends retaining the current policy while devoting more attention to the Continuing Disability Review (CDR) process.

## Chapter 7

1.  The sociopolitical structure may also discourage disabled individuals from having romantic relationships. For example, individuals with disabilities who receive Social Security income may lose financial support if they marry (Nemeth 2000). Likewise, institutions tend to segregate the sexes and to make no provision for the privacy of couples (Hwang 1997; Lifchez 1983).

2.  Women with SCI are more likely to have had physically disabled partners post-injury (24%) than pre-injury (8%) (Sipski and Alexander 1993). Of the women in Donohue and Gebhard's (1995) study, the largest group (44%) had engaged in intimate relationships only with nondisabled partners; 28% had been intimate with both able-bodied partners and those with spinal cord injuries, and 14% had been intimate with both able-bodied partners and those with disabilities other than SCI. Among the men, separate figures are provided for quadriplegics and paraplegics. Nearly 75% of quadriplegics and 66% of paraplegics had been intimate only with able-bodied partners. Fifteen percent of quadriplegics and 11% of paraplegics had been intimate with both able-bodied partners and those with SCI.

3.  The actual number of individuals involved in these relationships may have been higher, since I did not specifically solicit this information from all study participants.

4.  Crewe (1993) has been critical of the tendency for spouses to serve as caregivers for individuals with SCI—a trend that is encouraged by financial constraints and the fact that many rehabilitation agencies automatically identify the spouse as the caregiver. Intimacy may be diluted when one partner is perceived of as needy and helpless, and it is therefore important for couples who resume sexual relations to maintain separation between the roles of caregiver and intimate partner (Ducharme et al. 1988). On the other hand, sexual expression can be enhanced by the sense of comfort that is achieved when the caregiver is also a lover (Knight 1989), and some evidence suggests that sexual intimacy is not necessarily disrupted when one spouse assumes caregiving responsibilities (Kester 1986).

5.  Guttmann (1964) reports contrary results, finding that marriages established pre-injury have higher success rates.

6.  In a study of 579 men with SCI (Comarr 1973), 1% of those with complete upper motor neuron lesions and 10% of those with incomplete lower motor neuron lesions were able to father children. The success rates for those with other spinal cord injuries were generally around 6%.

7.  Vibratory stimulation, electrostimulation by rectal probe, and vas aspiration are the most effective techniques for aiding men with SCI who cannot ejaculate on their own (Seager and Halstead 1993). The ejaculate may then be used to impregnate a

woman by either (1) in utero insemination (insertion of the semen into the women's uterus), (2) in vitro fertilization, or (3) intracytoplasmic sperm injection (Sipski 1997c). With intracytoplasmic sperm injection, an individual sperm is used to fertilize an individual egg outside of the woman's body (Sipski 1997c). As a result, few sperm are needed and low motility is not a problem (Linsenmeyer 1997). For a review of the success rates and complications associated with electroejaculation and/ or vibration, see DeForge et al. (2004).

8. Some women may experience delays of two or three years (Comarr 1973), but this is relatively rare. Donohue and Gebhard (1995) conclude that more than half of all women with SCI report no changes whatsoever in their menstrual cycles.

9. Alexander and associates (1993) report that nearly half of the men with SCI feel that their condition negatively affects their ability to raise children. One-third of the women with SCI would rather not become pregnant due to the difficulties they feel they are likely to experience during childrearing (Charlifue et al. 1992).

10. While it is often assumed that the quality of the ejaculate, as judged by motility and sperm count, decreases with increasing time since injury, Seager and Halstead (1993) found that this is not necessarily the case. Their research showed that semen quality in the weeks after the onset of an SCI may not be as good as that obtained two to three years post-injury. Recent research indicates that the advantage of early freezing of sperm is outweighed by the loss of sperm motility during the procedure (DeForge et al. 2004).

## Chapter 8

1. See Boekamp, Overholser, and Schubert (1996); Bracken and Shepard (1980); Brenner (1990); Chwalisz and Vaux (2000); Clayton (1992); Coca (1990); Coyle et al. (1993); Crisp (1990); Danner and Radnitz (2000); Decker and Schulz (1985); DeLoach and Greer (1981); Drew (1997); Elliott et al. (1992a, 1992b); Elliott, Godshall, et al. (1991); Elliott, Herrick, et al. (1991); Fuhrer et al. (1992); Harris et al. (1973); Kemp and Vash (1971); Kennedy et al. (1995); Kishi, Robinson, and Forrester (1994); Krause et al. (1999); Livneh (2000); Mackelprang (1986); May (1999); McColl, Lei, and Skinner (1995); McCormick (1995); Mills (1989); Morgan, Patrick, and Charlston (1984); Pelletier, Alfano, and Fink (1994); Pollets (1975); Povolny (1993); Rintala et al. (1992); Roberts (1996); Rodriguez (1991); Schulz and Decker (1985); Sherman, DeVinney, and Sperling (2004); Smith (1984); White (1983); and Zirpolo (1986).

2. Disability may also promote social connectivity. One study of college students found that wheelchair users had more extensive friendship networks, more relationships involving casual conversation and entertainment, and more relationships providing transportation and housekeeping than their nondisabled counterparts (Stephens and Norris-Baker 1984).

3. However, the extent of organizational involvement among individuals with SCI may be overrepresented in my study, since many of the participants were recruited through the local SCI association.

4. Within my sample, 81% of paraplegics and 67% of quadriplegics who used manual wheelchairs reported that they drove a vehicle. Only 14% of quadriplegics who used power wheelchairs reported that they drove a vehicle.

5. See, for example, Albrecht (1976); Bogdan and Biklen (1993); Cole (2004); Dunn (2000); Fichten et al. (1989); Fine and Asch (1988a, 1988b, 1993); Fisher and Galler (1988); Goffman (1963); Henderson and Bryan (1984); Hundley (1985); Katz, Hass, and Bailey (1988); Kleck (1966, 1968); Lenney and Sercombe (2002); Makas (1988, 1993); Morris (1991, 1993b); Palmer, Kriegsman, and Palmer (2000); Safilios-Rothschild (1970); and Trieschmann (1980, 1988).

6. In understanding the stigmatization of individuals with disabilities, it may be helpful to evaluate what distinguishes nondisabled people who do not stereotype from those who do. Research indicates that individuals who are accepting of those with chronic disabilities are more likely to see them as individuals, view the other as reciprocating, and to define their disabled individuals as full and important members of their social units (Bogdan and Taylor 1993).

7. Approximately half a dozen participants asked me to define the word "stigmatization" during the course of the in-person interviews—despite the fact that all had answered the question on the survey. Goffman (1963: 3) uses the term *stigma* to refer to "an attribute that is deeply discrediting." When conducting the interviews, I generally defined *stigma* as "being treated as a social outcast."

8. A few study participants owned wheelchairs that allowed them to shift to standing positions. Todd demonstrated his chair at one meeting of the SCI association, but he wasn't using it when I interviewed him. He reported that it was much more cumbersome than his regular chair, although he acknowledged that the standing chair was "handy in the house."

9. Meanwhile, Tatum (1989) found that individuals with SCI exhibited levels of communication apprehension that were lower than those of the general population and reported no differences with regard to shyness and reticence.

10. Individuals with SCI who used computers pre-injury tend to use them in similar ways after becoming disabled—to shop, to find information, to meet new people, or to maintain previously established friendships (Frega 1996).

## Chapter 9

1. All cost data from Berkowitz and associates (1998) have been converted to 2004 dollars using the Consumer Price Index Inflation Calculator (National Aeronautics and Space Administration 2004).

2. Linear interpolation was used to estimate median personal and family income values, since income ranges rather than actual values were used in the questionnaire. Participants reported a median family income of $28,750. In comparison, the median annual income of all resident households in the area of my study was $33,235, and the median U. S. household income was $42,168 in 1999–2000 (United States Census Bureau 2001).While individuals with SCI are disadvantaged in comparison with the general population, they appear to have somewhat higher

incomes than other disabled individuals in the region (Wilder and Walters 2005). This finding may be related to the selectivity of my sample, and to the fact that several participants had received injury-related settlements.

3.  Spinlife.com sells wheelchairs at reduced prices. While the most basic unpowered wheelchair can be purchased for $135, the Quickie P200 Custom Power Wheelchair costs $5,125 (June 2005). A typical power wheelchair costs between $3,500 and $4,000.

4.  Two laws, Section 202 and Section 8, allow the U. S. Department of Housing and Urban Development to provide housing to disabled individuals at a substantially reduced cost. Under Section 202, private nonprofit corporations and consumer cooperatives may obtain government loans to construct or renovate apartments that are accessible to disabled individuals and senior citizens. The Housing Assistance Payments Program for Lower Income Families (Section 8) provides grants to public housing agencies in order to subsidize the rents of low-income tenants (Katz and Martin 1982). Individuals may be eligible for Section 8 housing if they have a disability, are low-income, or are at least 62 years old (Katz and Martin 1982).

5.  Katz and Martin (1982: 140) describe the various vocational rehabilitation services available: (1) physical and mental restoration services (e.g., surgery, psychological counseling, and the provision of appliances, prostheses, or special equipment); (2) general counseling and guidance during rehabilitation; (3) vocational guidance and training services (e.g., higher, technical, or remedial education); (4) maintenance subsidies to assist the client in becoming able to sustain and benefit from the rehabilitation program; (5) transportation services, with a similar aim; (6) telecommunications, sensory, and other technical aids (e.g., reader services, talking books, Braille instruction, and interpreter services); (7) assistance to the client's family in their efforts to promote the adjustment and rehabilitation of the client; (8) placement in suitable employment following rehabilitation; (9) tools, equipment, licenses, and supplies for the self-employed or small businessperson; and (10) post-employment services to help the client maintain suitable employment.

6.  The overwhelming majority of individuals with SCI (92%) are discharged to private residences. Only a small percentage are discharged to hospitals (1%) or nursing homes (4%) (Dijkers et al. 1995). At any given time, approximately 3% of individuals with SCI live in nursing homes or long-term care facilities (Dijkers 1996; Harvey et al. 1990, 1992). Quadriplegics are more than twice as likely as paraplegics to be discharged to a nursing home (Gordon and Brown 1997). Some of the variables that influence living arrangements include marital status, age at onset of injury, gender, education, transportation barriers, and economic disincentives (DeJong, Branch, and Corcoran 1984).

7.  Meanwhile, a healthy family environment seems to promote independence among individuals with SCI (McGowan and Roth 1987).

8.  Travis's father had been shot in Vietnam, and most of the muscle mass on the side of his leg was gone. Although he tried to walk without a limp (to "seem normal"), his disability had become more apparent as he aged.

## Chapter 10

1. For a comprehensive review of studies that have examined the relationship between SCI and post-injury employment, see Athanasou, Brown, and Murphy (1996); Trieschmann (1988); and Yasuda and associates (2002).

2. Using cohort data, Krause (1992c) demonstrated that 82% of research participants who had been injured for 25 or more years had worked at some point after becoming disabled. On the other hand, only 48% of all respondents in Krause's study were working at the time of the study. Many individuals with SCI successfully make the transition from full-time to part-time work (Berkowitz et al. 1998; Morris 1989; Schönherr et al. 2005a).

3. See, for example, Alfred, Fuhrer, and Rossi (1987); Berkowitz et al. (1998); DeVivo et al. (1987); Dijkers (1996); Dijkers et al. (1995); El Ghatit and Hanson (1978); Gordon and Brown (1997); Herron (1987); Inniss (1994); James, DeVivo, and Richards (1993); Jang, Wang, and Wang (2005); Krause (1992c); Krause and Anson (1996a), Krause et al. (1999); McShane and Karp (1993); Oliver et al. (1988); Schönherr et al. (2005b); Tomassen, Post, and van Asbeck (2000); Yoshida (1991); and Young et al. (1994). Some exceptions to these patterns have been observed, however. For example, Berkowitz and associates (1998) found that SCI restricts employment opportunities for men more than for women. Likewise, Krause and Anson (1996a) found that white women with SCI have higher rates of employment than white men—a finding that may be attributable to the higher educational levels of the women. Meanwhile, Herron (1987) found no significant relationship between level of injury and employment.

4. Safilios-Rothschild (1970: 233) identified five broad groups of variables that influence the likelihood of return to employment among individuals with disabilities. They include (1) demographic variables (age, sex, etc.), (2) socio-psychological variables (reaction to disability, level of aspiration, etc.), (3) vocational variables (work stability, job skill level, etc.), (4) medical variables·(severity of disability, presence of secondary disabilities, etc.), and (5) psychological variables (motivation to work, intelligence, etc.).

5. The term *high-level quadriplegia* describes a person who has sustained an injury between the C-1 and C-4 level of the spinal cord (Lathem, Gregorio, and Garber 1985).

6. Although an early study of individuals with SCI in Great Britain revealed that perceptions of occupational therapists are "almost universally negative" (Oliver et al. 1988: 80), an unmet need for occupational therapy has been linked to restrictive living arrangements following release from rehabilitation (DeJong, Branch, and Corcoran 1984).

7. Individuals with disabilities are at increased risk for occupational injuries (Zwerling et al. 2000). One Japanese study found, however, that paraplegics have especially low rates of absenteeism (Ikata 1987).

8. There are several barriers to computer use among individuals with high-level quadriplegia, however. For example, an individual who does not have voluntary control of his or her upper limbs may be able to use a mouthstick to strike keys, but

may be unable to operate a mouse, access power switches on the computer, or insert and remove disks (Frega 1996).

## Chapter 11

1. See, for example, Barnes and Mercer (2003); Fine and Asch (1993); Finkelstein (1980); Hevey (1993); Marinelli and Dell Orto (1999); Marks (1999); Oliver (1983, 1993c, 1996a); Weinberg and Williams (1978); and Wright (1960).

2. Weinberg (1988) asked 30 individuals with physical disabilities, "If there were a surgery available that was guaranteed to completely cure your disability (with no risk), would you be willing to undergo the surgery?" Forty-six percent said they would opt for the surgery, 43% would not, and 10% were undecided. While only half of those who had been injured since birth or prior to age seven said they would have chosen the surgery, all those who had been injured later in life said they would have chosen the surgery if it had been offered when they were newly disabled. Many of those injured early in life feared that they would no longer be the same person if they had the surgery.

3. Cole (2004) describes the experiences of two women with different functional electrical devices, one for walking and another for standing.

# Bibliography

Abberley, Paul. 1987. "The Concept of Oppression and the Development of a Social Theory of Disability." *Disability & Society* 2 (1): 5–19.

Abberley, Paul. 1996. "Work, Utopia, and Impairment." Chapter 4 in *Disability and Society: Emerging Issues and Insights,* edited by Len Barton, pp. 61–79. New York: Longman.

Adams, Martha, and Phil Beatty. 1998. "Consumer-Directed Personal Assistance Services: Independent Living, Community Integration and the Vocational Rehabilitation Process." *Journal of Vocational Rehabilitation* 10 (2): 93–101.

Aiello, Barbara. 1988. "The Kids on the Block and Attitude Change: A 10-Year Perspective." Chapter 16 in *Attitudes toward Persons with Disabilities,* edited by Harold E. Yuker, pp. 223–29. New York: Springer.

Albrecht, Gary L. 1976. "Socialization and the Disability Process." Chapter 1 in *The Sociology of Physical Disability and Rehabilitation,* edited by Gary L. Albrecht, pp. 3–38. Pittsburgh: University of Pittsburgh Press.

Albrecht, Gary L. 1992. *The Disability Business: Rehabilitation in America.* Newbury Park, CA: Sage.

Alexander, Craig J., Karen Hwang, and Marca L. Sipski. 2001. "Mothers with Spinal Cord Injuries: Impact on Family Division of Labor, Family Decision Making, and Rearing of Children." *Topics in Spinal Cord Injury Rehabilitation* 7 (1) : 25–36.

Alexander, Craig J., Karen Hwang, and Marca L. Sipski. 2002. "Mothers with Spinal Cord Injuries: Impact on Marital, Family, and Children's Adjustment." *Archives of Physical Medicine and Rehabilitation* 83 (1): 24–30.

Alexander, Craig J., Marca L. Sipski, and Thomas W. Findley. 1993. "Sexual Activities, Desire, and Satisfaction in Males Pre- and Post-Spinal Cord Injury." *Archives of Sexual Behavior* 22 (3): 217–28.

Alexander, Karl L. 1976. "Disability and Stratification Processes." Chapter 7 in *The Sociology of Physical Disability and Rehabilitation,* edited by Gary L. Albrecht, pp. 169–200. Pittsburgh: University of Pittsburgh Press.

Alfano, Dennis P., Patricia M. Neilson, and Milo P. Fink. 1993. "Long-Term Psychosocial Adjustment Following Head or Spinal Cord Injury." *Neuropsychiatry, Neuropsychology, and Behavioral Neurology* 6 (2): 117–25.

Alfano, Dennis P., Patricia M. Neilson, and Milo P. Fink. 1994. "Sources of Stress in Family Members Following Head or Spinal Cord Injury." *Applied Neuropsychology* 1 (1–2): 57–62.

Alfred, Wayne G., Marcus J. Fuhrer, and Charles D. Rossi. 1987. "Vocational Development Following Severe Spinal Cord Injury: A Longitudinal Study." *Archives of Physical Medicine and Rehabilitation* 68 (12): 854–57.

Allden, Phyllis. 1992. "Psychological Aspects of Spinal Cord Injury." *Educational & Child Psychology* 9 (1): 34–48.

Alston, Reginald J. 1994. "Sensation Seeking as a Psychological Trait of Drug Abuse among Persons with Spinal Cord Injury." *Rehabilitation Counseling Bulletin* 38 (2): 154–63.

Althof, Stanley E., and Stephen B. Levine. 1993. "Clinical Approach to the Sexuality of Patients with Spinal Cord Injury." *Urologic Clinics of North America* 20 (3): 527–34.

Anderson, Melissa. 1982. *The Relationship between Involvement in Social Sports and Independence in Self-Care in Persons with Spinal Cord Injury.* Unpublished master's thesis. University of North Carolina at Chapel Hill.

Anderson, Thomas P., and Marcia M. Andberg. 1979. "Psychosocial Factors Associated with Pressure Sores." *Archives of Physical Medicine and Rehabilitation* 60 (8): 341–46.

Anson, Carol A., Douglas J. Stanwyck, and J. Stuart Krause. 1993. "Social Support and Health Status in Spinal Cord Injury." *Paraplegia* 31 (10): 632–38.

Anspach, Renee. 1979. "From Stigma to Identity Politics: Political Activism among the Physically Disabled and Former Mental Patients." *Social Science and Medicine* 13A (6): 765–73.

Anthony, Walter, Jr. 1985. *An Evaluation of Meditation as a Stress Reduction Technique for Persons with Spinal Cord Injury.* Unpublished doctoral dissertation. University of Michigan.

Apple, David F., Rayden Cody, and Anne Allen. 1996. "Overuse Syndrome of the Upper Limb in People with Spinal Cord Injury." Chapter 5 in *Physical Fitness: A Guide For Individuals with Spinal Cord Injury,* edited by Tamara T. Sowell, pp. 97–107. Washington, DC: Department of Veterans Affairs, Veterans Health Administration, Rehabilitation Research and Development Service, Scientific and Technical Publications Section.

Arnold, Ruth. 1998. "Employment and Disability" (Letter). *Psychiatric Services* 49 (10): 1361.

Asch, Morton J. 1970. "The Psychologist in the Spinal Cord Injury Center." *Psychological Aspects of Disability* 17 (2): 79–82.

Athanasou, James A., Douglas J. Brown, and Gregory C. Murphy. 1996. "Vocational Achievements Following Spinal Cord Injury in Australia." *Disability and Rehabilitation* 18 (4): 191–96.

Athelstan, Gary T., and Nancy M. Crewe. 1979. "Psychological Adjustment to Spinal Cord Injury as Related to Manner of Onset of Disability." *Rehabilitation Counseling Bulletin* 22 (4): 311–19.

Axel, Suzanne J. 1982. "Spinal Cord Injured Women's Concerns: Menstruation and Pregnancy." *Rehabilitation Nursing* 7 (5): 10–15.

Baker, Emily R., and Diana D. Cardenas. 1996. "Pregnancy in Spinal Cord Injured Women." *Archives of Physical Medicine and Rehabilitation* 77 (5): 501–7.

Baldwin, Marjorie L. 2000. "Estimating the Potential Benefits of the ADA on the Wages and Employment of Persons with Disabilities." Chapter 10 in *Employment, Disability, and the Americans with Disability Act,* edited by Peter David Blanck, pp. 258–81. Evanston: Northwestern University Press.

Bamford, Erica, David Grundy, and John Russell. 1986. "ABC of Spinal Cord Injury: Social Needs of the Patient and His Family." *British Medical Journal* 292 (6519): 546–48.

Bardach, J. L., and F. J. Padrone. 1982. "Psychosexual Adjustment to Spinal Cord Injury." Chapter 20 in *Spinal Cord Injury,* edited by N. Eric Naftchi, pp. 253–66. Jamaica, NY: Spectrum.

Barnes, Colin. 1990. *"Cabbage Syndrome": The Social Construction of Dependence.* New York: Falmer.

Barnes, Colin. 1996. "Theories of Disability and the Origins of the Oppression of Disabled People in Western Society." Chapter 3 in *Disability and Society: Emerging Issues and Insights,* edited by Len Barton, pp. 43–60. New York: Longman.

Barnes, Colin. 1998. "The Social Model of Disability: A Sociological Phenomenon Ignored by Sociologists?" Chapter 5 in *The Disability Studies Reader,* edited by Tom Shakespeare, pp. 65–78. New York: Cassell.

Barnes, Colin, and Geof Mercer. 2003. *Disability.* Malden, MA: Blackwell.

Barnes, Colin, Geof Mercer, and Tom Shakespeare. 1999. *Exploring Disability: A Sociological Introduction.* Malden, MA: Blackwell.

Barone, Stacey Hoffman. 1993. *Adaptation to Spinal Cord Injury.* Unpublished doctoral dissertation. Boston College.

Barrett, Helen, Joan M. McClelland, Susan B. Rutkowski, and Philip J. Siddall. 2003. "Pain Characteristics in Patients Admitted to Hospital with Complications after Spinal Cord Injury." *Archives of Physical Medicine and Rehabilitation* 84 (6): 789–95.

Barton, Len, editor. 1996. *Disability and Society: Emerging Issues and Insights.* New York: Longman.

Barton, Len. 1998. "Sociology, Disability Studies and Education: Some Observations." Chapter 4 in *The Disability Studies Reader,* edited by Tom Shakespeare, pp. 53–64. New York: Cassell.

Batavia, Andrew I. 1997. "Disability and Physician-Assisted Suicide." *New England Journal of Medicine* 336 (23): 1671–73.

Batavia, Andrew I. 1998. "Unsustainable Growth: Preserving Disability Programs for Americans with Disabilities." In *Growth in Disability Benefits: Explanations and Policy Implications,* edited by Kalman Rupp and David C. Stapleton, pp. 325–36. Kalamazoo, MI: W. E. Upjohn Institute for Employment Research.

Becker, Elle Friedman. 1978. *Female Sexuality Following Spinal Cord Injury.* Bloomington, IL: Cheever.

Belgrave, Faye Z., and S. Lisbeth Jarama. 2002. "Culture and the Disability and Rehabilitation Experience: An African American Example." Chapter 28 in *Handbook of Rehabilitation Psychology,* edited by Robert G. Frank and Timothy R. Elliott, pp. 585–600. Washington, DC: American Psychological Association.

Beneš, Vladimír. 1968. *Spinal Cord Injuries.* London: Baillière, Tindall & Cassell.

Bennett, Tess, Deborah A. Deluca, and Robin W. Allen. 1995. "Religion and Children with Disabilities.*" Journal of Religion and Health* 34 (4): 301–11.

Benrud-Larson, Lisa M., and Stephen T. Wegener. 2000. "Chronic Pain in Neurorehabilitation Populations: Prevalence, Severity and Impact." *NeuroRehabilitation* 14 (3): 127–37.

Bérard, E. J. J. 1989. "The Sexuality of Spinal Cord Injured Women: Physiology and Pathophysiology. A Review." *Paraplegia* 27 (2): 99–112.

Berghammer, A., M. Gramm, L. Volger, and H-H. Schmitt-Dannert. 1997. "Investigation of the Social Status of Paraplegic Individuals after Medical Rehabilitation." *Spinal Cord* 35 (8): 493–97.

Berkman, Anne H., Rae Weissman, and Maxwell H. Frielich. 1978. "Sexual Adjustment of Spinal Cord Injured Veterans Living in the Community." *Archives of Physical Medicine and Rehabilitation* 59 (1): 29–33.

Berkowitz, Monroe, Carol Harvey, Carolyn G. Greene, and Sven E. Wilson. 1992. *The Economic Consequences of Traumatic Spinal Cord Injury.* New York: Demos.

Berkowitz, Monroe, Paul K. O'Leary, Douglas L. Kruse, and Carol Harvey. 1998. *Spinal Cord Injury: An Analysis of Medical and Social Costs.* New York: Demos.

Bermond, B., B. Nieuwenhuyse, L. Fasotti, and J. Schuerman. 1991. "Spinal Cord Lesions, Peripheral Feedback, and Intensities of Emotional Feelings." *Cognition and Emotion* 5 (3): 201–20.

Bielunis, Pamela J. 1995. *New Horizons in Sexuality after a Spinal Cord Injury.* Bloomington, IL: Cheever.

Blaska, Joan. 1993. "The Power of Language: Speak and Write Using 'Person First.'" In *Perspectives on Disability,* 2nd Edition, edited by Mark Nagler, pp. 25–32. Palo Alto, CA: Health Markets Research.

Blatt, Burton. 1985. "Faith, Science and Disability." *Journal of Learning Disabilities* 18 (2): 122–23.

Blissitt, Patricia Ann. 1990. "Nutrition in Acute Spinal Cord Injury." *Critical Care Nursing Clinics of North America* 2 (3): 375–84.

Boekamp, John Richard. 1998. *Interpersonal and Family Factors in the Course of Depression Following Acute Spinal Injury: An Investigation Across Hospital Rehabilitation and 4 Week Postdischarge Follow-up.* Unpublished doctoral dissertation. Case Western Reserve University.

Boekamp, John R., James C. Overholser, and Daniel S. P. Schubert. 1996. "Depression Following a Spinal Cord Injury." *International Journal of Psychiatry in Medicine* 26 (3): 329–49.

Bogdan, Robert, and Douglas Biklen. 1993. "Handicapism." In *Perspectives on Disability,* 2nd Edition, edited by Mark Nagler, pp. 69–76. Palo Alto, CA: Health Markets Research.

Bogdan, Robert, and Steven J. Taylor. 1993. "Relationships with Severely Disabled People: The Social Construction of Humanness." In *Perspectives on Disability,* 2nd Edition, edited by Mark Nagler, pp. 97–108. Palo Alto, CA: Health Markets Research.

Bogle, Jane Elder, and Susan L. Shaul. 1981. "Body Image and the Woman with a Disability." Chapter 14 in *Sexuality and Physical Disability,* edited by David G. Bullard and Susan E. Knight, pp. 91–95. St. Louis: C. V. Mosby.

Bombardier, Charles H. 2000. "Alcohol and Traumatic Disability." Chapter 19 in *Handbook of Rehabilitation Psychology,* edited by Robert G. Frank and Timothy R. Elliott, pp. 399–416. Washington, DC: American Psychological Association.

Bombardier, Charles H., J. Scott Richards, James S. Krause, David Tulsky, and Denise G. Tate. 2004. "Symptoms of Major Depression in People with Spinal Cord Injury: Implications for Screening." *Archives of Physical Medicine and Rehabilitation* 85 (11): 1749–56.

Bombardier, Charles H., Michael W. Stroud, Peter C. Esselman, and Carl T. Rimmele. 2004. "Do Preinjury Alcohol Problems Predict Poorer Rehabilitation Progress in Persons with Spinal Cord Injury?" *Archives of Physical Medicine and Rehabilitation* 85 (9): 1488–92.

Bonwich, Emily. 1985. "Sex Role Attitudes and Role Reorganization in Spinal Cord Injured Women." Chapter 5 in *Women and Disability: The Double Handicap,* edited by Mary Jo Deegan and Nancy A. Brooks, pp. 56–67. New Brunswick: Transaction Books.

Borman, Patricia D., and David N. Dixon. 1998. "Spirituality and the 12 Steps of Substance Abuse Recovery." *Journal of Psychology and Theology* 26 (3): 287–91.

Bors, Ernest, and A. Estin Comarr. 1960. "Neurological Disturbances of Sexual Function with Special Reference to 529 Patients with Spinal Cord Injury." *Urological Survey* 10 (February): 191–222.

Boschen, Kathryn A. 1996. "Correlates of Life Satisfaction, Residential Satisfaction, and Locus of Control among Adults with Spinal Cord Injuries." *Rehabilitation Counseling Bulletin* 39 (4): 230–43.

Boschen, Kathryn A., Mark Tonack, and Judith Gargaro. 2003. "Long-Term Adjustment and Community Reintegration Following Spinal Cord Injury." *International Journal of Rehabilitation Research* 26 (3): 157–64.

Boyer, Bret A., Michelle L. Knolls, Christina M. Kafkalas, Lawrence G. Tollen, and Mercedes Swartz. 2000. "Prevalence and Relationships of Posttraumatic Stress in Families Experiencing Pediatric Spinal Cord Injury." *Rehabilitation Psychology* 45 (4): 339–55.

Bozzacco, Victoria. 1993. "Long-Term Psychosocial Effects of Spinal Cord Injury." *Rehabilitation Nursing* 18 (2): 82–87.

Bracken, M. B., and M. Bernstein. 1980. "Adaptation to and Coping with Disability One Year after Spinal Cord Injury: An Epidemiological Study." *Social Psychiatry* 15 (1): 33–41.

Bracken, Michael B., and Mary Jo Shepard. 1980. "Coping and Adaptation Following Acute Spinal Cord Injury: A Theoretical Analysis." *Paraplegia* 18 (2): 74–85.

Bray, Grady P. 1978. "Rehabilitation of the Spinal Cord Injury: A Family Approach." *Journal of Applied Rehabilitation Counseling* 9 (3): 70–78.

Breasted, James Henry. 1930. *The Edwin Smith Surgical Papyrus: Volume One.* Chicago: University of Chicago Press.

Bregman, Sue. 1978. "Sexual Adjustment of Spinal Cord Injured Women." *Sexuality and Disability* 1 (2): 85–92.

Bregman, Sue, and Robert G. Hadley. 1976. "Sexual Adjustment and Feminine Attractiveness among Spinal Cord Injured Women." *Archives of Physical Medicine and Rehabilitation* 57 (9): 448–50.

Brenner, Helene Gail. 1990. *Cognitive Adaptation to Spinal Cord Injury: The Role of Interpretive Control, Mental Imagery and Social Support.* Unpublished doctoral dissertation. University of Denver.

Breslin, Mary Lou. 2002. "Introduction." In *Disability Rights Law and Policy: International and National Perspectives,* edited by Mary Lou Breslin and Silvia Yee, pp. xxi–xxx. Ardsley: Transnational Publishers.

Bricout, John C. 2004. "Using Telework to Enhance Return to Work Outcomes for Individuals with Spinal Cord Injuries." *NeuroRehabilitation* 19 (2): 147–59.

Brillhart, Barbara. 2004. "Studying the Quality of Life and Life Satisfaction among Persons with Spinal Cord Injury Undergoing Urinary Management." *Rehabilitation Nursing* 29 (4): 122–26.

Brillhart, Barbara. 2005. "A Study of Spirituality and Life Satisfaction among Persons with Spinal Cord Injury." *Rehabilitation Nursing* 30 (1): 31–34.

Brisenden, Simon. [1986] 1998. "Independent Living and the Medical Model of Disability." Chapter 2 in *The Disability Studies Reader,* edited by Tom Shakespeare, pp. 20–26. New York: Cassell.

Bristo, Marc, and Robert L. Burgdorf, Jr. 1998. "Assisted Suicide: A Disability Perspective." *Issues in Law & Medicine* 14 (3): 273–300.

Brown, Julia S., and Barbara Giesy. 1986. "Marital Status of Persons with Spinal Cord Injury." *Social Science and Medicine* 23 (3): 313–22.

Bryant, M. Darrol. 1993. "Religion and Disability: Some Notes on Religious Attitudes and Views." In *Perspectives on Disability,* 2nd Edition, edited by Mark Nagler, pp. 91–95. Palo Alto, CA: Health Markets Research.

Buck, Frances Marks, and George W. Hohmann. 1981. "Personality, Behavior, Values, and Family Relations of Children of Fathers with Spinal Cord Injury." *Archives of Physical Medicine and Rehabilitation* 62 (9): 432–38.

Buck, Frances Marks, and George W. Hohmann. 1984. "Child Adjustment as Related to Financial Security and Employment Status of Fathers with Spinal Cord Injuries." *Archives of Physical Medicine and Rehabilitation* 65 (6): 327–33.

Buckelew, Susan P., Karen E. Baumstark, Robert G. Frank, and John E. Hewett. 1990. "Adjustment Following Spinal Cord Injury." *Rehabilitation Psychology* 35 (2): 101–9.

Bulman, Ronnie Janoff, and Camille B. Wortman. 1977. "Attributions of Blame and Coping in the 'Real World': Severe Accident Victims Respond to their Lot." *Journal of Personality and Social Psychology* 35 (5): 351–63.

Bury, Michael R. 1979. "Disablement in Society: Towards an Integrated Perspective." *International Journal of Rehabilitation Research* 2 (1): 33–40.

Bury, Michael R. 1982. "Chronic Illness as Biographical Disruption." *Sociology of Health and Illness* 4 (2): 167–82.

Byrd, E. Keith. 1997. "Concepts Related to Inclusion of the Spiritual Component in Services to Persons with Disability and Chronic Illness." *Journal of Applied Rehabilitation Counseling* 28 (4): 26–29.

Cairns, Douglas, and John Baker. 1993. "Adjustment to Spinal Cord Injury: A Review of Coping Styles Contributing to the Process." *Journal of Rehabilitation* 59 (4): 30–33.

Cardenas, Diana D., Lisa Farrell-Roberts, Marca L. Sipski, and Deborah Rubner. 1995. "Management of Gastrointestinal, Genitourinary, and Sexual Function." Chapter 7 in *Spinal Cord Injury: Clinical Outcomes from the Model Systems,* edited by Samuel L. Stover, Joel A. DeLisa, and Gale G. Whiteneck, pp. 120–44. Gaithersburg, MD: Aspen.

Carroll, Douglas G. 1970. "History of Treatment of Spinal Cord Injuries." *Maryland State Medical Journal* 19 (January): 109–12.

Carroll, Annemarie. 1999. *The Relationship between Control Beliefs, Coping Strategies, Time Since Injury and Quality of Life among Persons with Spinal Cord Injuries.* Unpublished doctoral dissertation. Kent State University.

Castle, R. 1994. "An Investigation Into the Employment and Occupation of Patients with a Spinal Cord Injury." *Paraplegia* 32 (3): 182–87.

Cecka, Carl David. 1981. *Psychological Acceptance of Spinal Cord Injury as Related to Manner of Onset of Disability.* Unpublished master's thesis. University of Utah.

Chan, Raymond C. K. 2000. "How Does Spinal Cord Injury Affect Marital Relationship? A Story from Both Sides of the Couple." *Disability and Rehabilitation* 22 (17): 764–75.

Chapin, Martha H., and Donald G. Kewman. 2001. "Factors Affecting Employment Following Spinal Cord Injury: A Qualitative Study." *Rehabilitation Psychology* 46 (4): 400–16.

Charlifue, Susan W., and Kenneth A. Gerhart. 1991. "Behavioral and Demographic Predictors of Suicide after Traumatic Spinal Cord Injury." *Archives of Physical Medicine and Rehabilitation* 72 (7): 488–92.

Charlifue, Susan W., and Kenneth A. Gerhart. 2004. "Changing Psychosocial Morbidity in People Aging with Spinal Cord Injury." *NeuroRehabilitation* 19 (1): 15–23.

Charlifue, S. W., K. A. Gerhart, R. R. Menter, G. G. Whiteneck, and M. Scott Manley. 1992. "Sexual Issues of Women with Spinal Cord Injuries." *Paraplegia* 30 (3): 192–99.

Charlton, James I. 1998. *Nothing About Us without Us: Disability Oppression and Empowerment.* Berkeley: University of California Press.

Chase, Brent W. 1998. *An Examination of Factors Associated with Life Satisfaction of Persons with Spinal Cord Injury and their Spouses.* Unpublished doctoral dissertation. Florida State University.

Chesler, Mark A., and Barbara K. Chesney. 1988. "Self-Help Groups: Empowerment Attitudes and Behaviors of Disabled or Chronically Ill Persons." Chapter 17 in *Attitudes toward Persons with Disabilities,* edited by Harold E. Yuker, pp. 230–45. New York: Springer.

Chicano, Lois A. 1989. "Humanistic Aspects of Sexuality as Related to Spinal Cord Injury." *Journal of Neuroscience Nursing* 21 (6): 366–69.

Chigier, Emanuel. 1981. "Sexuality and Disability: The International Perspective." Chapter 18 in *Sexuality and Physical Disability,* edited by David G. Bullard and Susan E. Knight, pp. 134–43. St. Louis: C. V. Mosby.

Chipouras, Sophia. 1979. "Ten Sexuality Programs for Spinal Cord Injured Persons." *Sexuality and Disability* 2 (4): 301–21.

Chubon, Robert A., Karen S. Clayton, and David V. Vandergriff. 1995. "An Exploratory Study Comparing the Quality of Life of South Carolinians with Mental Retardation and Spinal Cord Injury." *Rehabilitation Counseling Bulletin* 39 (2): 107–18.

Chwalisz, Kathleen, Ed Diener, and Dennis Gallagher. 1988. "Autonomic Arousal Feedback and Emotional Experience: Evidence from the Spinal Cord Injured." *Journal of Personality and Social Psychology* 54 (5): 820–28.

Chwalisz, Kathleen, and Alan Vaux. 2000. "Social Support and Adjustment to Disability." Chapter 25 in *Handbook of Rehabilitation Psychology,* edited by Robert G. Frank and Timothy R. Elliott, pp. 537–52. Washington, DC: American Psychological Association.

Clayton, Karen Shepard. 1992. *Determinants of Quality of Life in Individuals with Spinal Cord Injury.* Unpublished doctoral dissertation. University of South Carolina.

Clayton, Karen S., and Robert A. Chubon. 1994. "Factors Associated with the Quality of Life of Long-Term Spinal Cord Injured Persons." *Archives of Physical Medicine and Rehabilitation* 75 (6): 633–38.

Cleveland, Martha. 1980. "Family Adaptation to Traumatic Spinal Cord Injury: Response to Crisis." *Family Relations* 29 (4): 558–65.

Coates, Rosemary, and Paola A. Ferroni. 1991. "Sexual Dysfunction and Marital Disharmony as a Consequence of Chronic Lumbar Spinal Pain." *Sexual and Marital Therapy* 6 (1): 65–69.

Cobos, Pilar, María Sánchez, Nieves Pérez, and Jaime Vila. 2004. "Effects of Spinal Cord Injuries on the Subjective Component of Emotions." *Cognition and Emotion* 18 (2): 281–87.

Coca, Beatriz. 1990. *Coping Strategies, Social Support and Acceptance of Disability among Persons with Spinal Cord Injury.* Unpublished doctoral dissertation. California School of Professional Psychology.

Cockerill, Rhonda, and Nancy Durham. 1992. "Attendant Care and Its Role in Independent Living, as Developed in Transitional Living Centres." *New England Journal of Human Services* 11 (2): 17–22.

Cohen, Michael J., David L. McArthur, Michael Vulpe, Steve L. Schandler, and Kenneth E. Gerber. 1988. "Comparing Chronic Pain from Spinal Cord Injury to Chronic Pain of Other Origins." *Pain* 35 (1): 57–63.

Cole, Jonathan. 2004. *Still Lives: Narratives of Spinal Cord Injury.* Cambridge: MIT Press.

Cole, Theodore M. 1975. "Sexuality and Physical Disabilities." *Archives of Sexual Behavior* 4 (4): 389–403.

Cole, Theodore M., Richard Chilgren, and Pearl Rosenberg. 1973. "A New Programme of Sex Education and Counselling for Spinal Cord Injured Adults and Health Care Professionals." *Paraplegia* 11 (2): 111–24.

Coleman, Diane. 2000. "Assisted Suicide and Disability." *Human Rights: Journal of the Section of Individuals Rights & Responsibilities* 27 (1): 6–9.

Coleman, D., and S. Drake. 2005. "A Disability Perspective from the United States on the Case of Ms. B." *Journal of Medical Ethics* 28 (4): 240–42.

Comarr, A. Estin. 1970. "Sexual Functioning among Patients with Spinal Cord Injury." *Urologia Internationalis* 25 (2): 134–68.

Comarr, A. Estin. 1973. "Sex among Patients with Spinal Cord and/or Cauda Equina Injuries." *Medical Aspects of Human Sexuality* 7 (3): 222–38.

Comarr, A. Estin, and Marjorie Vigue. 1978a. "Sexual Counseling among Male and Female Patients with Spinal Cord and/or Cauda Equina Injury. Part I." *American Journal of Physical Medicine* 57 (3): 107–22.

Comarr, A. Estin, and Marjorie Vigue. 1978b. "Sexual Counseling among Male and Female Patients with Spinal Cord and/or Cauda Equina Injury. Part II." *American Journal of Physical Medicine* 57 (5): 215–27.

Comfort, Alex. 1975. "Foreword." In *Sexual Options for Paraplegics and Quadriplegics,* edited by Thomas O. Mooney, Theodore M. Cole, and Richard A. Chilgren, pp. vii–ix. Boston: Little, Brown, and Company.

Conant, Lisa L. 1995. *A Causal Analysis of Psychological Variables Associated with Chronic Spinal Cord Injury Pain.* Unpublished doctoral dissertation. Ohio State University.

Conant, Lisa L. 1998. "Psychological Variables Associated with Pain Perceptions among Individuals with Chronic Spinal Cord Injury Pain." *Journal of Clinical Psychology in Medical Settings* 5 (1): 71–90.

Connell, R. W. 1995. *Masculinities.* Berkeley: University of California Press.

Cook, Daniel W. 1976. "Psychological Aspects of Spinal Cord Injury." *Rehabilitation Counseling Bulletin* 19 (4): 535–43.

Cook, Daniel W. 1979. "Psychological Adjustment to Spinal Cord Injury: Incidence of Denial, Depression, and Anxiety." *Rehabilitation Psychology* 26 (3): 97–104.

Cook, Daniel W. 1982. "Dimensions and Correlates of Postservice Adjustment to Spinal Cord Injury: A Longitudinal Inquiry." *International Journal of Rehabilitation Research* 5 (3): 373–75.

Corbet, Barry. 1993. "What Price Independence?" Chapter 17 in *Aging with Spinal Cord Injury,* edited by Gale G. Whiteneck, Susan W. Charlifue, Kenneth A. Gerhart, Daniel P. Lammertse, Scott Manley, Robert R. Menter, and Kathie R. Seedroff, pp. 219–27. New York: Demos.

Corcoran, James R. 1985. *The Interpersonal Influence of Depression Following Spinal Cord Injury.* Unpublished doctoral dissertation. University of Missouri-Columbia.

Coulter, David L. 1988. "Beyond Baby Doe: Does Infant Transplantation Justify Euthanasia." *Journal of the Association for Persons with Severe Handicaps* 13 (2): 71–75.

Courtois, F. J., K. F. Charvier, A. Leriche, and D. P. Raymond. 1993. "Sexual Function in Spinal Cord Injury Men. I. Assessing Sexual Capability." *Paraplegia* 31 (12): 771–84.

Cox, Ruth J., Delena I. Amsters, and Kiley J. Pershouse. 2001. "The Need for a Multidisciplinary Outreach Service for People with Spinal Cord Injury Living in the Community." *Clinical Rehabilitation* 15 (6): 600–606.

Coyle, Catherine P., Susanne Lesnik-Emas, and Walter B. Kinney. 1994. "Predicting Life Satisfaction among Adults with Spinal Cord Injuries." *Rehabilitation Psychology* 39 (2): 95–112.

Coyle, Catherine P., John W. Shank, Walter (Terry) Kinney, and Deborah A. Hutchins. 1993. "Psychosocial Functioning and Changes in Leisure Lifestyle among Individuals with Chronic Secondary Health Problems Related to Spinal Cord Injury." *Therapeutic Recreation Journal* 27 (4): 239–52.

Craig, A. R., K. Hancock, and E. Chang. 1994. "The Influence of Spinal Cord Injury on Coping Styles and Self-Perceptions Two Years after the Injury." *Australian and New Zealand Journal of Psychiatry* 28 (2): 307–12.

Craig, Ashley, Karen Hancock, Esther Chang, and Hugh Dickson. 1998. "The Effectiveness of Group Psychological Intervention in Enhancing Perceptions of Control Following Spinal Cord Injury." *Australian & New Zealand Journal of Psychiatry* 32 (1): 112–18.

Craig, Ashley R., Karen M. Hancock, and Hugh G. Dickson. 1994. "Spinal Cord Injury: A Search for the Determinants of Depression Two Years after the Event." *British Journal of Clinical Psychology* 33 (2): 221–30.

Craig, A. R., K. M. Hancock, H. Dickson, J. Martin, and E. Chang. 1990. "Psychological Consequences of Spinal Injury: A Review of the Literature." *Australian & New Zealand Journal of Psychiatry* 24 (3): 418–25.

Craigie, Frederic C., Jr., Ingrid Y. Liu, David B. Larson, and John S. Lyons. 1988. "A Systematic Analysis of Religious Variables in *The Journal of Family Practice,* 1976–1986." *The Journal of Family Practice* 27 (5): 509–13.

Crewe, Nancy M. 1993. "Spousal Relationships and Disability." Chapter 13 in *Reproductive Issues for Persons with Physical Disabilities,* edited by Florence P. Haseltine, Sandra S. Cole, and David B. Gray, pp. 141–51. Baltimore: Paul H. Brookes.

Crewe, Nancy M. 1997. "Life Stories of People with Long-Term Spinal Cord Injury." *Rehabilitation Counseling Bulletin* 41 (1): 26–42.

Crewe, Nancy M. 2000. "A 20-Year Longitudinal Perspective on the Vocational Experience of Persons with Spinal Cord Injury." *Rehabilitation Counseling Bulletin* 43 (3): 122–33, 141.

Crewe, Nancy M., Gary T. Athelstan, and John Krumberger. 1979. "Spinal Cord Injury: A Comparison of Preinjury and Postinjury Marriages." *Archives of Physical Medicine and Rehabilitation* 60 (6): 252–56.

Crewe, Nancy M., and James S. Krause. 1988. "Marital Relationships and Spinal Cord Injury." *Archives of Physical Medicine and Rehabilitation* 69 (6): 435–38.

Crewe, Nancy M., and James S. Krause. 1990. "An Eleven-Year Follow-Up of Adjustment to Spinal Cord Injury." *Rehabilitation Psychology* 35 (4): 205–10.

Crisp, Ross. 1990. "The Long-Term Adjustment of 60 Persons with Spinal Cord Injury." *Australian Psychologist* 27 (1): 43–47.

Cross, Leland L., Jay M. Meythaler, Stephen M. Tuel, and Audrey L. Cross. 1991. "Pregnancy Following Spinal Cord Injury." *The Western Journal of Medicine* 154 (5): 607–11.

Crow, Liz. 1996. "Including All Our Lives: Renewing the Social Model of Disability." Chapter 4 in *Exploring the Divide: Illness and Disability,* edited by Colin Barnes and Geof Mercer, pp. 55–73. Leeds: Disability Press.

Cunningham, Nancy E. 1986. *Adjustment to Spinal Cord Injury: A Strategic Approach.* Unpublished doctoral dissertation. Wright State University.

Dallmeijer, A. J., and L. H. V. van der Woude. 2001. "Health Related Functional Status in Men with Spinal Cord Injury: Relationship with Lesion Level and Endurance Capacity." *Spinal Cord* 39 (11): 577–83.

Daniel, Anna, and C. Manigandan. 2005. "Efficacy of Leisure Intervention Groups and their Impact on Quality of Life among People with Spinal Cord Injury." *International Journal of Rehabilitation Research* 28 (1): 43–48.

Daniels, Susan M., and Jane West. 1998. "Return to Work for SSI and DI Beneficiaries: Employment Policy Challenges." In *Growth in Disability Benefits: Explanations and Policy Implications,* edited by Kalman Rupp and David C. Stapleton, pp. 359–64. Kalamazoo, MI: W. E. Upjohn Institute for Employment Research.

Danner, Gina, and Cynthia L. Radnitz. 2000. "Protective Factors and Posttraumatic Stress Disorder in Veterans with Spinal Cord Injury." *International Journal of Rehabilitation and Health* 5 (3): 195–203.

Dattilo, John, Linda Caldwell, Youngkhill Lee, and Douglas A. Kleiber. 1998. "Returning to the Community with a Spinal Cord Injury: Implications for Therapeutic Recreation Specialists." *Therapeutic Recreation Journal* 32 (1): 13–27.

David, Amnon, Samuel Gur, and Raphael Rozin. 1977–1978. "Survival in Marriage in the Paraplegic Couple: Psychological Study." *Paraplegia* 15 (3): 198–201.

Davies, Brian Meredith. 1982. *The Disabled Child and Adult.* London: Baillière Tindall.

Davis, Estelle L. 1995. "What a Psychiatrist Needs to Know about Spinal Cord Injury." *Psychiatric Annals* 25 (6): 329–37.

Davis, Fred. 1961. "Deviance Disavowal: The Management of Strained Interaction by the Visibly Handicapped." *Social Problems* 9 (2): 120–32.

Davis, Ken. 1996. "Disability and Legislation: Rights and Equality." Chapter 12 in *Beyond Disability: Towards an Enabling Society,* edited by Gerald Hales, pp. 124–33. Thousand Oaks, CA: Sage.

Decker, Susan D., and Richard Schulz. 1985. "Correlates of Life Satisfaction and Depression in Middle-Aged and Elderly Spinal Cord-Injured Persons." *American Journal of Occupational Therapy* 39 (11): 740–45.

Deegan, Mary Jo, and Nancy A. Brooks. 1985. "Women and Disability: The Double Handicap." Chapter 1 in *Women and Disability: The Double Handicap,* edited by Mary Jo Deegan and Nancy A. Brooks, pp. 1–5. New Brunswick: Transaction Books.

DeForge, Dan, Jeff Blackmer, David Moher, Chantelle Garritty, Fatemeh Yazdi, Valerie Cronin, Nick Barrowman, Vasil Mamaladze, Li Zhang, and Margaret Sampson. 2004. *Sexuality and Reproductive Health Following Spinal Cord Injury.* Evidence Report/Technology Assessment No. 109. AHRQ Publication No. 05-E003–2. Rockville, MD: Agency for Healthcare Research and Quality.

Defrin, Ruth, Avi Ohry, Nava Blumen, and Gideon Urca. 2001. "Characterization of Chronic Pain and Somatosensory Function in Spinal Cord Injury Subjects." *Pain* 89 (2–3): 253–63.

DeJong, Gerben. 1979. *The Movement for Independent Living: Origins, Ideology, and Implications for Disability Research.* Occasional Paper No. 2. Published in Collaboration with The University Centers for International Rehabilitation, Michigan State University.

DeJong, Gerben. 1983. "Defining and Implementing the Independent Living Concept." Chapter 1 in *Independent Living for Physically Disabled People: Developing, Implementing and Evaluating Self-Help Rehabilitation Programs,* edited by Nancy M. Crewe and Irving Kenneth Zola, and associates, pp. 4–27. San Francisco: Jossey-Bass.

DeJong, Gerben, Laurence G. Branch, and Paul J. Corcoran. 1984. "Independent Living Outcomes in Spinal Cord Injury: Multivariate Analyses." *Archives of Physical Medicine and Rehabilitation* 65 (2): 66–73.

DeJong, Gerben, Ruth W. Brannon, and Andrew I. Batavia. 1993. "Financing Health and Personal Care." Chapter 22 in *Aging with Spinal Cord Injury,* edited by Gale G. Whiteneck, Susan W. Charlifue, Kenneth A. Gerhart, Daniel P. Lammertse, Scott Manley, Robert R. Menter, and Kathie R. Seedroff, pp. 275–94. New York: Demos.

DeLoach, Charlene, and Bobby G. Greer. 1981. *Adjustment to Severe Physical Disability: A Metamorphosis.* New York: McGraw-Hill.

Derry, F. A., W. W. Dinsmore, M. Fraser, B. P. Gardner, C. A. Glass, M. C. Maytom, and M. D. Smith. 1998. "Efficacy and Safety of Oral Sildenafil (Viagra) in Men with Erectile Dysfunction Caused by Spinal Cord Injury." *Neurology* 51 (6): 1629–33.

DeVivo, M. J., K. J. Black, J. Scott Richards, and S. L. Stover. 1991. "Suicide Following Spinal Cord Injury." *Paraplegia* 29 (9): 620–27.

DeVivo, Michael J., and Philip R. Fine. 1985. "Spinal Cord Injury: Its Short-term Impact on Marital Status." *Archives of Physical Medicine and Rehabilitation* 66 (8): 501–4.

DeVivo, Michael J., Paula L. Kartus, Samuel L. Stover, Richard D. Rutt, and Philip R. Fine. 1989. "Cause of Death for Patients with Spinal Cord Injuries." *Archives of Internal Medicine* 149 (8): 1761–66.

DeVivo, Michael J., Richard D. Rutt, Samuel L. Stover, and Philip R. Fine. 1987. "Employment after Spinal Cord Injury." *Archives of Physical Medicine and Rehabilitation* 68 (8): 494–98.

DeVivo, Michael J., and Samuel L. Stover. 1995. "Long-Term Survival and Causes of Death." Chapter 14 in *Spinal Cord Injury: Clinical Outcomes from the Model Systems,* edited by Samuel L. Stover, Joel A. DeLisa, and Gale G. Whiteneck, pp. 289–316. Gaithersburg, MD: Aspen.

DeVivo, Michael J., Gale G. Whiteneck, and Edgar D. Charles, Jr. 1995. "The Economic Impact of Spinal Cord Injury." Chapter 12 in *Spinal Cord Injury: Clinical Outcomes from the Model Systems,* edited by Samuel L. Stover, Joel A. DeLisa, and Gale G. Whiteneck, pp. 234–71. Gaithersburg, MD: Aspen.

Dew, Mary Amanda, Kathleen Lynch, Jeffrey Ernst, and Robert Rosenthal. 1983. "Reaction and Adjustment to Spinal Cord Injury: A Descriptive Study." *Journal of Applied Rehabilitation Counseling* 14 (1): 32–39.

Dew, Mary Amanda, Kathleen A. Lynch, Jeffrey Ernst, Robert Rosenthal, and Charles M. Judd. 1985. "A Causal Analysis of Factors Affecting Adjustment to Spinal Cord Injury." *Rehabilitation Psychology* 30 (1): 39–46.

Deyoe, Frank S. 1972. "Marriage and Family Patterns with Long-Term Spinal Cord Injury." *Paraplegia* 10 (3): 219–24.

Dias de Carvalho, Serafim Armindo, Maria João Andrade, Maria Assunção Tavares, and João Luís Sarmento de Freitas. 1998. "Spinal Cord Injury and Psychological Response." *General Hospital Psychiatry* 20 (6): 353–59.

Dijkers, Marcel. 1996. "Quality of Life after Spinal Cord Injury." *American Rehabilitation* 22 (3): 18–22.

Dijkers, Marcel P., Michelle Buda Abela, Bruce M. Gans, and Wayne A. Gordon. 1995. "The Aftermath of Spinal Cord Injury." Chapter 10 in *Spinal Cord Injury: Clinical Outcomes from the Model Systems,* edited by Samuel L. Stover, Joel A. DeLisa, and Gale G. Whiteneck, pp. 185–212. Gaithersburg, MD: Aspen.

Dinardo, Quentin E. 1971. *Psychological Adjustment to Spinal Cord Injury.* Unpublished doctoral dissertation. University of Houston.

Do Rozario, Loretta. 1997. "Spirituality in the Lives of People with Disability and Chronic Illness: A Creative Paradigm of Wholeness and Reconstitution." *Disability and Rehabilitation* 19 (10): 427–34.

Dodd, Jann E. 1991. *Case Studies of Wives who are Caregivers of Husbands with Spinal Cord Injury.* Unpublished doctoral dissertation. University of Houston.

Donatucci, Craig F., and Tom F. Lue. 1993. "Pathophysiology of Sexual Dysfunction in Males with Physical Disabilities." Chapter 26 in *Reproductive Issues for Persons with Physical Disabilities,* edited by Florence P. Haseltine, Sandra S. Cole, and David B. Gray, pp. 291–310. Baltimore: Paul H. Brookes.

Donelson, Earle. 1997. *The Relationship of Sexual Self-Concept to the Level of Spinal Cord Injury and Other Factors.* Unpublished doctoral dissertation. Kent State University.

Donohue, John, and Paul Gebhard. 1995. "The Kinsey Institute/Indiana University Report on Sexuality and Spinal Cord Injury." *Sexuality and Disability* 13 (1): 7–85.

Donovan, William H., Susan L. Garber, Steven M. Hamilton, Thomas A. Krouskop, Gladys P. Rodriguez, and Samuel Stal. 1988. "Pressure Ulcers." Chapter 25 in *Rehabilitation Medicine: Principles and Practices,* edited by Joel A. DeLisa, pp. 476–91. New York: J. B. Lippincott.

Dowler, Denetta, Linda Batiste, and Eddie Whidden. 1998. "Accommodating Workers with Spinal Cord Injury." *Journal of Vocational Rehabilitation* 10 (2): 115–22.

Drainoni, Mari-Lynn, Bethlyn Houlihan, Steve Williams, Mark Vedrani, David Esch, Elizabeth Lee-Hood, and Cheryl Weiner. 2004. "Patterns of Internet Use by Persons with Spinal Cord Injuries and Relationship to Health-Related Quality of Life." *Archives of Physical Medicine and Rehabilitation* 85 (11): 1872–79.

Dreifus, Claudia. 2004. "Defying Irreversibility in Spinal Cord Injuries." *The New York Times* 153 (52790): F3.

Drench, Meredith E. 1992. "Impact of Altered Sexuality and Sexual Function in Spinal Cord Injury: A Review." *Sexuality and Disability* 10 (1): 3–14.

Drew, Jana Brittain. 1997. *The Development of Perceived Social Support: Predictors in a Rehabilitation Population.* Unpublished doctoral dissertation. Wayne State University.

Drew-Cates, Jessie. 1989. *Adjustment in Spinal Cord Injury: A Partial Transcendence.* Unpublished doctoral dissertation. University of Rochester.

Ducharme, Stanley, Kathleen Gill, Susan Biener-Bergman, and Louisa Fertitta. 1988. "Sexual Functioning: Medical and Psychological Aspects." Chapter 27 in *Rehabilitation Medicine: Principles and Practices,* edited by Joel A. DeLisa, pp. 519–36. New York: J. B. Lippincott.

Ducharme, Stanley H., and Jacqueline Ducharme. 1985. "Psychological Adjustment to Spinal Cord Injury. Chapter 12 in *Emotional Rehabilitation of Physical Trauma and Disability,* edited by David W. Krueger, pp. 149–56. New York: Pergamon.

Ducharme, Stanley H., and Kathleen M. Gill. 1997. *Sexuality after Spinal Cord Injury.* Baltimore: Paul H. Brookes.

Duggan, Colette Hillebrand, and Marcel Dijkers. 1999. "Quality of Life—Peaks and Valleys: A Qualitative Analysis of the Narratives of Persons with Spinal Cord Injuries." *Canadian Journal of Rehabilitation* 12 (3): 181–91.

Duggan, Colette Hillebrand, and Marcel Dijkers. 2001. "Quality of Life after Spinal Cord Injury: A Qualitative Study." *Rehabilitation Psychology* 46 (1): 3–27.

Dunn, Dana S. 2000. "Social Psychological Issues in Disability." Chapter 27 in *Handbook of Rehabilitation Psychology,* edited by Robert G. Frank and Timothy R. Elliott, pp. 565–84. Washington, DC: American Psychological Association.

Dunn, Michael E. 1975a. "Psychological Interventions in a Spinal Cord Injury Center: An Introduction." *Rehabilitation Psychology* 22 (4): 165–78.

Dunn, Michael E. 1975b. "Thoughts on 'Psychological Intervention in a Spinal Cord Injury Center: An Introduction.'" *Rehabilitation Psychology* 22 (4): 206–11.

Dunn, Michael. 1977. "Social Discomfort in the Patient with Spinal Cord Injury." *Archives of Physical Medicine and Rehabilitation* 58 (6): 257–60.

Eaton, Bill, Ellen Condon, and Melinda Mast. 2001. "Making Employment a Reality." *Journal of Vocational Rehabilitation* 16 (1): 9–14.

Echols, Karen Ann. 1978. *The Importance of Sexual Functioning In Relation to Other Functional Losses of the Person with Spinal Cord Injury.* Unpublished master's thesis. University of Alabama at Birmingham.

Eisenberg, Myron G., and L. C. Rustad. 1974. *Sex and the Spinal Cord Injured: Some Questions and Answers.* Cleveland, OH: Veterans Administration Hospital.

El Ghatit, Ahmed Z., and Richard W. Hanson. 1976. "Marriage and Divorce after Spinal Cord Injury." *Archives of Physical Medicine and Rehabilitation* 57 (10): 470–72.

El Ghatit, Ahmed Z., and Richard W. Hanson. 1978. "Variables Associated with Obtaining and Sustaining Employment among Spinal Cord Injured Males: A Follow-up of 760 Veterans." *Journal of Chronic Diseases* 31 (5): 363–69.

Ell, Kathleen. 1996. "Social Networks, Social Support and Coping with Serious Illness: The Family Connection." *Social Science and Medicine* 42 (2): 173–83.

Elliott, Timothy Raymond. 1987. *Social and Interpersonal Responses to Spinal Cord Injury and Depression.* Unpublished doctoral dissertation. University of Missouri-Columbia.

Elliott, Timothy R. 1999. "Social Problem-Solving Abilities and Adjustment to Recent-Onset Spinal Cord Injury." *Rehabilitation Psychology* 44 (4): 315–32.

Elliott, Timothy R., and Robert G. Frank. 1996. "Depression Following Spinal Cord Injury." *Archives of Physical Medicine and Rehabilitation* 77 (8): 816–23.

Elliott, Timothy R., Frank J. Godshall, Stephen M. Herrick, Thomas E. Witty, and Michael Spruell. 1991. "Problem-Solving Appraisal and Psychological Adjustment Following Spinal Cord Injury." *Cognitive Therapy and Research* 15 (5): 387–98.

Elliott, Timothy R., Stephen M. Herrick, Anne M. Patti, Thomas E. Witty, Frank J. Godshall, and Michael Spruell. 1991. "Assertiveness, Social Support, and Psychological Adjustment Following Spinal Cord Injury." *Behaviour Research and Therapy* 29 (5): 485–93.

Elliott, Timothy R., Stephen M. Herrick, Thomas E. Witty, Frank Godshall, and Michael Spruell. 1992a. "Social Support and Depression Following Spinal Cord Injury." *Rehabilitation Psychology* 37 (1): 37–48.

Elliott, Timothy R., Stephen M. Herrick, Thomas E. Witty, Frank Godshall, and Michael Spruell. 1992b. "Social Relationships and Psychosocial Impairment of Persons with Spinal Cord Injury." *Psychology and Health* 7 (1): 55–67.

Elliott, Timothy R., and Paul Kennedy. 2004. "Treatment of Depression Following Spinal Cord Injury: An Evidence-Based Review." *Rehabilitation Psychology* 49 (2): 134–39.

Elliott, Timothy R., and Richard M. Shewchuk. 1995. "Social Support and Leisure Activities Following Severe Physical Disability: Testing the Mediating Effects of Depression." *Basic and Applied Social Psychology* 16 (4): 471–87.

Elliott, Timothy R., and Richard M. Shewchuk. 1998. "Recognizing the Family Caregiver: Integral and Formal Members of the Rehabilitation Process." *Journal of Vocational Rehabilitation* 10 (2): 123–32.

Elliott, Timothy R., and Richard M. Shewchuk. 2002. "Using the Nominal Group Technique to Identify the Problems Experienced by Persons Living with Severe Physical Disabilities." *Journal of Clinical Psychology in Medical Settings* 9 (2): 65–76.

Elliott, Timothy R., Richard M. Shewchuk, and J. Scott Richards. 2001. "Family Caregiver Social Problem-Solving Abilities and Adjustment During the Initial Year of the Caregiving Role." *Journal of Counseling Psychology* 48 (2): 223–32.

Elliott, Timothy R., Thomas E. Witty, Stephen Herrick, and Josephine T. Hoffman. 1991. "Negotiating Reality after Physical Loss: Hope, Depression, and Disability." *Journal of Personality and Social Psychology* 61 (4): 608–13.

Ellis, Albert. 1997. "Using Rational Emotive Behavior Therapy Techniques to Cope with Disability." *Professional Psychology: Research and Practice* 28 (1): 17–22.

Ellison, Christopher G., Jason D. Boardman, David R. Williams, and James S. Jackson. 2001. "Religious Involvement, Stress, and Mental Health: Findings from the 1995 Detroit Area Study." *Social Forces* 80 (1): 215–49.

Ernst, Jeffrey L., and Elizabeth H. Day. 1998. "Reducing the Penalties of Long-Term Employment: Alternatives in Vocational Rehabilitation and Spinal Cord Injury." *Journal of Vocational Rehabilitation* 10 (2): 133–39.

Estores, Irene M. 2003. "The Consumer's Perspective and the Professional Literature: What Do Persons with Spinal Cord Injury Want?" *Journal of Rehabilitation Research and Development* 40 (4): 93–98.

Evans, Joseph H. 1976. "Changing Attitudes toward Disabled Persons: An Experimental Study." *Rehabilitation Counseling Bulletin* 19 (4): 572–79.

Evans, Ron L., Robert D. Hendricks, Richard T. Connis, Jodie K. Haselkorn, Karen R. Ries, and Tamara E. Mennet. 1994. "Quality of Life after Spinal Cord Injury: A Literature Critique and Meta-analysis (1983–1992)." *Journal of the American Paraplegia Society* 17 (2): 60–66.

Fadem, Pamela, Meredith Minkler, Martha Perry, Klaus Blum, Leroy F. Moore, Jr., Judi Rogers, and Lee Williams. 2003. "Attitudes of People with Disabilities toward Physician-Assisted Suicide Legislation: Broadening the Dialogue." *Journal of Health Politics, Policy and Law* 28 (6): 977–1001.

Farrow, Jeff. 1990. "Sexuality Counseling with Clients Who Have Spinal Cord Injuries." *Rehabilitation Counseling Bulletin* 33 (3): 251–59.

Feigin, Rena. 1994. "Spousal Adjustment to Postmarital Disability in One Partner." *Family Systems Medicine* 12 (3): 235–47.

Ferington, Felicitus E. 1986. "Personal Control and Coping Effectiveness in Spinal Cord Injured Persons." *Research in Nursing and Health* 9 (3): 257–65.

Ferreiro-Velasco, M. E., A. Barca-Buyo, S. Salvador de la Barrera, A. Montoto-Marqués, X. Miguéns Vázquez, and A. Rodríguez-Sotillo. 2005. "Sexual Issues in a Sample of Women with Spinal Cord Injury." *Spinal Cord* 43 (1): 51–55.

Fichten, Catherine S., Kristen Robillard, Darlene Judd, and Rhonda Amsel. 1989. "College Students with Physical Disabilities: Myths and Realities." *Rehabilitation Psychology* 34 (4): 243–57.

Fine, Michelle, and Adrienne Asch. 1985. "Disabled Women: Sexism without the Pedestal." Chapter 2 in *Women and Disability: The Double Handicap,* edited by Mary Jo Deegan and Nancy A. Brooks, pp. 6–22. New Brunswick: Transaction Books.

Fine, Michelle, and Adrienne Asch. 1988a. "Disability Beyond Stigma: Social Interaction, Discrimination, and Activism." *Journal of Social Issues* 44 (1): 3–21.

Fine, Michelle, and Adrienne Asch. 1988b. "Introduction: Beyond Pedestals." Chapter 1 in *Women with Disabilities: Essays in Psychology, Culture, and Politics,* edited by Michelle Fine and Adrienne Asch, pp. 1–37. Philadelphia: Temple University Press.

Fine, Michelle, and Adrienne Asch, editors. 1988c. *Women with Disabilities: Essays in Psychology, Culture, and Politics.* Philadelphia: Temple University Press.

Finkelstein, Victor. 1980. *Attitudes and Disabled People.* New York: World Rehabilitation Fund.

Finkelstein, Vic. 1993. "The Commonality of Disability." Chapter 1.1 in *Disabling Bar-*

riers—*Enabling Environments,* edited by John Swain, Vic Finkelstein, Sally French, and Mike Oliver, pp. 9–16. Newbury Park, CA: Sage.

Finkelstein, Vic, and Sally French. 1993. "Towards a Psychology of Disability." Chapter 1.3 in *Disabling Barriers—Enabling Environments,* edited by John Swain, Vic Finkelstein, Sally French, and Mike Oliver, pp. 26–33. Newbury Park, CA: Sage.

Finkelstein, Vic, and Ossie Stuart. 1996. "Developing New Services." Chapter 17 in *Beyond Disability: Towards an Enabling Society,* edited by Gerald Hales, pp. 170–87. Thousand Oaks, CA: Sage.

Finnerup, N. B., and T. S. Jensen. 2004. "Spinal Cord Injury Pain—Mechanisms and Treatment." *European Journal of Neurology* 11 (2): 73–82.

Fisher, Bernice, and Roberta Galler. 1988. "Friendship and Fairness: How Disability Affects Friendship between Women." Chapter 6 in *Women with Disabilities: Essays in Psychology, Culture, and Politics,* edited by Michelle Fine and Adrienne Asch, pp. 172–94. Philadelphia: Temple University Press.

Fisher, Gilbert, and Melinda Upp. 1998. "Growth in Federal Disability Programs and Implications for Policy." In *Growth in Disability Benefits: Explanations and Policy Implications,* edited by Kalman Rupp and David C. Stapleton, pp. 288–97. Kalamazoo, MI: W. E. Upjohn Institute for Employment Research.

Fitchett, George, Bruce D. Rybarczyk, Gail A. DeMarco, and John J. Nicholas. 1999. "The Role of Religion in Medical Rehabilitation Outcomes: A Longitudinal Study." *Rehabilitation Psychology* 44 (4): 333–53.

Fitting, Melinda Dell, Susan Salisbury, Norma H. Davies, and Dan K. Mayclin. 1978. "Self-concept and Sexuality of Spinal Cord Injured Women." *Archives of Sexual Behavior* 7 (2): 143–56.

Fitzgerald, Denise Bonga. 1983. *Relationship between Depression and Adjustment in Spinal Cord Injury.* Unpublished doctoral dissertation. Nova University.

Fitzgerald, Jennifer. 1997. "Reclaiming the Whole: Self, Spirit, and Society." *Disability and Rehabilitation* 19 (10): 407–13.

Fordyce, Wilbert E. 1976. "A Behavioral Perspective on Rehabilitation." Chapter 4 in *The Sociology of Physical Disability and Rehabilitation,* edited by Gary L. Albrecht, pp. 73–95. Pittsburgh: University of Pittsburgh Press.

Formal, Christopher. 1992. "Metabolic and Neurologic Changes after Spinal Cord Injury." *Physical Medicine and Rehabilitation Clinics of North America* 3 (4): 783–95.

Fouad, Karim, and Keir Pearson. 2004. "Restoring Walking after Spinal Cord Injury." *Progress in Neurobiology* 73 (2): 107–26.

Fow, Neil R., and Linda S. Rockey. 1995. "A Preliminary Conceptualization of the Influence of Personality and Psychological Development on Group Therapy with Spinal Cord Patients." *Journal of Applied Rehabilitation Counseling* 26 (1): 30–32.

Fox, Amy Jo. 1999. *The Assessment of Independence and Personality in Adults with Spina Bifida and Spinal Cord Injury.* Unpublished doctoral dissertation. Fairleigh Dickinson University.

Fox, Sherry W., Barbara J. Anderson, and William O. McKinley. 1996. "Case Management and Critical Pathways: Links to Quality Care for Persons with Spinal Cord Injury." *American Rehabilitation* 22 (4): 20–25.

Frank, Robert G., Timothy R. Elliott, James R. Corcoran, and Stephen Wonderlich.

1987. "Depression after Spinal Cord Injury: Is it Necessary?" *Clinical Psychology Review* 7 (6): 611–30.

Frank, Robert G., Javad H. Kashani, Stephen A. Wonderlich, Alexander Lising, and Luis R. Visot. 1985. "Depression and Adrenal Function in Spinal Cord Injury." *American Journal of Psychiatry* 142 (2): 252–53.

Frank, Robert G., Robert L. Umlauf, Stephen A. Wonderlich, Glenn S. Askanazi, Susan P. Buckelew, and Timothy R. Elliott. 1987. "Differences in Coping Styles among Persons with Spinal Cord Injury: A Cluster-Analytic Approach." *Journal of Consulting and Clinical Psychology* 55 (5): 727–31.

Frank, Roger A. 1992. *Structured Group Psychotherapy for Individuals with Spinal Cord Injury.* Unpublished doctoral dissertation. Oregon State University.

Frankl, Viktor E. 1959. *Man's Search for Meaning: An Introduction to Logotherapy.* Boston: Beacon Press.

Freehafer, Alvin A. 1997. *Endless Struggle: Spinal Cord Injury.* Pittsburgh: Dorrance.

Frega, Donald L. 1996. *Computer Use Prior to and Following a Spinal Cord Injury.* Unpublished master's thesis. Rush University.

Freijat, Hashem Ahmed. 2000. *The Lived Experience of Spirituality of Jordanian Spinal Cord Injured Patients.* Unpublished doctoral dissertation. Catholic University.

French, Sally. 1993a. "Disability, Impairment or Something in Between?" Chapter 1.2 in *Disabling Barriers—Enabling Environments,* edited by John Swain, Vic Finkelstein, Sally French, and Mike Oliver, pp. 17–25. Newbury Park, CA: Sage.

French, Sally. 1993b. "Experiences of Disabled Health and Caring Professionals." Chapter 4.2 in *Disabling Barriers—Enabling Environments,* edited by John Swain, Vic Finkelstein, Sally French, and Mike Oliver, pp. 201–10. Newbury Park, CA: Sage.

French, Sally. 1996. "The Attitudes of Health Professionals towards Disabled People." Chapter 15 in *Beyond Disability: Towards an Enabling Society,* edited by Gerald Hales, pp. 151–62. Thousand Oaks, CA: Sage.

Frieden, Lex, and Jean A. Cole. 1985. "Independence: The Ultimate Goal of Rehabilitation for Spinal Cord-Injured Persons." *The American Journal of Occupational Therapy* 39 (11): 734–39.

Frost, Frederick. 1993. "Role of Rehabilitation after Spinal Cord Injury." *Urologic Clinics of North America* 20 (3): 549–59.

Fuhrer, Marcus J., Susan L. Garber, Diana H. Rintala, Rebecca Clearman, and Karen A. Hart. 1993. "Pressure Ulcers in Community-Resident Persons with Spinal Cord Injury: Prevalence and Risk Factors." *Archives of Physical Medicine and Rehabilitation* 74 (11): 1172–77.

Fuhrer, Marcus J., Diana H. Rintala, Karen A. Hart, Rebecca Clearman, and Mary Ellen Young. 1992. "Relationship of Life Satisfaction to Impairment, Disability, and Handicap among Persons with Spinal Cord Injury Living in the Community." *Archives of Physical Medicine and Rehabilitation* 73 (6): 552–57.

Fuhrer, Marcus J., Diana H. Rintala, Karen A. Hart, Rebecca Clearman, and Mary Ellen Young. 1993. "Depression Symptomatology in Persons with Spinal Cord Injury Who Reside in the Community." *Archives of Physical Medicine and Rehabilitation* 74 (3): 255–60.

Fullerton, Donald T., Richard F. Harvey, Marjorie H. Klein, and Timothy Howell. 1981.

"Psychiatric Disorders in Patients with Spinal Cord Injuries." *Archives of General Psychiatry* 38 (12): 1369–71.

Galvin, L. R., and H. P. D. Godfrey. 2001. "The Impact of Coping on Emotional Adjustment to Spinal Cord Injury (SCI): Review of the Literature and Application of a Stress Appraisal and Coping Formulation." *Spinal Cord* 39 (12): 615–27.

Garden, Fae H. 1991. "Incidence of Sexual Dysfunction in Neurologic Disability." *Sexuality and Disability* 9 (1): 39–47.

Gatens, Cynthia Ellen. 1980. *Sexuality and the Woman with a Spinal Cord Injury.* Unpublished master's thesis. University of Washington.

Geiger, Robert C. 1979. "Neurophysiology of Sexual Response in Spinal Cord Injury." *Sexuality and Disability* 2 (4): 257–66

Geisler, W. O., A. T. Jousse, Megan Wynne-Jones, and D. Breithaupt. 1983. "Survival in Traumatic Spinal Cord Injury." *Paraplegia* 21 (6): 364–73.

Gerhart, Kenneth A., Susan W. Charlifue, Robert R. Menter, David A. Weitzenkamp, and Gale G. Whiteneck. 1997. "Aging with Spinal Cord Injury." *American Rehabilitation* 23 (1): 19–25.

Giardino, Nicholas D., Mark P. Jensen, Judith A. Turner, Dawn M. Edhe, and Diana D. Cardenas. 2003. "Social Environment Moderates the Association between Catastrophizing and Pain among Persons with Spinal Cord Injury." *Pain* 106 (1–2): 19–25.

Ginis, Kathleen A. Martin, Amy E. Latimer, Kyle McKechnie, David S. Ditor, Neil McCartney, Audrey L. Hicks, Joanne Bugaresti, and B. Catharine Craven. 2003. "Using Exercise to Enhance Subjective Well-Being among People with Spinal Cord Injury: The Mediating Influences of Stress and Pain." *Rehabilitation Psychology* 48 (3): 157–64.

Glaser, Roger M., Thomas W. J. Janssen, Agaram G. Suryaprasad, Satyendra C. Gupta, and Thomas Mathews. 1996. "The Physiology of Exercise." Chapter 1 in *Physical Fitness: A Guide For Individuals with Spinal Cord Injury,* edited by Tamara T. Sowell, pp. 3–23. Washington, DC: Department of Veterans Affairs, Veterans Health Administration, Rehabilitation Research and Development Service, Scientific and Technical Publications Section.

Glass, Edward J. 1980–1981. "Problem Drinking among the Blind and Visually Impaired." *Alcohol Health and Research World* 5 (2): 20–25.

Glickman, Scott, and Michael Kamm. 1996. "Bowel Dysfunction in Spinal-Cord-Injury Patients." *The Lancet* 347 (9016): 1651–53.

Gliedman, John, and William Roth. 1980. *The Unexpected Minority: Handicapped Children in America.* New York: Harcourt Brace Jovanovich.

Glow, Benita Anne. 1989. "Alcohol, Drugs and the Disabled." Chapter 4 in *Alcoholism and Substance Abuse in Special Populations,* edited by Gary W. Lawson and Ann W. Lawson, pp. 65–93. Rockville, MD: Aspen.

Go, Bette K., Michael J. DeVivo, and J. Scott Richards. 1995. "The Epidemiology of Spinal Cord Injury." Chapter 3 in *Spinal Cord Injury: Clinical Outcomes from the Model Systems,* edited by Samuel L. Stover, Joel A. DeLisa, and Gale G. Whiteneck, pp. 21–55. Gaithersburg, MD: Aspen.

Godshall, Frank J. 1989. *Psychological Adjustment as a Function of Problem Solving Self-Appraisal among Persons with Spinal Cord Injury.* Unpublished master's thesis. Virginia Commonwealth University.

Goffman, Erving. 1963. *Stigma: Notes on the Management of Spoiled Identity.* Englewood Cliffs, NJ: Prentice-Hall.

Gold, Judy R. 1983. *The Relationship among Selected Personality Characteristics, Activity Patterns of Adjustment, and Manner of Onset of Spinal Cord Injury.* Unpublished doctoral dissertation. New York University.

Goldman, Howard H. 1998. "Policy Implications of Recent Growth in Beneficiaries with Mental Illness." In *Growth in Disability Benefits: Explanations and Policy Implications,* edited by Kalman Rupp and David C. Stapleton, pp. 337–41. Kalamazoo, MI: W. E. Upjohn Institute for Employment Research.

Goldstein, Marlene. 1996. *An Ethnographic Study of Leisure Participation among People with Spinal Cord Injury.* Unpublished doctoral dissertation. New York University.

Goodrich, James Tait. 2004. "History of Spine Surgery in the Ancient and Medieval Worlds." *Neurosurgical Focus* 16 (1): 1–13.

Gordon, Wayne A., and Margaret Brown. 1997. "Community Integration of Individuals with Spinal Cord Injuries." *American Rehabilitation* 23 (1): 11–14.

Gordon, Wayne A., Stefan Harasymiw, Susan Bellile, Laurie Lehman, and Biddy Sherman. 1982. "The Relationship between Pressure Sores and Psychosocial Adjustment in Persons with Spinal Cord Injury." *Rehabilitation Psychology* 27 (3): 185–91.

Gove, Walter. 1976. "Societal Reaction Theory and Disability." Chapter 3 in *The Sociology of Physical Disability and Rehabilitation,* edited by Gary L. Albrecht, pp. 57–71. Pittsburgh: University of Pittsburgh Press.

Green, Brian C., Clara C. Pratt, and Tom E. Grigsby. 1984. "Self-Concept among Persons with Long-Term Spinal Cord Injury." *Archives of Physical Medicine and Rehabilitation* 65 (12): 751–54.

Green, Stacy. 1996. "Specific Exercise Programs." Chapter 4 in *Physical Fitness: A Guide For Individuals with Spinal Cord Injury,* edited by Tamara T. Sowell, pp. 45–96. Washington, DC: Department of Veterans Affairs, Veterans Health Administration, Rehabilitation Research and Development Service, Scientific and Technical Publications Section.

Greer, Bobby G. 1986. "Substance Abuse among People with Disabilities: A Problem of Too Much Accessibility." *Journal of Rehabilitation* 52 (1): 34–38.

Griffith, Ernest R., Michael A. Tomko, and Robert J. Timms. 1973. "Sexual Function in Spinal Cord-Injured Patients: A Review." *Archives of Physical Medicine and Rehabilitation* 54 (12): 539–43.

Griffith, Ernest R., and Roberta B. Trieschmann. 1975. "Sexual Functioning in Women with Spinal Cord Injury." *Archives of Physical Medicine and Rehabilitation* 56 (1): 18–21.

Griffith, Ernest R., and Roberta B. Trieschmann. 1976. "Treatment of Sexual Dysfunction in Patients with Physical Disorders." Chapter 10 in *Clinical Management of Sexual Disorders,* edited by Jon K. Meyer, pp. 206–25. Baltimore: Williams and Wilkins.

Grundy, David, and John Russell. 1986. "ABC of Spinal Cord Injury: Later Management and Complications." *British Medical Journal* 292 (6521): 677–80.

Gutierrez, Paul A., Robert R. Young, and Michael Vulpe. 1993. "Spinal Cord Injury: An Overview." *Urologic Clinics of North America* 20 (3): 373–82.

Guttmann, L. 1964. "The Married Life of Paraplegics and Tetraplegics." *Paraplegia* 2: 182–88.

Haber, Lawrence D., and Richard T. Smith. 1971. "Disability and Deviance: Normative Adaptations of Role Behavior." *American Sociological Review* 36 (1): 87–97.

Hadley, Robert G., and Martin G. Brodwin. 1988. "Language About People with Disabilities." *Journal of Counseling and Development* 67 (3): 147–49.

Hahn, Harlan. 1986. "Disability and the Urban Environment: A Perspective on Los Angeles." *Society and Space* 4: 273–88.

Hahn, Harlan. 1988a. "Can Disability Be Beautiful?" *Social Policy* 18 (3): 26–32.

Hahn, Harlan. 1988b. "The Politics of Physical Differences: Disability and Discrimination." *Journal of Social Issues* 44 (1): 39–47.

Hahn, Harlan. 1993. "The Political Implications of Disability Definitions and Data." *Journal of Disability Policy Studies* 4 (2): 41–52.

Hahn, Harlan. 1994. "The Minority Group Model of Disability: Implications for Medical Sociology." *Research in Sociology of Health Care* 11: 3–24.

Hahnstadt, William Arl. 1985. *Physiological and Subjective Responses to Emotional Incidents as Related to Level of Spinal Cord Injury.* Unpublished doctoral dissertation. University of Kansas.

Halstead, Lauro S. 1985. "Sexuality and Disability." Chapter 18 in *Emotional Rehabilitation of Physical Trauma and Disability,* edited by David W. Krueger, pp. 235–52. New York: Spectrum Publications.

Halstead, Lauro S., and S. W. J. Seager. 1993. "Electroejaculation and Its Techniques in Males with Neurologic Impairments." Chapter 27 in *Reproductive Issues for Persons with Physical Disabilities,* edited by Florence P. Haseltine, Sandra S. Cole, and David B. Gray, pp. 311–30. Baltimore: Paul H. Brookes.

Hamilton, Kenneth W. 1950. *Counseling the Handicapped in the Rehabilitation Process.* New York: Ronald Press.

Hammell, Karen R. Whalley. 1994. "Establishing Objectives in Occupational Therapy Practice, Part 1." *British Journal of Occupational Therapy* 57 (1): 9–14.

Hammell, K. Whalley. 2004a. "Exploring Quality of Life Following High Spinal Cord Injury: A Review and Critique." *Spinal Cord* 42 (9): 491–502.

Hammell, K. Whalley. 2004b. "Quality of Life among People with High Spinal Cord Injury Living in the Community." *Spinal Cord* 42 (11): 607–20.

Hammond, Margaret C., Robert L. Umlauf, Brenda Matteson, and Sonya Perduta-Fulginiti, editors. 1992. *Yes, You Can! A Guide to Self-Care for Persons with Spinal Cord Injury.* Washington, DC: Paralyzed Veterans of America.

Hampton, Nan Zhang. 2004. "Subjective Well-Being among People with Spinal Cord Injuries." *Rehabilitation Counseling Bulletin* 48 (1): 31–37.

Hanak, Marcia, and Anne Scott. 1983. *Spinal Cord Injury: An Illustrated Guide for Health Care Professionals.* New York: Springer.

Hancock, K. M., A. R. Craig, H. G. Dickson, E. Chang, and J. Martin. 1993. "Anxiety and Depression Over the First Year of Spinal Cord Injury: A Longitudinal Study." *Paraplegia* 31 (6): 349–57.

Hancock, Karen, Ashley Craig, Chris Tennant, and Esther Chang. 1993. "The Influence of Spinal Cord Injury on Coping Styles and Self-Perceptions: A Controlled Study." *Australian and New Zealand Journal of Psychiatry* 27 (3): 450–56.

Haney, Maureen Ann. 1982. *Modifying Attitudes toward the Disabled while Resocializing*

*Spinal Cord Injury Patients.* Unpublished master's thesis. California State University at Long Beach.

Hanks, Jane R., and L. M. Hanks, Jr. 1948. "The Physically Handicapped in Certain Non-Occidental Societies." *Journal of Social Issues* 4 (3): 11–20.

Hanna, William John, and Betsy Rogovsky. 1993. "Women with Disabilities: Two Handicaps Plus." In *Perspectives on Disability,* 2nd Edition, edited by Mark Nagler, pp. 109–19. Palo Alto, CA: Health Markets Research.

Hanson, Richard W., and Michael R. Franklin. 1976. "Sexual Loss in Relation to Other Functional Losses for Spinal Cord Injured Males." *Archives of Physical Medicine and Rehabilitation* 57 (6): 291–93.

Hanson, Stephanie, Susan P. Buckelew, John Hewett, and Grant O'Neal. 1993. "The Relationship between Coping and Adjustment after Spinal Cord Injury: A 5-Year Follow-Up Study." *Rehabilitation Psychology* 38 (1): 41–52.

Hardy, Richard E., and John G. Cull. 1983. "Counseling with Severely Disabled Persons: A Basic Component in Independent Living Services." Chapter 28 in *Vocational Evaluation, Work Adjustment, and Independent Living for Severely Disabled People,* edited by Robert A. Lassiter, Martha Hughes Lassiter, Richard E. Hardy, J. William Underwood, and John G. Cull, pp. 344–75. Springfield, IL: Charles C. Thomas.

Harris, Phillip, S. S. Patel, Wendy Greer, and J. A. L. Naughton. 1973. "Psychological and Social Reactions to Acute Spinal Paralysis." *Paraplegia* 11 (2): 132–36.

Hart, Geraldine. 1981. "Spinal Cord Injury: Impact on Clients' Significant Others." *Rehabilitation Nursing* 6 (1): 11–15.

Harvey, C., B. B. Rothschild, A. J. Asmann, and T. Stripling. 1990. "New Estimates of Traumatic SCI Prevalence: A Survey-based Approach." *Paraplegia* 28 (9): 537–44.

Harvey, C., S. E. Wilson, C. G. Greene, M. Berkowitz, and T. E. Stripling. 1992. "New Estimates of the Direct Costs of Traumatic Spinal Cord Injuries: Results of a Nationwide Survey." *Paraplegia* 30 (12): 834–50.

Hawkins, Darlene A., and Allen W. Heinemann. 1998. "Substance Abuse and Medical Complications Following Spinal Cord Injury." *Rehabilitation Psychology* 43 (3): 219–31.

Hayes, Richard L., Carol G. Potter, and Camille Hardin. 1995. "Counseling the Client on Wheels: A Primer for Mental Health Service Counselors New to Spinal Cord Injury." *Journal of Mental Health Counseling* 17 (1): 18–30.

Heinemann, Allen W. 1993. "Prevalence and Consequences of Alcohol and Other Drug Problems Following Spinal Cord Injury." Chapter 5 in *Substance Abuse and Physical Disability,* edited by Allen W. Heinemann, pp. 63–78. New York: Haworth.

Heinemann, Allen W., Matthew Doll, and Sidney Schnoll. 1989. "Treatment of Alcohol Abuse in Persons with Recent Spinal Cord Injuries." *Alcohol Health and Research World* 13 (2): 110–17.

Heinemann, Allen W., Nancy Goranson, Karen Ginsburg, and Sidney Schnoll. 1989. "Alcohol Use and Activity Patterns Following Spinal Cord Injury." *Rehabilitation Psychology* 34 (3): 191–205.

Heinemann, Allen W., Brian Mamott, Mary Keen, and Sidney Schnoll. 1987. *Substance Use by Persons with Recent Spinal Cord Injuries.* Washington, DC: U. S. Department of Education.

Heinemann, Allen W., Brian D. Mamott, and Sidney Schnoll. 1990. "Substance Use by Persons with Recent Spinal Cord Injuries." *Rehabilitation Psychology* 35 (4): 217–28.

Heinemann, Allen W., Mary F. Schmidt, and Patrick Semik. 1994. "Drinking Patterns, Drinking Expectancies, and Coping after Spinal Cord Injury." *Rehabilitation Psychology* 38 (2): 134–53.

Heinrich, Robert K., and Denise G. Tate. 1996. "Latent Variable Structure of the Brief Symptom Inventory in a Sample of Persons with Spinal Cord Injury." *Rehabilitation Psychology* 41 (2): 131–47.

Henderson, George, and Willie V. Bryan. 1984. *Psychosocial Aspects of Disability.* Springfield, IL: Charles C. Thomas.

Henderson, Karla A., Leandra A. Bedini, and Lynn Hecht. 1994. "'Not Just a Wheelchair, Not Just a Woman': Self-Identity and Leisure." *Therapeutic Recreation Journal* 28 (2): 73–86.

Hendrick, Susan S. 1981. "Spinal Cord Injury: A Special Kind of Loss." *Personnel and Guidance Journal* 59 (6): 355–59.

Henwood, Penelope, and Jacqueline A. Ellis. 2004. "Chronic Neuropathic Pain in Spinal Cord Injury: The Patient's Perspective." *Pain Research and Management* 9 (1): 39–45.

Herrick, Stephen, Timothy R. Elliott, and Frank Crow. 1994a. "Self-Appraised Problem-Solving Skills and the Prediction of Secondary Complications among Persons with Spinal Cord Injuries." *Journal of Clinical Psychology in Medical Settings* 1 (3): 269–83.

Herrick, Stephen, Timothy R. Elliott, and Frank Crow. 1994b. "Social Support and the Prediction of Health Complications among Persons with Spinal Cord Injuries." *Rehabilitation Psychology* 39 (4): 231–50.

Herron, Carolyn Paula. 1987. *Vocational Needs, Locus of Control, and Demographic Variables as Related to Productivity Following Spinal Cord Injury.* Unpublished doctoral dissertation. University of Minnesota.

Heslinga, K., A. M. C. M. Schellen, and A. Verkuyl. 1974. *Not Made of Stone: The Sexual Problems of Handicapped People.* Springfield, IL: Charles C. Thomas.

Hevey, David. 1993. "The Tragedy Principle: Strategies for Change in the Representation of Disabled People." Chapter 2.7 in *Disabling Barriers—Enabling Environments,* edited by John Swain, Vic Finkelstein, Sally French, and Mike Oliver, pp. 117–21. Newbury Park, CA: Sage.

Higgins, Glenn E., Jr. 1979. "Sexual Response in Spinal Cord Injured Adults: A Review of the Literature." *Archives of Sexual Behavior* 8 (2): 173–96.

Hingley, Audrey T. 1993. "Spinal Cord Injuries." *FDA Consumer* 27 (6): 14–18.

Hohmann, George W. 1966. "Some Effects of Spinal Cord Lesions on Experienced Emotional Feelings." *Psychophysiology* 3 (2): 143–56.

Hohmann, George W. 1972. "Considerations in Management of Psychosexual Readjustment in the Cord Injured Male." *Rehabilitation Psychology* 19 (2): 50–58.

Hohmann, George W. 1975. "Psychological Interventions in the Spinal Cord Injury Center: Some Cautions." *Rehabilitation Psychology* 22 (4): 194–96.

Hopkins, Mary T. 1971. "Patterns of Self-Destruction among the Orthopedically Disabled." *Rehabilitation Research and Practice Review* 3 (1): 5–16.

Horton, Trudi Venters. 1999. *The Role of Religion in the Adjustment of Mothers of Children with Chronic Physical Conditions.* Unpublished doctoral dissertation. University of Alabama at Birmingham.

Houda, Barbara. 1993. "Evaluation of Nutritional Status in Persons with Spinal Cord Injury: A Prerequisite for Successful Rehabilitation." *SCI Nursing* 10 (1): 4–7.

Houle, John D., and Alan Tessler. 2003. "Repair of Chronic Spinal Cord Injury." *Experimental Neurology* 182 (2): 247–60.

Houlihan, Bethlyn Vergo, Mari-Lynn Drainoni, Grace Warner, Shanker Nesathurai, Jane Wierbicky, and Steven Williams. 2003. "The Impact of Internet Access for People with Spinal Cord Injuries: A Descriptive Analysis of a Pilot Study." *Disability and Rehabilitation* 25 (8): 422–31.

Houston, Eva M. 1999. *What Are the Roles of Spiritual and Religious Practices, Attitudes, and Beliefs in the Lives of People with Acquired Physical Disabilities?* Unpublished doctoral dissertation. University of Wisconsin at Madison.

Howard, Brenda S., and Jay R. Howard. 1997. "Occupation as Spiritual Activity." *American Journal of Occupational Therapy* 51 (3): 181–85.

Howell, Timothy, Donald T. Fullerton, Richard F. Harvey, and Marjorie Klein. 1981. "Depression in Spinal Cord Injured Patients." *Paraplegia* 19 (5): 284–88.

Hudson, Megan Louise. 1990. *Family Adjustment Following Closed Head Injury or Spinal Cord Injury.* Unpublished doctoral dissertation. George Washington University.

Hundley, Jo Ann. 1985. *Social Competence and Pressure Sores in Spinal Cord Injury.* Unpublished doctoral dissertation. University of North Carolina at Chapel Hill.

Hutchinson, Susan L., and Douglas A. Kleiber. 2000. "Heroic Masculinity Following Spinal Cord Injury: Implications for Therapeutic Recreation Practice and Research." *Therapeutic Recreation Journal* 34 (1): 42–54.

Hwang, Karen. 1997. "Living with a Disability: A Woman's Perspective." Chapter 7 in *Sexual Function in People with Disability and Chronic Illness: A Health Professional's Guide,* edited by Marca L. Sipski and Craig J. Alexander, pp. 119–30. Gaithersburg, MD: Aspen.

Idler, Ellen. 1994. *Cohesiveness and Coherence: Religion and the Health of the Elderly.* New York: Garland.

Idler, Ellen L. and Stanislav V. Kasl. 1992. "Religion, Disability, Depression, and the Timing of Death." *American Journal of Sociology* 97 (4): 1052–79.

Idler, Ellen L. and Stanislav V. Kasl. 1997a. "Religion among Disabled and Nondisabled Persons I: Cross-sectional Patterns in Health Practices, Social Activities, and Well-Being." *Journal of Gerontology: Social Sciences* 52b (6): S294–S305.

Idler, Ellen L. and Stanislav V. Kasl. 1997b. "Religion among Disabled and Nondisabled Persons II: Attendance at Religious Services as a Predictor of the Course of Disability." *Journal of Gerontology: Social Sciences* 52b (6): S306–S316.

Ikata, Takaaki. 1987. "Resettlement and Employment of Paraplegic Patients in Japan." *Paraplegia* 25 (3): 308–9.

Inge, Katherine J., Paul Wehman, John Kregel, and Pam Sherron Targett. 1996. "Vocational Rehabilitation for Persons with Spinal Cord Injuries and Other Severe Physical Disabilities." *American Rehabilitation* 22 (4): 2–12.

Inge, Katherine J., Paul Wehman, Wendy Strobel, Deanie Powell, and Jennifer Todd. 1998. "Supported Employment and Assistive Technology for Persons with Spinal Cord Injury: Three Illustrations of Successful Work Supports." *Journal of Vocational Rehabilitation* 10 (2): 141–52.

Ingstad, Benedicte, and Susan Reynolds Whyte. 1995. "Disability and Culture: An Overview." Chapter 1 in *Disability and Culture,* edited by Susan Reynolds Whyte and Benedicte Ingstad, pp. 3–32. Berkeley: University of California Press.

Inniss, Patrick. 1994. *A Study of Daily Life Activities of Spinal Cord Injured Women.* Unpublished doctoral dissertation. New York University.

Isaacson, June, and Harriet E. Delgado. 1974. "Sex Counseling for Those with Spinal Cord Injuries." *Social Casework* 55 (10): 622–27.

Jackson, Amie B., Marcel Dijkers, Michael J. DeVivo, and Robert B. Poczatek. 2004. "A Demographic Profile of New Traumatic Spinal Cord Injuries: Change and Stability Over 30 Years." *Archives of Physical Medicine and Rehabilitation* 85 (11): 1740–48.

Jackson, Amie B., Virginia G. Wadley, J. Scott Richards, and Michael J. DeVivo. 1995. "Sexual Behavior and Function among Spinal Cord Injured Women." *The Journal of Spinal Cord Medicine* 18: 141.

Jackson, R. W. 1987. "Sport for the Spinal Paralysed Person." *Paraplegia* 25 (3): 301–4.

James, Magna, Michael J. DeVivo, and J. Scott Richards. 1993. "Postinjury Employment Outcomes among African-Americans and White Persons with Spinal Cord Injury." *Rehabilitation Psychology* 38 (3): 151–64.

Jang, Yuh, Yen-Ho Wang, and Jung-Der Wang. 2005. "Return to Work after Spinal Cord Injury in Taiwan: The Contribution of Functional Independence." *Archives of Physical Medicine and Rehabilitation* 86 (4): 681–86.

Johnston, Mark V., Kenneth Wood, Scott Millis, Steve Page, and David Chen. 2004. "Perceived Quality of Care and Outcomes Following Spinal Cord Injury: Minority Status in the Context of Multiple Predictors." *The Journal of Spinal Cord Medicine* 27 (3): 241–51.

Jubala, John A., and Gilbert Brenes. 1988. "Spinal Cord Injuries." Chapter 25 in *Handbook of Developmental and Physical Disabilities,* edited by Vincent B. Van Hasselt, Phillip S. Strain, and M. Hersen, pp. 423–38. Oxford: Pergamon.

Judd, Fiona K., and Douglas J. Brown. 1992. "Psychiatric Consultation in a Spinal Injuries Unit." *Australian & New Zealand Journal of Psychiatry* 26 (2): 218–22.

Judd, Fiona K., Jillian Stone, John E. Webber, Douglas J. Brown, and Graham D. Burrows. 1989. "Depression Following Spinal Cord Injury: A Prospective In-patient Study." *British Journal of Psychiatry* 154 (May): 668–71.

Kailes, June Isaacson. 1985. "Watch Your Language, Please!" *Journal of Rehabilitation* 51 (1): 68–69.

Kallianes, Virginia, and Phyllis Rubenfeld. 1997. "Disabled Women and Reproductive Rights." *Disability & Society* 12 (2): 203–21.

Kanellos, Margaret Carrol. 1985. "Enhancing Vocational Outcomes of Spinal Cord-Injured Persons: The Occupational Therapist's Role." *American Journal of Occupational Therapy* 39 (11): 726–33.

Karp, Gary, and Stanley D. Klein, editors. 2004. *From There to Here: Stories of Adjustment to Spinal Cord Injury.* Horsham, PA: No Limits Communication.

Kasprzyk, Danuta Maria. 1983. *Psychological Factors Associated with Responses to Hypertension or Spinal Cord Injury: An Investigation of Coping with a Chronic Illness or Disability.* Unpublished doctoral dissertation. University of Washington.

Katz, Alfred H., and Knute Martin. 1982. *A Handbook of Services for the Handicapped.* Westport, CT: Greenwood.

Katz, Irwin, R. Glen Hass, and Joan Bailey. 1988. "Attitudinal Ambivalence and Behavior toward People with Disabilities." Chapter 4 in *Attitudes toward Persons with Disabili-ties,* edited by Harold E. Yuker, pp. 47–57. New York: Springer.

Katz, Jonathan F., Joan C. Adler, Nicholas J. Mazzarella, and Laurence P. Ince. 1985. "Psychological Consequences of an Exercise Training Program for a Paraplegic Man: A Case Study." *Rehabilitation Psychology* 30 (1): 53–58.

Katz, Shlomo, and Shlomo Kravetz. 1987. "Rehabilitation Status of Spinal Cord Injured Persons." *International Journal of Rehabilitation Research* 10 (4): 428–30.

Keller, Sandra, and Denton C. Buchanan. 1993. "Sexuality and Disability: An Overview." In *Perspectives on Disability,* 2nd Edition, edited by Mark Nagler, pp. 227–34. Palo Alto, CA: Health Markets Research.

Kemp, Bryan J., Jason S. Kahan, James S. Krause, Rodney H. Adkins, and Gabriel Nava. 2005. "Treatment of Major Depression in Individuals with Spinal Cord Injury." *The Journal of Spinal Cord Medicine* 27 (1): 22–28.

Kemp, Bryan J., and J. Stuart Krause. 1999. "Depression and Life Satisfaction among People Ageing with Post-Polio and Spinal Cord Injury." *Disability and Rehabilitation* 21 (5–6): 241–49.

Kemp, Bryan, J. Stuart Krause, and Rodney Adkins. 1999. "Depression among Afri-can Americans, Latinos, and Caucasians with Spinal Cord Injury: An Exploratory Study." *Rehabilitation Psychology* 44 (3): 235–47.

Kemp, Bryan J., and Carolyn L. Vash. 1971. "Productivity after Injury in a Sample of Spinal Cord Injured Persons: A Pilot Study." *Journal of Chronic Disease* 24 (4): 259–75.

Kennedy, Paul. 2001. "Spinal Cord Injuries." Chapter 8.19 in *Health Psychology, Volume 8: Comprehensive Clinical Psychology,* edited by Derek W. Johnston and Marie John-ston, pp. 445–62. Amsterdam: Elsevier Science Publishers.

Kennedy, P., J. Duff, M. Evans, and A. Beedie. 2003. "Coping Effectiveness Training Reduces Depression and Anxiety Following Traumatic Spinal Cord Injury." *British Journal of Clinical Psychology* 42 (1): 41–52.

Kennedy, Paul, Keren Fisher, and Eileen Pearson. 1988. "Ecological Evaluation of a Re-habilitative Environment for Spinal Cord Injured People: Behavioural Mapping and Feedback." *British Journal of Clinical Psychology* 27 (3): 239–46.

Kennedy, Paul, Nicola Gorsuch, and Neal Marsh. 1995. "Childhood Onset of Spinal Cord Injury: Self-Esteem and Self-Perception." *British Journal of Clinical Psychology* 34 (4): 581–88.

Kennedy, Paul, Mal Hopwood, and Jane Duff. 2001. "Psychological Management of Chronic Illness and Disability." Chapter 7 in *Psychology and Psychiatry: Integrating Medical Practice,* edited by Jeannette Milgrom and Graham D. Burrows, pp. 183–211. New York: John Wiley & Sons.

Kennedy, Paul, Robert Lowe, Nick Grey, and Emma Short. 1995. "Traumatic Spinal Cord Injury and Psychological Impact: A Cross-sectional Analysis of Coping Strate-gies." *British Journal of Clinical Psychology* 34 (4): 627–39.

Kennedy, Paul, Neal Marsh, Rob Lowe, Nick Grey, Emma Short, and Ben Rogers. 2000. "A Longitudinal Analysis of Psychological Impact and Coping Strategies Following Spinal Cord Injury." *British Journal of Health Psychology* 5 (Part 2): 157–72.

Kennedy, Paul, Nicola M. Taylor, and Jane Duff. 2005. "Characteristics Predicting Ef-fective Outcomes after Coping Effectiveness Training for Patients with Spinal Cord Injuries." *Journal of Clinical Psychology in Medical Settings* 12 (1): 93–98.

Kester, Barbara Lynn. 1986. *Long-Term Spouse Adjustment to Spinal Cord Injury.* Unpublished doctoral dissertation. University of Vermont.

Kester, Barbara L., Esther D. Rothblum, Debra Lobato, and Raymond L. Milhous. 1988. "Spouse Adjustment to Spinal Cord Injury: Long-term Medical and Psychosocial Factors." *Rehabilitation Counseling Bulletin* 32 (1): 4–21.

Kettl, Paul, Sue Zarefoss, Kevin Jacoby, Christine Garman, Cindy Hulse, Fran Rowley, Robin Corey, Michelle Sredy, Edward Bixler, and Kathy Tyson. 1991. "Female Sexuality after Spinal Cord Injury." *Sexuality and Disability* 9 (4): 287–95.

Kewman, Donald G., and Denise G. Tate. 1998. "Suicide in SCI: A Psychological Autopsy." *Rehabilitation Psychology* 43 (2): 143–51.

Killen, Joan Marie. 1987. *Parental and Spousal Role Changes after Spinal Cord Injury of a Child or Spouse.* Unpublished doctoral dissertation. University of Texas at Austin.

King, Charles, and Paul Kennedy. 1999. "Coping Effectiveness Training for People with Spinal Cord Injury: Preliminary Results of a Controlled Trial." *British Journal of Clinical Psychology* 38 (1): 5–14.

King, Sharon V. 1998. "The Beam In Thine Own Eye: Disability and the Black Church." *The Western Journal of Black Studies* 22 (1): 37–48.

Kirkby, Robert J., Julia Cull, and Peter Foreman. 1996. "Association of Prelesion Sports Participation and Involvement in Wheelchair Sports Following Spinal Cord Injury." *Perceptual and Motor Skills* 82 (2): 481–82.

Kirubakaran, Vellore R., V. Nanda Kumar, Barbara J. Powell, Alan J. Tyler, and Philip J. Armatas. 1986. "Survey of Alcohol and Drug Misuse in Spinal Cord Injured Veterans." *Journal of Studies on Alcohol* 47 (3): 223–27.

Kishi, Yasuhiro, and Robert G. Robinson. 1996. "Suicidal Plans Following Spinal Cord Injury: A Six-Month Study." *Journal of Neuropsychiatry and Clinical Neurosciences* 8 (4): 442–45.

Kishi, Yasuhiro, Robert G. Robinson, and Alfred W. Forrester. 1994. "Prospective Longitudinal Study of Depression Following Spinal Cord Injury." *Journal of Neuropsychiatry and Clinical Neurosciences* 6 (3): 237–44.

Kishi, Yasuhiro, Robert G. Robinson, and Alfred W. Forrester. 1995. "Comparison between Acute and Delayed Onset Major Depression after Spinal Cord Injury." *The Journal of Nervous and Mental Disease* 183 (5): 286–92.

Kishi, Yasuhiro, Robert G. Robinson, and James T. Kosier. 2001. "Suicidal Ideation among Patients with Acute Life-Threatening Physical Illness: Patients with Stroke, Traumatic Brain Injury, Myocardial Infarction, and Spinal Cord Injury." *Psychosomatics* 42 (5): 382–90.

Kjorsvig, Joan Marie. 1994. *Psychosocial Predictors of Longevity Following a Spinal Cord Injury: A Prospective Approach.* Unpublished doctoral dissertation. University of Minnesota.

Kleck, Robert. 1966. "Emotional Arousal in Interactions with Stigmatized Persons." *Psychological Reports* 19 (3): 1226.

Kleck, Robert. 1968. "Physical Stigma and Nonverbal Cues Emitted in Face-to-Face Interaction." *Human Relations* 21 (1): 19–28.

Kleiber, Douglas A., Stephen C. Brock, Youngkhill Lee, John Dattilo, and Linda Caldwell. 1995. "The Relevance of Leisure in an Illness Experience: Realities of Spinal Cord Injury." *Journal of Leisure Research* 27 (3): 283–99.

Knight, Susan E. 1981. "Consumer-Based Sex Education: A Different Look at the Peer Counselor." Chapter 32 in *Sexuality and Physical Disability,* edited by David G. Bullard and Susan E. Knight, pp. 269–75. St. Louis: C. V. Mosby.

Knight, Susan E. 1989. "Sexual Concerns of the Physically Disabled." Chapter 11 in *Psychosocial Interventions with Physically Disabled Persons,* edited by Bruce W. Heller, Louis M. Flohr, and Leonard S. Zegans, pp. 183–99. New Brunswick: Rutgers University Press.

Knorr, Norman J., and John C. Bull. 1970. "Spinal Cord Injury: Psychiatric Considerations." *Maryland State Medical Journal* 19 (4): 105–8.

Knox, Marie, and Trevor R. Parmenter. 1993. "Social Networks and Support Mechanisms for Mild Intellectual Disability in Competitive Employment." *International Journal of Rehabilitation Research* 16 (1): 1–12.

Kocan, Mary Jo. 1990. "Pulmonary Considerations in the Critical Care Phase." *Critical Care Nursing Clinics of North America* 2 (3): 369–74.

Koenig, Harold G., Linda K. George, Keith G. Meador, Dan G. Blazer, and P. B. Dyck. 1994. "Religious Affiliation and Psychiatric Disorder among Protestant Baby Boomers." *Hospital and Community Psychiatry* 45 (6): 586–96.

Kolakowsky-Hayner, Stephanie A., Eugene V. Gourley III, Jeffrey S. Kreutzer, Jennifer H. Marwitz, David X. Cifu, and William O. McKinley. 1999. "Pre-Injury Substance Abuse among Persons with Brain Injury and Persons with Spinal Cord Injury." *Brain Injury* 13 (8): 571–81.

Krassioukov, Andrei V., Julio C. Furlan, and Michael G. Fehlings. 2003. "Autonomic Dysreflexia in Acute Spinal Cord Injury: An Under-Recognized Clinical Entity." *Journal of Neurotrauma* 20 (8): 707–16.

Krause, Elliott A. 1976. "The Political Sociology of Rehabilitation." Chapter 8 in *The Sociology of Physical Disability and Rehabilitation,* edited by Gary L. Albrecht, pp. 201–21. Pittsburgh: The University of Pittsburgh Press.

Krause, James S. 1990. "The Relationship between Productivity and Adjustment Following Spinal Cord Injury." *Rehabilitation Counseling Bulletin* 33 (3): 188–99.

Krause, James S. 1991. "Survival Following Spinal Cord Injury: A Fifteen-Year Prospective Study." *Rehabilitation Psychology* 36 (2): 89–98.

Krause, James S. 1992a. "Adjustment to Life after Spinal Cord Injury: A Comparison among Three Participant Groups Based on Employment Status." *Rehabilitation Counseling Bulletin* 35 (4): 218–29.

Krause, James S. 1992b. "Life Satisfaction after Spinal Cord Injury: A Descriptive Study." *Rehabilitation Psychology* 37 (1): 61–70.

Krause, James S. 1992c. "Employment after Spinal Cord Injury." *Archives of Physical Medicine and Rehabilitation* 73 (2): 163–69.

Krause, J. Stuart. 1996. "Employment after Spinal Cord Injury: Transition and Life Adjustment." *Rehabilitation Counseling Bulletin* 39 (4): 244–55.

Krause, J. Stuart. 1997. "Personality and Traumatic Spinal Cord Injury: Relationship to Participation in Productive Activities." *Journal of Applied Rehabilitation Counseling* 28 (2): 15–20.

Krause, J. Stuart. 1998a. "Changes in Adjustment after Spinal Cord Injury: A 20-Year Longitudinal Study." *Rehabilitation Psychology* 43 (1): 41–55.

Krause, J. Stuart. 1998b. "Subjective Well-Being after Spinal Cord Injury: Relationship to

Gender, Race-Ethnicity, and Chronologic Age." *Rehabilitation Psychology* 43 (4): 282–96.

Krause, James S. 2003. "Years to Employment after Spinal Cord Injury." *Archives of Physical Medicine and Rehabilitation* 84 (9): 1282–89.

Krause, James S. 2004. "Factors Associated with Risk for Subsequent Injuries after Traumatic Spinal Cord Injury." *Archives of Physical Medicine and Rehabilitation* 85 (9): 1503–8.

Krause, J. Stuart, and Carol A. Anson. 1996a. "Employment after Spinal Cord Injury: Relation to Selected Participant Characteristics." *Archives of Physical Medicine and Rehabilitation* 77 (8): 737–43.

Krause, J. Stuart, and Carol A. Anson. 1996b. "Self-Perceived Reasons for Unemployment Cited by Persons with Spinal Cord Injury: Relationships to Gender, Race, Age, and Level of Injury." *Rehabilitation Counseling Bulletin* 39 (3): 217–27.

Krause, J. Stuart, and Carol A. Anson. 1997a. "Adjustment after Spinal Cord Injury: Relationship to Participation in Employment or Educational Activities." *Rehabilitation Counseling Bulletin* 40 (3): 202–14.

Krause, J. Stuart, and Carol A. Anson. 1997b. "Adjustment after Spinal Cord Injury: Relationship to Gender and Race." *Rehabilitation Psychology* 42 (1): 31–46.

Krause, James S., and Lynne Broderick. 2004. "Outcomes after Spinal Cord Injury: Comparisons as a Function of Gender and Race and Ethnicity." *Archives of Physical Medicine and Rehabilitation* 85 (3): 355–62.

Krause, James S., Lynne E. Broderick, and Joy Broyles. 2004. "Subjective Well-Being among African-Americans with Spinal Cord Injury: An Exploratory Study between Men and Women." *NeuroRehabilitation* 19 (2): 81–89.

Krause, J. Stuart, Jennifer Coker, Susan Charlifue, and Gale G. Whiteneck. 1999. "Depression and Subjective Well-Being among 97 American Indians with Spinal Cord Injury: A Descriptive Study." *Rehabilitation Psychology* 44 (4): 354–72.

Krause, James S., and Nancy M. Crewe. 1987. "Prediction of Long-Term Survival of Persons with Spinal Cord Injury: An 11-Year Prospective Study." *Rehabilitation Psychology* 32 (4): 205–13.

Krause, James S., and Nancy M. Crewe. 1991. "Chronologic Age, Time Since Injury, and Time of Measurement: Effect on Adjustment after Spinal Cord Injury." *Archives of Physical Medicine and Rehabilitation* 72 (2): 91–100.

Krause, James S., and Rene V. Dawis. 1992. "Prediction of Life Satisfaction after Spinal Cord Injury: A Four-Year Longitudinal Approach." *Rehabilitation Psychology* 37 (1): 49–60.

Krause, James S., Michael J. DeVivo, and Amie B. Jackson. 2004. "Health Status, Community Integration, and Economic Risk Factors for Mortality after Spinal Cord Injury." *Archives of Physical Medicine and Rehabilitation* 85 (11): 1764–73.

Krause, J. Stuart, Donald Kewman, Michael J. DeVivo, Frederick Maynard, Jennifer Coker, Mary Joan Roach, and Stanley Ducharme. 1999. "Employment after Spinal Cord Injury: An Analysis of Cases from the Model Spinal Cord Injury Systems." *Archives of Physical Medicine and Rehabilitation* 80 (11): 1492–1500.

Krause, J. Stuart, and Daniel E. Rohe. 1998. "Personality and Life Adjustment after Spinal Cord Injury: An Exploratory Study." *Rehabilitation Psychology* 43 (2): 118–30.

Krause, J. Stuart, Carol Anson Stanwyck, and Joseph Maides. 1998. "Locus of Control and Life Adjustment: Relationship among People with Spinal Cord Injury." *Rehabilitation Counseling Bulletin* 41 (3): 162–72.

Krause, James S., Joan Saari, and Dennis Dykstra. 1990. "Quality of Life and Survival after SCI." *SCI Psychosocial Process* 3 (3): 4–8.

Krause, J. Stuart, and Maya Sternberg. 1997. "Aging and Adjustment to Spinal Cord Injury: The Roles of Chronologic Age, Time Since Injury, and Environmental Change." *Rehabilitation Psychology* 42 (4): 287–302.

Kreuter, M., M. Sullivan, and A. Siösteen. 1994a. "Sexual Adjustment after Spinal Cord Injury (SCI) Focusing on Partner Experiences." *Paraplegia* 32 (4): 225–35.

Kreuter, M., M. Sullivan, and A. Siösteen. 1994b. "Sexual Adjustment after Spinal Cord Injury—Comparison of Partner Experiences in Pre- and Postinjury Relationships." *Paraplegia* 32 (11): 759–70.

Kroll-Smith, Steve. 2004. *Diseased or Disabled? Two Strategies for the Social Representation of Contested Bodies.* Unpublished manuscript. University of North Carolina at Greensboro.

Kruse, Douglas, Alan Krueger, and Susan Drastal. 1996. "Computer Use, Computer Training, and Employment: Outcomes among People with Spinal Cord Injuries." *Spine* 21 (7): 891–96.

Kutner, Nancy G. 1987. "Social Ties, Social Support, and Perceived Health Status among Chronically Disabled People." *Social Science and Medicine* 25 (1): 29–34.

La Forge, Jan. 1991. "Preferred Language Practice in Professional Rehabilitation Journals." *Journal of Rehabilitation* 57 (1): 49–51.

Laatsch, Linda, and Bhagwan T. Shahani. 1996. "The Relationship between Age, Gender and Psychological Distress in Rehabilitation Inpatients." *Disability and Rehabilitation* 18 (12): 604–8.

Langer, Karen G. 1994. "Depression and Denial in Psychotherapy of Persons with Disabilities." *Journal of Psychotherapy* 48 (2): 181–94.

Lanig, Indira S., and Daniel P. Lammertse. 1992. "The Respiratory System in Spinal Cord Injury." *Physical Medicine and Rehabilitation Clinics of North America* 3 (4): 725–40.

Lasfargues, J. E., D. Custis, F. Morrone, J. Carswell, and T. Nguyen. 1995. "A Model for Estimating Spinal Cord Injury Prevalence in the United States." *Paraplegia* 33 (2): 62–68.

Lassiter, Robert A. 1983. "Adjustment to Work: Exploring Special Needs of the Severely Physically Disabled Person." Chapter 19 in *Vocational Evaluation, Work Adjustment, and Independent Living for Severely Disabled People,* edited by Robert A. Lassiter, Martha Hughes Lassiter, Richard E. Hardy, J. William Underwood, and John G. Cull, pp. 231–42. Springfield, IL: Charles C. Thomas.

Lathem, Pamela A., Theresa L. Gregorio, and Susan Lipton Garber. 1985. "High-Level Quadriplegia: An Occupational Therapy Challenge." *The American Journal of Occupational Therapy* 39 (11): 705–14.

Leach, Bernard. 1996. "Disabled People and the Equal Opportunities Movement." Chapter 8 in *Beyond Disability: Towards an Enabling Society,* edited by Gerald Hales, pp. 88–95. Thousand Oaks, CA: Sage.

Leduc, Bernard E., and Yves Lepage. 2002. "Health-Related Quality of Life after Spinal Cord Injury." *Disability and Rehabilitation* 24 (4): 196–202.

Lee, Youngkhill, Stephen Brock, John Dattilo, and Douglas Kleiber. 1993. "Leisure and

Adjustment to Spinal Cord Injury: Conceptual and Methodological Suggestions." *Therapeutic Recreation Journal* 27 (3): 200–11.

Lee, Youngkhill, John Dattilo, Douglas A. Kleiber, and Linda Caldwell. 1996. "Exploring the Meaning of Continuity of Recreation Activity in the Early Stages of Adjustment for People with Spinal Cord Injury." *Leisure Sciences* 18 (3): 209–25.

Lee, Youngkhill, and Bryan McCormick. 2004. "Subjective Well-Being of People with Spinal Cord Injury: Does Leisure Contribute?" *Journal of Rehabilitation* 70 (3): 5–12.

Lemon, Marilynn A. 1993. "Sexual Counseling and Spinal Cord Injury." *Sexuality and Disability* 11 (1): 73–97.

Lenney, Michael, and Howard Sercombe. 2002. "'Did You See That Guy in the Wheelchair Down in the Pub?' Interactions across Difference in a Public Place." *Disability and Society* 17 (1): 5–18.

Leonard, Jonathan S. 1986. "Labor Supply Incentives and Disincentives for Disabled Persons." In *Disability and the Labor Market: Economic Problems, Policies, and Programs,* edited by Monroe Berkowitz and M. Anne Hill, pp. 64–94. Ithaca: ILR Press.

Leonard, Jonathan S. 1991. "Disability Policy and the Return to Work." Chapter 4 in *Disability and Work: Incentives, Rights, and Opportunities,* edited by Carolyn L. Weaver, pp. 46–55. Washington, DC: AEI Press.

Levin, Jeff. 2001a. *God, Faith and Health: Exploring the Spirituality-Healing Connection.* New York: John Wiley and Sons.

Levin, Jeff. 2001b. "God, Love, and Health: Findings from a Clinical Study." *Review of Religious Research* 42 (3): 277–93.

Levin, Jeff. 2002. "Is Depressed Affect a Function of One's Relationship with God? Findings from a Study of Primary Care Patients." *International Journal of Psychiatry in Medicine* 32 (4): 379–93.

Levin, Jeffrey S., and Harold Y. Vanderpool. 1987. "Is Frequent Religious Attendance Really Conducive to Better Health? Toward an Epidemiology of Religion." *Social Science and Medicine* 24 (7): 589–600.

Levin, Jeffrey S., and Harold Y. Vanderpool. 1989. "Is Religion Therapeutically Significant for Hypertension?" *Social Science and Medicine* 29 (1): 69–78.

Levitt, Rona. 1980. "Understanding Sexuality and Spinal Cord Injury." *Journal of Neurosurgical Nursing* 12 (2): 88–89.

Li, Li, and Dennis Moore. 1998. "Acceptance of Disability and Its Correlates." *The Journal of Social Psychology* 138 (1): 13–25.

Lifchez, Raymond. 1983. "Designing Supportive Physical Environments." Chapter 8 in *Independent Living for Physically Disabled People: Developing, Implementing, and Evaluating Self-Help Rehabilitation Programs,* edited by Nancy M. Crewe, Irving Kenneth Zola, and associates, pp. 130–56. San Francisco: Jossey-Bass.

Lifshutz, Jason, and Austin Colohan. 2004. "A Brief History of Therapy for Traumatic Spinal Cord Injury." *Neurosurgical Focus* 16 (1): 1–8.

Linsenmeyer, Todd A. 1997. "Management of Male Infertility." Chapter 24 in *Sexual Function in People with Disability and Chronic Illness: A Health Professional's Guide,* edited by Marca L. Sipski and Craig J. Alexander, pp. 487–508. Gaithersburg, MD: Aspen.

Linton, Simi S. 1985. *Sexual Satisfaction Following Spinal Cord Injury as a Function of Locus of Control.* Unpublished doctoral dissertation. New York University.

Linton, Simi S. 1990. "Sexual Satisfaction in Males Following Spinal Cord Injury as a Function of Locus of Control." *Rehabilitation Psychology* 35 (1): 19–27.

Linton, Simi. 1998. *Claiming Disability: Knowledge and Identity.* New York: New York University Press.

Livneh, Hanoch. 2000. "Psychosocial Adaptation to Spinal Cord Injury: The Role of Coping Strategies." *Journal of Applied Rehabilitation Counseling* 31 (2): 3–10.

Livneh, Hanoch, and Richard F. Antonak. 1997. *Psychosocial Adaptation to Chronic Illness and Disability.* Gaithersburg, MD: Aspen.

Livneh, Hanoch, and Erin Martz. 2003. "Psychosocial Adaptation to Spinal Cord Injury as a Function of Time Since Injury." *International Journal of Rehabilitation Research* 26 (3): 191–200.

Loeser, John D. 2002. "Pain after Spinal Cord Injury." Chapter 1 in *Spinal Cord Injury Pain: Assessment, Mechanisms, Management,* edited by Robert P. Yezierski and Kim J. Burchiel, pp. 3–8. Seattle: IASP Press.

Lohne, Vibeke, and Elisabeth Severinsson. 2003. "Hope During the First Months after Acute Spinal Cord Injury." *Journal of Advanced Nursing* 47 (3): 279–86.

Longmore, Paul K. 1996. "Disability Community Leaders Denounce Jack Kevorkian." Independent Living Institute. Retrieved August 9, 2005, at www.independentliving.org.

Longmore, Paul. 1997. "Reasons to Oppose PAS." ZNet. Retrieved October 3, 2005, at www.zmag.org.

Longo, Daniele A., and Stephanie M. Peterson. 2002. "The Role of Spirituality in Psychosocial Rehabilitation." *Psychiatric Rehabilitation Journal* 25 (4): 333–40.

Loughead, Richard M. 1983. *Males' Perception of Changes in their Sex Role Orientation as a Function of Spinal Cord Injury.* Unpublished doctoral dissertation. Kent State University.

Lovitt, Robert. 1970. "Sexual Adjustment of Spinal Cord Injury Patients." *Rehabilitation Research and Practice Review* 1 (3): 25–29.

Low, Jacqueline. 1996. "Negotiating Identities, Negotiating Environments: An Interpretation of the Experiences of Students with Disabilities." *Disability & Society* 11 (2): 235–48.

Lowe, Judith, and Douglas Carroll. 1985. "The Effect of Spinal Injury on the Intensity of Emotional Experience." *British Journal of Clinical Psychology* 24 (2): 135–36.

Loy, David P., John Dattilo, and Douglas A. Kleiber. 2003. "Exploring the Influence of Leisure on Adjustment: Development of the Leisure and Spinal Cord Injury Adjustment Model." *Leisure Sciences* 25 (2–3): 231–55.

Lude, P., P. Kennedy, M. Evans, Y. Lude, and A. Beedie. 2005. "Post Traumatic Distress Symptoms Following Spinal Cord Injury: A Comparative Review of European Samples." *Spinal Cord* 43 (2): 102–8.

Lundqvist, C., A. Siösteen, C. Blomstrand, B. Lind, and M. Sullivan. 1991. "Spinal Cord Injuries: Clinical, Functional, and Emotional Status." *Spine* 16 (1): 78–83.

Lustig, Daniel C. 2005. "The Adjustment Process for Individuals with Spinal Cord Injury: The Effect of Perceived Premorbid Sense of Coherence." *Rehabilitation Counseling Bulletin* 48 (3): 146–56.

Lynch, Ruth Torkelson, and Kenneth R. Thomas. 1994. "People with Disabilities as Victims: Changing an Ill-Advised Paradigm." *Journal of Rehabilitation* 60 (1): 8–11.

Lyons, Renee Felice. 1985. "Are We Still Friends? The Impact of Chronic Illness on Personal Relationships and Leisure." *Society and Leisure* 8 (2): 453–65.

Lys, K., and R. Pernice. 1995. "Perceptions of Positive Attitudes toward People with Spinal Cord Injury." *International Journal of Rehabilitation Research* 18 (1): 35–43.

Mackelprang, Romel W. 1986. *Social and Emotional Adjustment Following Spinal Cord Injury.* Unpublished doctoral dissertation. University of Utah.

Mackelprang, Romel W., and Dean H. Hepworth. 1990. "Sexual Adjustment Following Spinal Cord Injury: Empirical Findings and Clinical Implications." *Arrete* 15 (1): 1–13.

Macleod, A. D. 1988. "Self-Neglect of Spinal Injured Patients." *Paraplegia* 26 (5): 340–49.

Makas, Elaine. 1988. "Positive Attitudes toward Disabled People: Disabled and Nondisabled Persons' Perspectives." *Journal of Social Issues* 44 (1): 49–61.

Makas, Elaine. 1993. "Getting in Touch: The Relationship between Contact with and Attitudes toward People with Disabilities." In *Perspectives on Disability*, 2nd Edition, edited by Mark Nagler, pp. 121–36. Palo Alto, CA: Health Markets Research.

Malec, James, Richard F. Harvey, and Jay J. Cayner. 1982. "Cannibas Effect on Spasticity in Spinal Cord Injury." *Archives of Physical Medicine and Rehabilitation* 63 (3): 116–18.

Malec, James, and Robert Neimeyer. 1983. "Psychologic Prediction of Duration of Inpatient Spinal Cord Injury Rehabilitation and Performance of Self-Care." *Archives of Physical Medicine and Rehabilitation* 64 (8): 359–63.

Mariano, Anthony J. 1992. "Chronic Pain and Spinal Cord Injury." *The Clinical Journal of Pain* 8 (2): 87–92.

Marinelli, Robert P., and Arthur E. Dell Orto, editors. 1999. *The Psychological and Social Impact of Disability*, 4th Edition. New York: Springer

Marini, Irmo, Lee Rogers, John R. Slate, and Cheryl Vines. 1995. "Self-Esteem Differences among Persons with Spinal Cord Injury." *Rehabilitation Counseling Bulletin* 38 (3): 198–206.

Marks, Deborah. 1999. *Disability: Controversial Debates and Psychosocial Perspectives.* New York: Routledge.

Marti, Mollie Weighner, and Peter David Blanck. 2000. "Attitudes, Behavior, and ADA Title I." Chapter 14 in *Employment, Disability, and the Americans with Disabilities Act*, edited by Peter David Blanck, pp. 356–84. Evanston: Northwestern University Press.

Martin, Douglas. 2004. "Christopher Reeve, 52, Symbol of Courage, Dies." *The New York Times* 154 (53000): A1–A29.

Martin, E. Davis, Jr., and Gerald L. Gandy. 1990. *Rehabilitation and Disability: Psychosocial Case Studies.* Springfield, IL: Charles C. Thomas.

Martz, Erin. 2004. "Do Reactions of Adaptation to Disability Influence the Fluctuation of Future Time Orientation among Individuals with Spinal Cord Injuries?" *Rehabilitation Counseling Bulletin* 47 (2): 86–95.

Martz, E., and H. Livneh. 2003. "Death Anxiety as a Predictor of Future Time Orientation among Individuals with Spinal Cord Injuries." *Disability and Rehabilitation* 25 (18): 1024–32.

Mashaw, Jerry L. 1991. "In Search of the Disabled Under the Americans with Disabilities Act." Chapter 5 in *Disability and Work: Incentives, Rights, and Opportunities*, edited by Carolyn L. Weaver, pp. 61–71. Washington, DC: AEI Press.

Mathew, K. M., G. Ravichandran, K. May, and K. Morsley. 2001. "The Biopsychosocial Model and Spinal Cord Injury." *Spinal Cord* 39 (12): 644–49.

Maton, Kenneth I. 1989. "The Stress-Buffering Role of Spiritual Support: Cross-sectional and Prospective Investigations." *Journal for the Scientific Study of Religion* 28 (3): 310–23.

Mattlar, C. E., P. Tarkkanen, A. Carlsson, T. Aaltonen, and H. Helenius. 1993. "Personality Characteristics for 83 Paraplegic Patients." *British Journal of Projective Psychology* 38 (2): 20–30.

May, Laura Anne. 1999. *Measurement and Prediction of Quality of Life of Persons with Spinal Cord Injury.* Unpublished doctoral dissertation. University of Alberta.

Mayer, John D., and Myron G. Eisenberg. 1982. "Self-Concept and the Spinal-Cord-Injured: An Investigation Using the Tennessee Self-Concept Scale." *Journal of Consulting and Clinical Psychology* 50 (4): 604–5.

Mayer, Thomas, and Henry B. Andrews. 1981. "Changes in Self-Concept Following a Spinal Cord Injury." *Journal of Applied Rehabilitation Counseling* 12 (3): 135–37.

Mayers, Kathleen S. 1978. "Sexual and Social Concerns of the Disabled: A Group Counseling Approach." *Sexuality and Disability* 1 (2): 100–11.

Maynard, Frederick M., Rosalie S. Karunas, Rodney H. Adkins, J. Scott Richards, and William P. Waring III. 1995. "Management of the Neuromusculoskeletal Systems." Chapter 8 in *Spinal Cord Injury: Clinical Outcomes from the Model Systems,* edited by Samuel L. Stover, Joel A. DeLisa, and Gale G. Whiteneck, pp. 145–69. Gaithersburg, MD: Aspen.

McAweeney, Mary J., Denise G. Tate, and William McAweeney. 1997. "Psychosocial Interventions in the Rehabilitation of People with Spinal Cord Injury: A Comprehensive Methodological Inquiry." *SCI Psychosocial Process* 10 (2): 58–66.

McCarren, Marie. 1990. "Injection Erections: Risking Health for a Hard-on?" *Spinal Network Extra* (Spring): 18–21.

McCarthy, Henry. 1997. "Integrating Spirituality into Rehabilitation in a Technocratic Society." *Rehabilitation Education* 9 (2): 87–95.

McCarthy, Sharon Chamberlin. 1991. *Male Sexuality after Spinal Cord Injury.* Unpublished master's thesis. New Mexico State University.

McColl, Mary Ann, Hau Lei, and Harvey Skinner. 1995. "Structural Relationships between Social Support and Coping." *Social Science and Medicine* 41 (3): 395–407.

McColl, Mary Ann, and Harvey A. Skinner. 1996. "Spinal Cord Injury and Lifestyle Health Risks." *Canadian Journal of Rehabilitation* 9 (2): 69–82.

McCormick, Mercedes A. 1995. *Family Issues and Outcomes of Adjustment to Spinal Cord Injury.* Unpublished doctoral dissertation. Seton Hall University.

McDonald, Sylvia Eichner, Willa M. Lloyd, Donna Murphy, and Margaret Gretchen Russert. 1993. *Sexuality and Spinal Cord Injury.* Milwaukee, WI: Spinal Cord Injury Center, Froedtert Memorial Lutheran Hospital.

McDonnell, Dennis E., editor. 2004. "History of Spinal Surgery" (special volume). *Neurosurgical Focus* 16 (1).

McEver, Dan H. 1972. "Pastoral Care of the Spinal Cord Injury Patient." *Pastoral Psychology* 23 (221): 47–56.

McGowan, M. B., and S. Roth. 1987. "Family Functioning and Functional Independence in Spinal Cord Injury Adjustment." *Paraplegia* 25 (4): 357–65.

McMillen, J. Curtis, and Cynthia Loveland Cook. 2003. "The Positive By-products of Spinal Cord Injury and their Correlates." *Rehabilitation Psychology* 48 (2): 77–85.

McShane, Steven L., and Jeffrey Karp. 1993. "Employment Following Spinal Cord Injury: A Covariance Structure Analysis." *Rehabilitation Psychology* 38 (1): 27–40.

Meade, Michelle A., Allen Lewis, M. Njeri Jackson, and David W. Hess. 2004. "Race, Employment, and Spinal Cord Injury." *Archives of Physical Medicine and Rehabilitation* 84 (11): 1782–92.

Meade, Michelle A., Laura A. Taylor, Jeffrey S. Kreutzer, Jennifer H. Marwitz, and Vera Thomas. 2004. "A Preliminary Study of Acute Family Needs after Spinal Cord Injury: Analysis and Implications." *Rehabilitation Psychology* 49 (2): 150–55.

Melendez, Ruby. 1992. *The Relationship between Functional Independence and Psychosocial Adaptation in Spinal Cord Injury Individuals.* Unpublished master's thesis. Arizona State University.

Meyer, Therese Marie. 1998. *Coping and Adjustment During Acute Rehabilitation for Spinal Cord Injury.* Unpublished doctoral dissertation. Auburn University.

Meyerson, Lee. 1948. "Social Action for the Disabled." *Journal of Social Issues* 4 (4): 111–12.

Meyerson, Lee, and Thomas Scruggs. 1980. "Attitudes and Disabled People: A Supplementary View." Commentary in *Attitudes and Disabled People,* by Victor Finkelstein, pp. 59–67. New York: World Rehabilitation Fund.

Miller, Donald K. 1975. "Sexual Counseling with Spinal Cord-Injured Clients." *Journal of Sex & Marital Therapy* 1 (4): 312–18.

Miller, Paul Steven. 1993. "The Impact of Assisted Suicide on Persons with Disabilities: Is it a Right without Freedom?" *Issues in Law & Medicine* 9 (1): 47–61.

Miller, Paul Steven. 2000. "The Evolving ADA." Introduction to *Employment, Disability, and the Americans with Disabilities Act*, edited by Peter David Blanck, pp. 3–15. Evanston: Northwestern University Press.

Miller, Sue Barrick. 1988. "Spinal Cord Injury: Self-Perceived Sexual Information and Counseling Needs During the Acute, Rehabilitation, and Post-Rehabilitation Phases." Rehabilitation Psychology 33 (4): 221–26.

Milligan, Maureen S., and Alfred H. Neufeldt. 1998. "Postinjury Marriage to Men with Spinal Cord Injury: Women's Perspectives on Making a Commitment." *Sexuality and Disability* 16 (2): 117–32.

Mills, John Andrew. 1989. *Stress, Social Support, and Adjustment to Spinal Cord Injury.* Unpublished doctoral dissertation. State University of New York at Buffalo.

Moeller, Tamerra P., and David W. Hartman. 1985. "The Group Psychotherapy Process in Rehabilitation Settings." Chapter 17 in *Emotional Rehabilitation of Physical Trauma and Disability,* edited by David W. Krueger, pp. 219–33. Elmsford, NY: Pergamon.

Mona, Linda R., James S. Krause, Fran H. Norris, Rebecca P. Cameron, Seth C. Kalichman, and Linda M. Lesondak. 2000. "Sexual Expression Following Spinal Cord Injury." *NeuroRehabilitation* 15 (2): 121–31.

Money, John. 1993. "Orgasmology: Relevance for Persons with Physical Disabilities." Chapter 16 in *Reproductive Issues for Persons with Physical Disabilities,* edited by Florence P. Haseltine, Sandra S. Cole, and David B. Gray, pp. 187–95. Baltimore: Paul H. Brookes.

Montague, Drogo K., and Milton M. Lakin. 1994. "Penile Prosthesis Implantation in Men with Neurogenic Impotence." *Sexuality and Disability* 12 (1): 95–98.

Mooney, Thomas O., Theodore M. Cole, Richard A. Chilgren. 1975. *Sexual Options for Paraplegics and Quadriplegics.* Boston: Little, Brown and Company.

Moore, Dennis, and Lewis Polsgrove. 1991. "Disabilities, Developmental Handicaps, and Substance Misuse: A Review." *The International Journal of the Addictions* 26 (1): 65–90.

Morehouse, Pamela Jane. 1996. *The Process by which Individuals with Spinal Cord Injury Return to Employment after Injury.* Unpublished master's thesis. Smith College.

Morgan, Essie D., George W. Hohmann, and John E. Davis, Jr. 1974. "Psychosocial Rehabilitation in VA Spinal Cord Injury Centers." *Rehabilitation Psychology* 21 (1): 3–27.

Morgan, Myfanwy, Donald L. Patrick, and John R. Charlton. 1984. "Social Networks and Psychosocial Support among Disabled People." *Social Science and Medicine* 19 (5): 489–97.

Morris, Jenny, editor. 1989. *Able Lives: Women's Experience of Paralysis.* London: Women's Press.

Morris, Jenny. 1991. *Pride Against Prejudice: Transforming Attitudes to Disability.* Philadelphia: New Society.

Morris, Jenny. 1993a. "Gender and Disability." Chapter 2.3 in *Disabling Barriers—Enabling Environments,* edited by John Swain, Vic Finkelstein, Sally French, and Mike Oliver, pp. 85–92. Newbury Park, CA: Sage.

Morris, Jenny. 1993b. "Prejudice." Chapter 2.5 in *Disabling Barriers—Enabling Environments,* edited by John Swain, Vic Finkelstein, Sally French, and Mike Oliver, pp. 101–6. Newbury Park, CA: Sage.

Morris, Jenny. 1993c. "Housing, Independent Living and Physically Disabled People." Chapter 3.2 in *Disabling Barriers—Enabling Environments,* edited by John Swain, Vic Finkelstein, Sally French, and Mike Oliver, pp. 136–44. Newbury Park, CA: Sage.

Morse, Janice M., and Barbara Doberneck. 1995. "Delineating the Concept of Hope." *Image: Journal of Nursing Scholarship* 27 (4): 277–85.

Mulcahey, M. J. 1992. "Returning to School after a Spinal Cord Injury: Perspectives from Four Adolescents." *The American Journal of Occupational Therapy* 46 (4): 305–12.

Muller, L. Scott, and Peter M. Wheeler. 1998. "The Growth in Disability Programs as Seen by SSA Field Office Managers." In *Growth in Disability Benefits: Explanations and Policy Implications,* edited by Kalman Rupp and David C. Stapleton, pp. 207–22. Kalamazoo, MI: W. E. Upjohn Institute for Employment Research.

Myckatyn, Terence M., Susan E. Mackinnon, and John W. McDonald. 2004. "Stem Cell Transplantation and Other Novel Techniques for Promoting Recovery from Spinal Cord Injury." *Transplant Immunology* 12 (3–4): 343–58.

Nagler, Benedict. 1950. "Psychiatric Aspects of Cord Injury." *American Journal of Psychiatry* 107 (1): 49–56.

Nagler, Mark, editor. 1993a. *Perspectives on Disability,* 2nd Edition. Palo Alto, CA: Health Markets Research.

Nagler, Mark. 1993b. "The Disabled: The Acquisition of Power." In *Perspectives on Disability,* 2nd Edition, edited by Mark Nagler, pp. 33–36. Palo Alto, CA: Health Markets Research.

Nagumo, Naoji. 2000. "Relationships between Low-grade Chronic Depression, Pain and

Personality Traits among Community-Dwelling Persons with Traumatic Spinal Cord Injury." *The Japanese Journal of Psychology* 71 (3): 205–10.

Nash, Linda Barbara. 1988. *Causal Attributions and Adjustment to Spinal Cord Injury.* Unpublished doctoral dissertation. State University of New York at Buffalo.

National Aeronautics and Space Administration. 2004. "Consumer Price Index (CPI) Inflation Calculator." Retrieved June 17, 2005, at www.jsc.nasa.gov.

National Institutes of Health. 2005. "Charley Horse." Retrieved September 16, 2005, at www.nlm.nih.gov.

National Spinal Cord Injury Association. n.d. *Every Day More Than Thirty People Become Paralyzed* (Informational brochure).

National Spinal Cord Injury Association. 2005. "Fact Sheets." Retrieved August 9, 2005, at www.spinalcord.org.

National Spinal Cord Injury Statistical Center. 2003. "Spinal Cord Injury: Facts and Figures at a Glance." Retrieved July 23, 2004, at www.spinalcord.uab.edu.

National Spinal Cord Injury Statistical Center. 2004. "Spinal Cord Injury: Facts and Figures at a Glance." *The Journal of Spinal Cord Injury Medicine* 27 (1): S139–S140.

National Spinal Cord Injury Statistical Center. 2005. "Spinal Cord Injury: Facts and Figures at a Glance." Retrieved August 9, 2005, at www.spinalcord.uab.edu.

Neath, Jeanne. 1997. "Social Causes of Impairment, Disability, and Abuse." *Journal of Disability Policy Studies* 8 (1–2): 195–230.

Neilson, Patricia M. 1990. *Psychosocial Adjustment, Family Stress, and Ways of Coping after Neurotrauma.* Unpublished doctoral dissertation. University of Regina.

Nemeth, Sally A. 2000. "Society, Sexuality, and Disabled/Ablebodied Romantic Relationships." Chapter 2 in *Handbook of Communication and People with Disabilities: Research and Application,* edited by Dawn O. Braithwaite and Teresa L. Thompson, pp. 37–48. Mahwah, NJ: Lawrence Erlbaum Associates.

Nemiah, John C. 1957. "The Psychiatrist and Rehabilitation." *Archives of Physical Medicine and Rehabilitation* 38 (3): 143–47.

Neumann, Robert J. 1978. "Sexuality and the Spinal Cord Injured: High Drama or Improvisational Theater?" *Sexuality and Disability* 1 (2): 93–99.

Nickerson, Eileen T. 1971. "Some Correlates of Adjustment by Paraplegics." *Perceptual and Motor Skills* 32 (1): 11–23.

Nielsen, Monica Stougaard. 2003. "Prevalence of Posttraumatic Stress Disorder in Persons with Spinal Cord Injuries: The Mediating Effect of Social Support." *Rehabilitation Psychology* 48 (4): 289–95.

Nielson, Warren R., and Michael R. MacDonald. 1988. "Attributions of Blame and Coping Following Spinal Cord Injury: Is Self-Blame Adaptive?" *Journal of Social and Clinical Psychology* 7 (2–3): 163–75.

Nierenberg, Barry, and Alissa Sheldon. 2001. "Psychospirituality and Pediatric Rehabilitation." *Journal of Rehabilitation* 67 (1): 15–19.

Noreau, Luc, and Patrick Fougeyrollas. 2000. "Long-term Consequences of Spinal Cord Injury on Social Participation: The Occurrence of Handicap Situations." *Disability and Rehabilitation* 22 (4): 170–80.

Northcott, Rebekah, and Gill Chard. 2000. "Sexual Aspects of Rehabilitation: The Client's Perspective." *British Journal of Occupational Therapy* 63 (9): 412–18.

Nosek, Margaret A., Marcus J. Fuhrer, Diana H. Rintala, and Karen A. Hart. 1993. "The

Use of Personal Assistance Services by Persons with Spinal Cord Injury." *Journal of Disability Policy Studies* 4 (1): 89–103.

Nosek, Margaret A., and Rosemary B. Hughes. 2001. "Psychospiritual Aspects of Sense of Self in Women with Physical Disabilities." *Journal of Rehabilitation* 67 (1): 20–25.

Not Dead Yet. n.d. "Argument." Retrieved July 19, 2005, at www.notdeadyet.org/argue1a.html.

Not Dead Yet. 2003. "Not Dead Yet: The Resistance." Retrieved August 16, 2004, at www.notdeadyet.org.

Nunchuck, Susan Kay. 1991. *Perceived Control and Health-Promoting Behaviors as Predictors of Life Satisfaction and Well-Being Outcomes of Women with Long-Term Spinal Cord Injury.* Unpublished doctoral dissertation. Texas Woman's University.

O'Brien, Ruth. 2001. *Crippled Justice: The History of Modern Disability Policy in the Workplace.* Chicago: University of Chicago Press.

O'Donnell, James J., Jonathan E. Cooper, John E. Gessner, Isabelle Shehan, and Judy Ashley. 1981–1982. "Alcohol, Drugs, and Spinal Cord Injury." *Alcohol Health and Research World* 6 (2): 27–29.

O'Hare, Pat, and Karyl M. Hall. 1997. "Preventing Spinal Cord Injuries Through Safety Education Programs." *American Rehabilitation* 23 (1): 15–18.

Occupational Therapy Direct. n.d. *OTdirect.* Retrieved August 15, 2001, at www.otdirect.co.uk/index.html

Ogden, Lane Gordon. 1983. *Pre- and Post-Injury Vocational Interests of Men with Spinal Cord Injury.* Unpublished doctoral dissertation. Texas Tech University.

Oliver, Michael. 1983. *Social Work with Disabled People.* London: Macmillan.

Oliver, Michael. 1990. *The Politics of Disablement: A Sociological Approach.* New York: St. Martin's.

Oliver, Michael. 1993a. "Disability and Dependency: A Creation of Industrial Societies?" Chapter 1.6 in *Disabling Barriers—Enabling Environments,* edited by John Swain, Vic Finkelstein, Sally French, and Mike Oliver, pp. 49–60. Newbury Park, CA: Sage.

Oliver, Michael. 1993b. "Re-defining Disability: A Challenge to Research." Chapter 1.7 in *Disabling Barriers—Enabling Environments,* edited by John Swain, Vic Finkelstein, Sally French, and Mike Oliver, pp. 61–67. Newbury Park, CA: Sage.

Oliver, Michael J. 1993c. "Societal Responses to Long-Term Disability." Chapter 20 in *Aging with Spinal Cord Injury,* edited by Gale G. Whiteneck, Susan W. Charlifue, Kenneth A. Gerhart, Daniel P. Lammertse, Scott Manley, Robert R. Menter, and Kathie R. Seedroff, pp. 251–62. New York: Demos.

Oliver, Michael. 1996a. *Understanding Disability: From Theory to Practice.* New York: St. Martin's.

Oliver, Mike. 1996b. "A Sociology of Disability or a Disabling Sociology?" Chapter 2 in *Disability and Society: Emerging Issues and Insights,* edited by Len Barton, pp. 18–42. New York: Longman.

Oliver, Mike. 1996c. "Defining Impairment and Disability: Issues at Stake." Chapter 3 in *Exploring the Divide: Illness and Disability,* edited by Colin Barnes and Geof Mercer, pp. 39–54. Leeds: The Disability Press.

Oliver, Mike, and Colin Barnes. 1993. "Discrimination, Disability and Welfare: From Needs to Rights." Chapter 5.2 in *Disabling Barriers—Enabling Environments,* edited by John Swain, Vic Finkelstein, Sally French, and Mike Oliver, pp. 267–77. Newbury Park, CA: Sage.

Oliver, M., G. Zarb, J. Silver, M. Moore, and V. Salisbury. 1988. *Walking Into Darkness: The Experience of Spinal Cord Injury.* London: Macmillan.

Overholser, James C., and Daniel S. P. Schubert. 1993. "Depression in Patients with Spinal Cord Injuries: A Synthesis of Cognitive and Somatic Processes." *Current Psychology* 12 (2): 172–83.

Overholser, James C., Daniel S. P. Schubert, Roland Foliart, and Fred Frost. 1993. "Assessment of Emotional Distress Following a Spinal Cord Injury." *Rehabilitation Psychology* 38 (3): 187–98.

Palmer, Sara, Kay Harris Kriegsman, and Jeffrey B. Palmer. 2000. *Spinal Cord Injury: A Guide For Living.* Baltimore: The Johns Hopkins University Press.

Parrott, Roxanne, Tricia Stuart, and Adrian Bennett Cairns. 2000. "Reducing Uncertainty Through Communication During Adjustment to Disability: Living with Spinal Cord Injury." Chapter 19 in *Handbook of Communication and People with Disabilities: Research and Application,* edited by Dawn O. Braithwaite and Teresa L. Thompson, pp. 339–52. Mahwah, NJ: Lawrence Erlbaum Associates.

Parsons, Donald O. 1991. "Measuring and Deciding Disability." Chapter 6 in *Disability and Work: Incentives, Rights, and Opportunities,* edited by Carolyn L. Weaver, pp. 72–82. Washington: AEI Press.

Patterson, Kathi A. 1989. *The Perceived Health of Individuals with New Spinal Cord Injury: A Longitudinal Study.* Unpublished master's thesis. University of Washington.

Pelletier, P. M., D. P. Alfano, and M. P. Fink. 1994. "Social Support, Locus of Control and Psychological Health in Family Members Following Head or Spinal Cord Injury." *Applied Neuropsychology* 1 (1–2): 38–44.

Perduta-Fulginiti, P. Sonya. 1992. "Sexual Functioning of Women with Complete Spinal Cord Injury: Nursing Implications." *Sexuality and Disability* 10 (2): 103–18.

Perlman, Robert. 1983. "Use of the Tax System in Home Care: A Brief Note." In *Family Home Care: Critical Issues for Services and Policies,* edited by Robert Perlman, pp. 280–83. New York: Haworth.

Pervin-Dixon, Lisa. 1988. "Sexuality and the Spinal Cord Injured." *Journal of Psychosocial Nursing* 26 (4): 31–34.

Phelps, Graham, Margaret Brown, Jeanette Chen, Michael Dunn, Elaine Lloyd, Marcia L. Stefanick, Julian M. Davidson, and Inder Perkash. 1983. "Sexual Experience and Plasma Testosterone Levels in Male Veterans after Spinal Cord Injury." *Archives of Physical Medicine and Rehabilitation* 64 (2): 47–52.

Piedmont, Ralph L. 2001. "Spiritual Transcendence and the Scientific Study of Spirituality." *Journal of Rehabilitation* 67 (1): 4–14.

Pollets, Dan Franklin. 1975. *Ego Development, Coping, Social Support in the Adjustment to Spinal Cord Injury.* Unpublished doctoral dissertation. Washington University.

Post, Marcel W. M., Luc P. de Witte, Floris W. A. van Asbeck, Alphons J. van Dijk, and August J. P. Schrijvers. 1998. "Predictors of Health Status and Life Satisfaction in Spinal Cord Injury." *Archives of Physical Medicine and Rehabilitation* 79 (4): 395–401.

Post, Marcel W. M., Alphons J. van Dijk, Floris W. A. van Asbeck, and August J. P. Schrijvers. 1998. "Life Satisfaction of Persons with Spinal Cord Injury Compared to a Population Group." *Scandinavian Journal of Rehabilitation Medicine* 30 (1): 23–30.

Post, Marcel W. M., Wynand J. G. Ros, and August J. P. Schrijvers. 1999. "Impact of Social Support on Health Status and Life Satisfaction in People with a Spinal Cord Injury." *Psychology and Health* 14 (4): 679–95.

Povolny, Mary Alice. 1993. *The Relationship between Perceived Social Support and Acceptance of Disability among Persons with Traumatic Spinal Cord Injury.* Unpublished doctoral dissertation. Illinois Institute of Technology.

Povolny, Mary Alice, Steven P. Kaplan, Michelle Marme, and Gwen Roldan. 1993. "Perceptions of Adjustment Issues Following a Spinal Cord Injury: A Case Study." *Journal of Applied Rehabilitation Counseling* 24 (3): 31–34.

Price, Robert James. 1983. *Spinal Cord Injury, Life Stage and Leisure Satisfaction.* Unpublished doctoral dissertation. University of Illinois at Urbana-Champaign.

Putzke, John D., John J. Barrett, John S. Richards, Andrew T. Underhill, and Steven G. LoBello. 2004. "Life Satisfaction Following Spinal Cord Injury: Long-Term Follow-Up." *The Journal of Spinal Cord Medicine* 27 (2): 106–10.

Putzke, John D., Timothy R. Elliott, and J. Scott Richards. 2001. "Marital Status and Adjustment 1 Year Post-Spinal-Cord-Injury." *Journal of Clinical Psychology in Medical Settings* 8 (2): 101–7.

Putzke, John David, J. Scott Richards, and Rachael Nicole Dowler. 2000. "The Impact of Pain in Spinal Cord Injury: A Case-Control Study." *Rehabilitation Psychology* 45 (4): 386–401.

Quigley, M. Claire. 1994. "Impact of Spinal Cord Injury on the Life Roles of Women." *American Journal of Occupational Therapy* 49 (8): 780–86.

Quinn, Kathleen S. 1985. *Communication Apprehension: A Social Skills Approach to Psychosocial-Vocational Adaptation to Recent Spinal Cord Injury.* Unpublished master's thesis. University of Wisconsin at Milwaukee.

Quintiliani, Steven. 2000. *Hearing their Voices: The Experience of Life after Spinal Cord Injury for Adult American Women.* Unpublished doctoral dissertation. Massachusetts School of Professional Psychology.

Radnitz, Cynthia. 1996. "The Prevalence of Psychiatric Disorders in Veterans with Spinal Cord Injury: A Controlled Comparison." *Journal of Nervous & Mental Disease* 184 (7): 431–33.

Radnitz, Cynthia L., Louis Hsu, Dennis D. Tirch, Jeffrey Willard, Lynn B. Lillian, Stacey Walczak, Joanne Festa, Lysandra Perez-Strumolo, Charles P. Broderick, Martin Binks, Ilana Schlein, Neil Bockian, Leon Green, and Arthur Cytryn. 1998. "A Comparison of Posttraumatic Stress Disorder in Veterans with and without Spinal Cord Injury." *Journal of Abnormal Psychology* 107 (4): 676–80.

Radnitz, Cynthia L., Louis Hsu, Jeffrey Willard, Lysandra Perez-Strumolo, Joanne Festa, Lynn B. Lillian, Stacey Walczak, Dennis D. Tirch, Ilana S. Schlein, Martin Binks, and Charles P. Broderick. 1998. "Posttraumatic Stress Disorder in Veterans with Spinal Cord Injury: Trauma-Related Risk Factors." *Journal of Traumatic Stress* 11 (3): 505–20.

Radnitz, Cynthia L. and Dennis Tirch. 1995. "Substance Misuse in Individuals with Spinal Cord Injury." *The International Journal of the Addictions* 30 (9): 1117–40.

Ragnarsson, Kristjan, and Wayne A. Gordon. 1992. "Rehabilitation after Spinal Cord Injury: The Team Approach." *Physical Medicine and Rehabilitation Clinics of North America* 3 (4): 853–78.

Randell, N., A. C. Lynch, A. Anthony, B. R. Dobbs, J. A. Roake, and F. A. Frizelle. 2001.

"Does a Colostomy Alter Quality of Life in Patients with Spinal Cord Injury? A Controlled Study." *Spinal Cord* 39 (5): 279–82.

Ray, Colette, and Julia West. 1983. "Spinal Cord Injury: The Nature of Its Implications and Ways of Coping." *International Journal of Rehabilitation Research* 6 (3): 364–65.

Ray, Colette, and Julia West. 1984. "Social, Sexual and Personal Implications of Paraplegia." *Paraplegia* 22 (2): 75–86.

Reinelt, Claire, and Mindy Fried. 1993. "'I Am This Child's Mother': A Feminist Perspective on Mothering with a Disability." In *Perspectives on Disability,* 2nd Edition, edited by Mark Nagler, pp. 195–202. Palo Alto, CA: Health Markets Research.

Reitz, A., V. Tobe, P. A. Knapp, and B. Schurch. 2004. "Impact of Spinal Cord Injury on Sexual Health and Quality of Life." *International Journal of Impotence Research* 16 (2): 167–74.

Richards, Eleanor, Mitchell Tepper, Beverly Whipple, and Barry R. Komisaruk. 1997. "Women with Complete Spinal Cord Injury: A Phenomenological Study of Sexuality and Relationship Experiences." *Sexuality and Disability* 15 (4): 271–83.

Richards, J. Scott. 1986. "Psychologic Adjustment to Spinal Cord Injury During First Postdischarge Year." *Archives of Physical Medicine and Rehabilitation* 67 (6): 362–65.

Richards, J. Scott. 1992. "Chronic Pain and Spinal Cord Injury: Review and Comment." *The Clinical Journal of Pain* 8 (2): 119–22.

Richards, J. Scott, Timothy R. Elliott, Richard M. Shewchuk, and Philip R. Fine. 1997. "Attribution of Responsibility for Onset of Spinal Cord Injury and Psychosocial Outcomes in First Year Post-Injury." *Rehabilitation Psychology* 42 (2): 115–24.

Richards, J. Scott, Donald G. Kewman, and Christopher A. Pierce. 2000. "Spinal Cord Injury." Chapter 1 in *Handbook of Rehabilitation Psychology,* edited by Robert G. Frank and Timothy R. Elliott, pp. 11–27. Washington, DC: American Psychological Association.

Richards, J. Scott, L. Keith Lloyd, Joseph W. James, and Jane Brown. 1992. "Treatment of Erectile Dysfunction Secondary to Spinal Cord Injury: Sexual and Psychosocial Impact on Couples." *Rehabilitation Psychology* 37 (3): 205–13.

Richards, J. Scott, Samuel L. Stover, and Theresa Jaworski. 1990. "Effect of Bullet Removal on Subsequent Pain in Persons with Spinal Cord Injury Secondary to Gunshot Wound." *Journal of Neurosurgery* 73 (3): 401–4.

Riggin, Ona Ziehli. 1976. *A Comparison of Individual and Group Therapy on Self Concept and Depression of Patients with Spinal Cord Injury.* Unpublished doctoral dissertation. Memphis State University.

Rintala, Diana H., Mary Ellen Young, Karen A. Hart, Rebecca R. Clearman, and Marcus J. Fuhrer. 1992. "Social Support and the Well-Being of Persons with Spinal Cord Injury Living in the Community." *Rehabilitation Psychology* 37 (3): 155–63.

Rintala, Diana H., Mary Ellen Young, Karen A. Hart, and Marcus J. Fuhrer. 1994. "The Relationship between the Extent of Reciprocity with Social Supporters and Measures of Depressive Symptomatology, Impairment, Disability, and Handicap in Persons with Spinal Cord Injury." *Rehabilitation Psychology* 39 (1): 15–27.

Rivas, David A., and Michael B. Chancellor. 1997. "Management of Erectile Dysfunction." Chapter 22 in *Sexual Function in People with Disability and Chronic Illness: A Health Professional's Guide,* edited by Marca L. Sipski and Craig J. Alexander, pp. 429–64. Gaithersburg, MD: Aspen.

Robbins, Kathleen H. 1985. "Traumatic Spinal Cord Injury & Its Impact Upon Sexuality." *Journal of Applied Rehabilitation Counseling* 16 (1): 24–27, 31.

Roberts, April Lee. 1996. *Identity Integration in Adults Following Spinal Cord Injury.* Unpublished master's thesis. University of Utah.

Roberts, Edward V. 1989. "A History of the Independent Living Movement: A Founder's Perspective." Chapter 14 in *Psychosocial Interventions with Physically Disabled Persons,* edited by Bruce W. Heller, Louis M. Flohr, and Leonard S. Zegans, pp. 231–44. New Brunswick: Rutgers University Press.

Rodriguez, A. Miguel. 1991. *Adjustment to Spinal Cord Injury as Related to Responsibility for Onset of Disability.* Unpublished doctoral dissertation. Wayne State University.

Roessler, Richard T. 1978. "Life Outlook, Hopes, and Fears of Persons with Spinal Cord Injury." *Journal of Applied Rehabilitation Counseling* 9 (3): 103–7.

Roessler, Richard, Tim Milligan, and Ann Ohlson. 1976. "Personal Adjustment Training for the Spinal Cord Injured." *Rehabilitation Counseling Bulletin* 19 (4): 544–50.

Rogers, Sandee Melton. 1996. "Factors that Influence Exercise Tolerance." Chapter 2 in *Physical Fitness: A Guide For Individuals with Spinal Cord Injury,* edited by Tamara T. Sowell, pp. 25–32. Washington, DC: Department of Veterans Affairs, Veterans Health Administration, Rehabilitation Research and Development Service, Scientific and Technical Publications Section.

Rogers-Dulan, Jeannette, and Jan Blacher. 1995. "African American Families, Religion, and Disability: A Conceptual Framework." *Mental Retardation* 33 (4): 226–38.

Rohe, Daniel E., and Gary T. Athelstan. 1982. "Vocational Interests of Persons with Spinal Cord Injury." *Journal of Counseling Psychology* 29 (3): 283–91.

Rohe, Daniel E., and Gary T. Athelstan. 1985. "Changes in Vocational Interests after Spinal Cord Injury." *Rehabilitation Psychology* 30 (3): 131–43.

Rohe, Daniel E., and Jeffrey R. Basford. 1989. "Traumatic Spinal Cord Injury, Alcohol, and the Minnesota Multiphasic Personality Inventory." *Rehabilitation Psychology* 34 (1): 25–32.

Rohe, Daniel E., and James S. Krause. 1999a. "The Five-Factor Model of Personality: Findings in Males with Spinal Cord Injury." *Assessment* 6 (3): 203–13.

Rohe, Daniel E., and J. Stuart Krause. 1999b. "Vocational Interests of Middle-Aged Men with Traumatic Spinal Cord Injury." *Rehabilitation Psychology* 44 (2): 160–75.

Rohrer, Katherine, Beth Adelman, Janet Puckett, Beverly Toomey, Deborah Talbert, and Ernest W. Johnson. 1980. "Rehabilitation in Spinal Cord Injury: Use of a Patient-Family Group." *Archives of Physical and Medical Rehabilitation* 61 (5): 225–29.

Romano, Mary D. 1978. "Sexuality and the Disabled Female." *Sexuality and Disability* 1 (1): 27–33.

Romeo, Allen Joseph. 1992. *Sexual Adjustment to Spinal-Cord Injury.* Unpublished doctoral dissertation. The California School of Professional Psychology at Berkeley/Alameda.

Romeo, Allen J., Richard Wanlass, and Silverio Arenas. 1993. "A Profile of Psychosexual Functioning in Males Following Spinal Cord Injury." *Sexuality and Disability* 11 (4): 269–76.

Rose, Avi. 1997. "'Who Causes the Blind to See': Disability and Quality of Religious Life." *Disability & Society* 12 (3): 395–405.

Rosenthal, Mitchell. 1989. "Psychosocial Evaluation of Physically Disabled Persons."

Chapter 3 in *Psychosocial Interventions with Physically Disabled Persons,* edited by Bruce W. Heller, Louis M. Flohr, and Leonard S. Zegans, pp. 43–57. New Brunswick: Rutgers University Press.

Rummery, Kirstein. 2002. *Disability, Citizenship and Community Care: A Case for Welfare Rights?* Burlington, VT: Ashgate.

Rupp, Kalman, and David C. Stapleton. 1998. "Introduction." In *Growth in Disability Benefits: Explanations and Policy Implications,* edited by Kalman Rupp and David C. Stapleton, pp. 1–27. Kalamazoo, MI: W. E. Upjohn Institute for Employment Research.

Russell, Marta. 1998. *Beyond Ramps: Disability at the End of the Social Contract.* Monroe, ME: Common Courage Press.

Safilios-Rothschild, Constantina. 1970. *The Sociology and Social Psychology of Disability and Rehabilitation.* New York: Random House.

Safilios-Rothschild, Constantina. 1976. "Disabled Persons' Self-Definitions and their Implications for Rehabilitation." Chapter 2 in *The Sociology of Physical Disability and Rehabilitation,* edited by Gary L. Albrecht, pp. 39–56. Pittsburgh: The University of Pittsburgh Press.

Samsa, Gregory P., Clifford H. Patrick, and John R. Feussner. 1993. "Long-Term Survival of Veterans with Traumatic Spinal Cord Injury." *Archives of Neurology* 50 (9): 909–14.

Sandowski, Carol L. 1976. "Sexuality and the Paraplegic." *Rehabilitation Literature* 37 (11–12): 322–27.

Santora, Joyce Marie. 1996. *To Stay or Not to Stay: The Effects of Social Support and Caregiver Burden on Life Satisfaction, Loss of Self and Social Participation of Wives of Spinal Cord Injured Persons.* Unpublished doctoral dissertation. State University of New York at Buffalo.

Sargant, Coletta, and Mary Ann Braun. 1986. "Occupational Therapy Management of the Acute Spinal Cord-Injured Patient." *The American Journal of Occupational Therapy* 40 (5): 333–37.

Scheid, Teresa L. 2000. "Compliance with the ADA and Employment of Those with Mental Disabilities." Chapter 6 in *Employment, Disability, and the Americans with Disabilities Act,* edited by Peter David Blanck, pp. 146–73. Evanston: Northwestern University Press.

Schönherr, M. C., J. W. Groothoff, G. A. Mulder, and W. H. Eisma. 2005a. "Participation and Satisfaction after Spinal Cord Injury: Results of a Vocational and Leisure Outcome Study." *Spinal Cord* 43 (4): 241–48.

Schönherr, M. C., J. W. Groothoff, G. A. Mulder, and W. H. Eisma. 2005b. "Vocational Perspectives after Spinal Cord Injury." *Clinical Rehabilitation* 19 (2): 200–208.

Schönherr, M. C., J. W. Groothoff, G. A. Mulder, T. Schoppen, and W. H. Eisma. 2004. "Vocational Reintegration Following Spinal Cord Injury: Expectations, Participation and Interventions." *Spinal Cord* 42 (3): 177–84.

Schuler, Mark. 1982. "Sexual Counseling for the Spinal Cord Injured: A Review of Five Programs." *Journal of Sex and Marital Therapy* 8 (3): 241–52.

Schultz, Ronald C. 1985. "Purpose in Life among Spinal Cord Injured Males." *Journal of Applied Rehabilitation Counseling* 16 (2): 45–47, 51.

Schulz, Richard, and Susan Decker. 1985. "Long-term Adjustment to Physical Disability:

The Role of Social Support, Perceived Control, and Self-Blame." *Journal of Personality and Social Psychology* 48 (5): 1162–72.

Schwartz, Howard D. 1988. "Further Thoughts on a 'Sociology of Acceptance' for Disabled People." *Social Policy* 19 (2): 36–39.

Schweinberg, Thomas A. 1995. *Depression Following Spinal Cord Injury.* Unpublished doctoral dissertation. Wright State University.

Scivoletto, Giorgio, Annelisa Petrelli, Lina Di Lucente, and Vincenzo Castellano. 1997. "Psychological Investigation of Spinal Cord Injured Patients." *Spinal Cord* 35 (8): 516–20.

Seager, S. W. J., and Lauro S. Halstead. 1993. "Fertility Options and Success after Spinal Cord Injury." *Urologic Clinics of North America* 20 (3): 543–48.

Selecki, B. R., G. Berry, B. Kwok, J. A. Mandryk, I. T . Ring, M. F. Sewell, D. A. Simpson, and G. K. Vanderfield. 1986. "Experience with Spinal Injures in New South Wales." *Australian and New Zealand Journal of Surgery* 56 (7): 567–76.

Seligman, Martin E. P. 1975. *Helplessness: On Depression, Development, and Death.* San Francisco: W. H. Freeman and Company.

Selway, Deborah, and Adrian F. Ashman. 1998. "Disability, Religion and Health: A Literature Review in Search of the Spiritual Dimensions of Disability." *Disability & Society* 13 (3): 429–39.

Senelick, Richard C. (with Karla Dougherty). 1998. *The Spinal Cord Injury Handbook for Patients and their Families.* Birmingham, AL: HealthSouth.

Seymour, Charlyne T. 1955. "Personality and Paralysis: I. Comparative Adjustment of Paraplegics and Quadriplegics." *Archives of Physical Medicine and Rehabilitation* 36 (11): 691–94.

Shadish, William R., Jr., Donald Hickman, and M. Carole Arrick. 1981. "Psychological Problems of Spinal Cord Injury Patients: Emotional Distress as a Function of Time and Locus of Control." *Journal of Consulting and Clinical Psychology* 49 (2): 297.

Shakespeare, Tom. 1993. "Disabled People's Self-Organisation: A New Social Movement?" *Disability, Handicap and Society* 8 (3): 249–64.

Shakespeare, Tom. 1996. "Disability, Identity and Difference." Chapter 6 in *Exploring the Divide: Illness and Disability,* edited by Colin Barnes and Geof Mercer, pp. 94–113. Leeds: Disability Press.

Shakespeare, Tom, editor. 1998. *The Disability Studies Reader.* New York: Cassell.

Shapiro, Joseph P. 1993. *No Pity: People with Disabilities Forging a New Civil Rights Movement.* New York: Times Books.

Shaul, Susan, Pamela Dowling, and Bernice F. Laden. 1981. "Like Other Women: Perspectives of Mothers with Physical Disabilities." *Journal of Sociology and Social Welfare* 8 (2): 364–75.

Shaul, Susan, Pamela J. Dowling, and Bernice F. Laden. 1985. "Like Other Women: Perspectives of Mothers with Physical Disabilities." Chapter 11 in *Women and Disability: The Double Handicap,* edited by Mary Jo Deegan and Nancy A. Brooks, pp. 133–42. New Brunswick: Transaction Books.

Sherman, J. E., D. J. DeVinney, and K. B. Sperling. 2004. "Social Support and Adjustment after Spinal Cord Injury: Influence of Past Peer-Mentoring Experiences and Current Live-in Partner." *Rehabilitation Psychology* 49 (2): 140–49.

Sherman, Jo, and Jerome M. Fischer. 2002. "Spirituality and Addiction Recovery for Rehabilitation Counseling." *Journal of Applied Rehabilitation Counseling* 33 (4): 27–31.

Shewchuk, Richard, and Timothy R. Elliott. 2000. "Family Caregiving in Chronic Disease and Disability." Chapter 26 in *Handbook of Rehabilitation Psychology,* edited by Robert G. Frank and Timothy R. Elliott, pp. 553–63. Washington, DC: American Psychological Association.

Shnek, Zachary M. 1995. *Predictors of Depression in Multiple Sclerosis and Spinal Cord Injury.* Unpublished doctoral dissertation. Yeshiva University.

Shnek, Zachary M., Frederick W. Foley, Nicholas G. LaRocca, Wayne A. Gordon, John DeLuca, Harlene G. Schwartzman, June Halper, Shelley Lennox, and Jane Irvine. 1997. "Helplessness, Self-Efficacy, Cognitive Distortions, and Depression in Multiple Sclerosis and Spinal Cord Injury." *Annals of Behavioral Medicine* 19 (3): 287–94.

Sholomskas, Diane E., Janice M. Steil, and Jack Plummer. 1990. "The Spinal Cord Injured Revisited: The Relationship between Self-Blame, Other-Blame and Coping." *Journal of Applied Social Psychology* 20 (7): 548–74.

Shrey, Donald E. 1983. "Independent Living, Job Placement, and the Work Environment: A Skill-Based Training Perspective." Chapter 24 in *Vocational Evaluation, Work Adjustment, and Independent Living for Severely Disabled People,* edited by Robert A. Lassiter, Martha Hughes Lassiter, Richard E. Hardy, J. William Underwood, and John G. Cull, pp. 290–304. Springfield, IL: Charles C. Thomas.

Siddall, Philip J., Robert P. Yezierski, and John D. Loeser. 2002. "Taxonomy and Epidemiology of Spinal Cord Injury Pain." Chapter 2 in *Spinal Cord Injury Pain: Assessment, Mechanisms, Management,* edited by Robert P. Yezierski and Kim J. Burchiel, pp. 9–24. Seattle: IASP Press.

Sidman, Janice M. 1977. "Sexual Functioning and the Physically Disabled Adult." *American Journal of Occupational Therapy* 31 (2): 81–85.

Silver, Roxane L., and Camille B. Wortman. 1980. "Coping with Undesirable Life Events." Chapter 12 in *Human Helplessness: Theory and Applications,* edited by Judy Garber and Martin E. P. Seligman, pp. 279–340. New York: Academic Press.

Simmons, Stephen. 1981. *Marital Adjustment and Self-Actualization among Couples with Spinal-Cord-Injured Husbands: A Comparison between Pre- and Post-Marriage Injury.* Unpublished doctoral dissertation. East Texas State University.

Simmons, Stephen, and Steven E. Ball. 1984. "Marital Adjustment and Self-actualization in Couples Married before and after Spinal Cord Injury." *Journal of Marriage and the Family* 46 (4): 943–45.

Singh, Roop, and Sansar C. Sharma. 2005. "Sexuality and Women with Spinal Cord Injury." *Sexuality and Disability* 23 (1): 21–33.

Singh, Silas P., and Tom Magner. 1975. "Sex and Self: The Spinal Cord-Injured." *Rehabilitation Literature* 36 (1): 2–10.

Singleton, Sharron M. 1985. "Crisis Intervention with the Spinal Cord Injured Individual." *Emotional First Aid* 2 (3): 29–35.

Sipski, Marca L. 1991. "Spinal Cord Injury: What is the Effect on Sexual Response?" *Journal of the American Paraplegia Society* 14 (2): 40–43.

Sipski, Marca L. 1997a. "Spinal Cord Injury and Sexual Function: An Educational Model." Chapter 9 in *Sexual Function in People with Disability and Chronic Illness: A*

*Health Professional's Guide,* edited by Marca L. Sipski and Craig J. Alexander, pp. 149–76. Gaithersburg, MD: Aspen.

Sipski, Marca L. 1997b. "The Impact of Spinal Cord Trauma on Female Sexual Function." Chapter 18 in *Reproductive Issues for Persons with Physical Disabilities,* edited by Florence P. Haseltine, Sandra S. Cole, and David B. Gray, pp. 209–20. Baltimore: Paul H. Brookes.

Sipski, Marca. 1997c. "Sexuality and Spinal Cord Injury: Where We Are and Where We Are Going." *American Rehabilitation* 23 (1): 26–30.

Sipski, Marca L., and Craig J. Alexander. 1991. "Sexual Activities, Desire and Satisfaction in Females Pre- and Post-Spinal Cord Injury." *Journal of the American Paraplegia Society* 14 (2): 72.

Sipski, Marca L., and Craig J. Alexander. 1992. "Sexual Function and Dysfunction after Spinal Cord Injury." *Physical Medicine and Rehabilitation Clinics of North America* 3 (4): 811–28.

Sipski, Marca L., and Craig J. Alexander. 1993. "Sexual Activities, Response and Satisfaction in Women Pre- and Post-Spinal Cord Injury." *Archives of Physical Medicine and Rehabilitation* 74 (10): 1025–29.

Sipski, Marca L., and Craig J. Alexander. 1995. "Spinal Cord Injury and Female Sexuality." *Annual Review of Sex Research* 6: 224–44.

Sipski, Marca L., Craig J. Alexander, and Raymond Rosen. 2001. "Sexual Arousal and Orgasm in Women: Effects of Spinal Cord Injury." *Annals of Neurology* 49 (1): 35–44.

Sipski, Marca L., Amie B. Jackson, Orlando Gómez-Marín, Irene Estores, and Adam Stein. 2004. "Effects of Gender on Neurologic and Functional Recovery after Spinal Cord Injury." *Archives of Physical Medicine and Rehabilitation* 85 (11): 1826–36.

Sipski, Marca L., Raymond C. Rosen, Craig J. Alexander, and Orlando Gómez-Marín. 2004. "Sexual Responsiveness in Women with Spinal Cord Injuries: Differential Effects of Anxiety-Eliciting Stimulation." *Archives of Sexual Behavior* 33 (3): 295–302.

Sishuba, J. E. 1992. "Sexuality and Spinal Cord Injury." *Social Work/Maatskaplike Werk* 28 (1): 73–77.

Sjögren, Kerstin, and Karin Egberg. 1983. "The Sexual Experience in Younger Males with Complete Spinal Cord Injury." *Scandinavian Journal of Rehabilitation Medicine* 9: 189–94.

Skinner, Amy L., Kevin J. Armstrong, and John Rich. 2003. "Depression and Spinal Cord Injury: A Review of Diagnostic Methods for Depression, 1985 to 2000." *Rehabilitation Counseling Bulletin* 46 (3): 174–75.

Slater, Daniel, and Michelle A. Meade. 2004. "Participation in Recreation and Sports for Persons with Spinal Cord Injury: Review and Recommendations." *Neuro-Rehabilitation* 19 (2): 121–29.

Smith, Barry S., and Leslie D. Porter. 1992. "Decubitus Ulcers and Skin and Nail Changes after Spinal Cord Injury." *Physical Medicine and Rehabilitation Clinics of North America* 3 (4): 797–809.

Smith, Eric M., and Donald R. Bodner. 1993. "Sexual Dysfunction after Spinal Cord Injury." *Urologic Clinics of North America* 20 (3): 535–42.

Smith, Patricia Ann. 1984. *Adjustment to Spinal Cord Injury: Social Support, Locus of Control, Time Since Onset of Injury.* Unpublished doctoral dissertation. Ohio State University.

Sobsey, Dick. 1994. *Violence and Abuse in the Lives of People with Disabilities: The End of Silent Acceptance?* Baltimore: Paul H. Brookes.

Soliz Debra. 1981. "Sexuality and Attendant Care: A Panel Discussion." Chapter 16 in *Sexuality and Physical Disability,* edited by David G. Bullard and Susan E. Knight, pp. 113–15. St. Louis: C. V. Mosby Company.

Song, Hee-Young. 2005. "Modeling Social Reintegration in Persons with Spinal Cord Injury." *Disability and Rehabilitation* 27 (3): 131–41.

Sparkes, Andrew C., and Brett Smith. 2002. "Sport, Spinal Cord Injury, Embodied Masculinities, and the Dilemmas of Narrative Identity." *Men and Masculinities* 4 (3): 258–85.

Spungen, Ann M., Peter L. Almenoff, Marvin Lesser, and William A. Bauman. 1995. "Prevalence of Cigarette Smoking in a Group of Male Veterans with Chronic Spinal Cord Injury." *Military Medicine* 160 (6): 308–11.

Staas, William E., Jr., and John F. Ditunno, Jr., editors. 1992. *Physical Medicine and Rehabilitation Clinics of North America.* Philadelphia: W. B. Saunders Company, Harcourt Brace Jovanovich.

Staas, William E., Jr., Christopher S. Formal, Arthur M. Gershkoff, Maureen Freda, Judith F. Hirschwald, Gail D. Miller, Leonard Forrest, and Beth A. Burkhard. 1988. "Rehabilitation of the Spinal-Cord Injured Patient." Chapter 32 in *Rehabilitation Medicine: Principles and Practices,* edited by Joel A. DeLisa, pp. 635–59. New York: J. B. Lippincott.

Starkloff, Max J. 1997. "Spinal Cord Injury and Centers for Independent Living." *American Rehabilitation* 23 (1): 7–10.

Steger, Jeffrey C., and Jo Ann Brockway. 1980. "Sexual Enhancement in Spinal Cord Injured Patients: Behavioral Group Treatment." *Sexuality and Disability* 3 (2): 84–96.

Stein, Mark, Joe W. Chamberlin, Seth E. Lerner, and Mark Gladshteyn. 1993. "The Evaluation and Treatment of Sexual Dysfunction in the Neurologically Impaired Patient." *Journal of Neurologic Rehabilitation* 7 (2): 63–71.

Steinglass, Peter, Scott Temple, Stephen A. Lisman, and David Reiss. 1982. "Coping with Spinal Cord Injury: The Family Perspective." *General Hospital Psychiatry* 4 (4): 259–64.

Stephens, Mary Ann Parris, and Carolyn Norris-Baker. 1984. "Social Support in College Life for Disabled Students." *Rehabilitation Psychology* 29 (2): 107–11.

Stern, Peter H., and Kathleen Slattery. 1975. "Spinal-Cord Injury Rehabilitation." *New York State Journal of Medicine* 75 (June): 1029–34.

Stewart, Thomas D. 1977. "Spinal Cord Injury: A Role for the Psychiatrist." *American Journal of Psychiatry* 134 (5): 538–41.

Stewart, Thomas D. 1988. "Psychiatric Diagnosis and Treatment Following Spinal Cord Injury." *Psychosomatics* 29 (2): 214–20.

Stewart, Thomas D., and Alain B. Rossier. 1978. "Psychological Considerations in the Adjustment to Spinal Cord Injury." *Rehabilitation Literature* 39 (3): 75–80.

Stiles, Beverly L., Robert E. Clark, and Emily E. LaBeff. 1997. "Sexuality and Paraplegia: Myths and Misconceptions among College Students." *Free Inquiry in Creative Sociology* 25 (2): 227–35.

Stohl, Ellen. 1987. "Meet Ellen Stohl." *Playboy* 34: 68–75.

Stone, Deborah A. 1984. *The Disabled State.* Philadelphia: Temple University Press.

Störmer, S., H. J. Gerner, W. Grüninger, K. Metzmacher, S. Föllinger, C. Wienke, W. Aldinger, N. Walker, N. Zimmermann, and V. Paeslack. 1997. "Chronic Pain/Dysaesthesiae in Spinal Cord Injury Patients: Results of a Multicentre Study." *Spinal Cord* 35 (7): 446–55.

Stover, Samuel L. 1996. "Facts, Figures, and Trends on Spinal Cord Injury." *American Rehabilitation* 22 (3): 25–32.

Stover, Samuel L., Joel A. DeLisa, and Gale G. Whiteneck, editors. 1995. *Spinal Cord Injury: Clinical Outcomes from the Model Systems.* Gaithersburg, MD: Aspen.

Strauss, Anselm L., and Barney G. Glaser. 1975. *Chronic Illness and the Quality of Life.* St. Louis: The C. V. Mosby Company.

Strawn, Martha. 1966. *A Study of Factors Affecting Marital Relationships before and after Spinal Cord Injury.* Unpublished master's thesis. San Diego State College.

Stubbins, Joseph. 1988. "The Politics of Disability." Chapter 2 in *Attitudes toward Persons with Disabilities,* edited by Harold E. Yuker, pp. 22–32. New York: Springer.

Sullivan, Jacqueline, editor. 1990a. *Critical Care Nursing Clinics of North America.* Philadelphia: W. B. Saunders Company.

Sullivan, Jacqueline. 1990b. "Individual and Family Responses to Acute Spinal Cord Injury." *Critical Care Nursing Clinics of North America* 2 (3): 407–14.

Summers, Jay D., Michael A. Rapoff, George Varghese, Kent Porter, and Richard E. Palmer. 1991. "Psychosocial Factors in Chronic Spinal Cord Injury Pain." *Pain* 47 (2): 183–89.

Susman, Joan. 1994. "Disability, Stigma and Deviance." *Social Science and Medicine* 38 (1): 15–22.

Sutherland, Mimi Watson. 1993. "The Prevention of Violent Spinal Cord Injuries." *SCI Nursing* 10 (3): 91–95.

Swain, John, Vic Finkelstein, Sally French, and Mike Oliver, editors. 1993. *Disabling Barriers—Enabling Environments.* Newbury Park, CA: Sage.

Swanson, Frank. 2000. *Physical Disability and Learned Helplessness and Depression.* Unpublished doctoral dissertation. United States International University.

Sweeney, Terence T., and Janis E. Foote. 1982. "Treatment of Drug and Alcohol Abuse in Spinal Cord Injury Veterans." *The International Journal of the Addictions* 17 (5): 897–904.

Szymanski, Edna Mora. 2000. "Disability and Vocational Behavior." Chapter 23 in *Handbook of Rehabilitation Psychology,* edited by Robert G. Frank and Timothy R. Elliott, pp. 499–517. Washington, DC: American Psychological Association.

Talbot, Herbert S. 1955. "The Sexual Function in Paraplegia." *Journal of Urology* 73 (1): 91–100.

Targett, Pam, Paul Wehman, and Cynthia Young. 2004. "Return to Work for Persons with Spinal Cord Injury: Designing Work Supports." *NeuroRehabilitation* 19 (2): 131–39.

Targett, Pam S., Kristi Wilson, Paul Wehman, and William O. McKinley. 1998. "Community Needs Assessment Survey of People with Spinal Cord Injury: An Early Follow-up Study." *Journal of Vocational Rehabilitation* 10 (2): 169–77.

Tasiemski, Tomasz, Paul Kennedy, Brian P. Gardner, and Rachel A. Blaikley. 2004. "Athletic Identity and Sports Participation in People with Spinal Cord Injury." *Adapted Physical Activity Quarterly* 21 (4): 364–78.

Tate, Denise G., Martin B. Forchheimer, James S. Krause, Michelle A. Meade, and Charles H. Bombardier. 2004. "Patterns of Alcohol and Substance Use and Abuse in Persons with Spinal Cord Injury: Risk Factors and Correlates." *Archives of Physical Medicine and Rehabilitation* 85 (11): 1837–47.

Tate, Denise G., Donald G. Kewman, and Frederick Maynard. 1990. "The Brief Symptom Inventory: Measuring Psychological Distress in Spinal Cord Injury." *Rehabilitation Psychology* 35 (4): 211–16.

Tate, Denise G., Frederick Maynard, and Martin Forchheimer. 1993. "Predictors of Psychologic Distress One Year after Spinal Cord Injury." *American Journal of Physical Medicine and Rehabilitation* 72 (5): 272–75.

Tatum, Bonnie White. 1989. *The Effect of Physical Disability on Communication Fear: A Study of Spinal Cord Injury.* Unpublished doctoral dissertation. University of Southern Mississippi.

Tayal, Poonam, Ravinder Dang, Radhey Shyam, and S. S. Gupta. 1997. "A Study of Deterioration in Various Areas of Adjustment in Spinal Cord Injured Patients." *Journal of Personality and Clinical Studies* 13 (1–2): 55–61.

Taylor, George P., Jr. 1967. *Predicted Versus Actual Response to Spinal Cord Injury: A Psychological Study.* Unpublished doctoral dissertation. University of Minnesota.

Teal, Jeffrey C., and Gary T. Athelstan. 1975. "Sexuality and Spinal Cord Injury: Some Psychosocial Considerations." *Archives of Physical Medicine and Rehabilitation* 56 (6): 264–68.

Tepper, Mitchell S. 1992. "Sexual Education in Spinal Cord Injury Rehabilitation: Current Trends and Recommendations." *Sexuality and Disability* 10 (1): 15–31.

Tepper, Mitchell S. 1997a. "Living with a Disability: A Man's Perspective." Chapter 8 in *Sexual Function in People with Disability and Chronic Illness: A Health Professional's Guide,* edited by Marca L. Sipski and Craig J. Alexander, pp. 131–46. Gaithersburg, MD: Aspen.

Tepper, Mitchell S. 1997b. "Providing Comprehensive Sexual Health Care in Spinal Cord Injury Rehabilitation: Implementation and Evaluation of a New Curriculum for Health Care Professionals." *Sexuality and Disability* 15 (3): 131–65.

Tepper, Mitchell S. 1997c. "Discussion Guide for the Sexually Explicit Educational Video *Sexuality Reborn: Sexuality Following Spinal Cord Injury.*" *Sexuality and Disability* 15 (3): 183–99.

Tepper, Mitchell S. 1997d. "Use of Sexually Explicit Films in Spinal Cord Rehabilitation Programs." *Sexuality and Disability* 15 (3): 167–81.

Thoits, Peggy A. 1995. "Stress, Coping, and Social Support Processes: Where Are We? What Next?" *Journal of Health and Social Behavior* 36 (5): 53–79.

Thompson, Nancy J., Jennifer Coker, James S. Krause, and Else Henry. 2003. "Purpose in Life as a Mediator of Adjustment after Spinal Cord Injury." *Rehabilitation Psychology* 48 (2): 100–108.

Thornton, Carla E. 1979. "Sexuality Counseling of Women with Spinal Cord Injuries." *Sexuality and Disability* 2 (4): 267–77.

Through the Looking Glass. 2005. "Parents with Disabilities." Retrieved July 14, 2005, at lookingglass.org.

Tighe, Cynthia Anne. 2001. "'Working at Disability': A Qualitative Study of the Mean-

ing of Health and Disability for Women with Physical Impairments." *Disability &
Society* 16 (4): 511–29.

Tomassen, P. C. D., M. W. M. Post, and F. W. A. van Asbeck. 2000. "Return to Work
after Spinal Cord Injury." *Spinal Cord* 38 (1): 51–55.

Traustadottir, Rannveig. 1993. "Mothers Who Care: Gender, Disability, and Family Life."
In *Perspectives on Disability,* 2nd Edition, edited by Mark Nagler, pp. 173–84. Palo
Alto, CA: Health Markets Research.

Travis, Roberta. 1997. "Like a Woman." *New Mobility: Disability Lifestyle, Culture &
Resources* 8 (41): 39.

Treloar, Linda L. 1998. *Perceptions of Spiritual Beliefs, Response to Disability, and the
Church.* Unpublished doctoral dissertation. Union Institute Graduate School.

Trieschmann, Roberta B. 1980. *Spinal Cord Injuries: Psychological, Social, and Vocational
Adjustment.* New York: Pergamon.

Trieschmann, Roberta B. 1988. *Spinal Cord Injuries: Psychological, Social, and Vocational
Adjustment,* 2nd Edition. New York: Demos.

Trieschmann, Roberta B. 1989. "Psychosocial Adjustment to Spinal Cord Injury." Chap-
ter 7 in *Psychosocial Interventions with Physically Disabled Persons,* edited by Bruce
W. Heller, Leonard S. Zegans, and Louis M. Flohr, pp. 117–36. New Brunswick:
Rutgers University Press.

Trieschmann, Roberta B. 2001. "Spirituality and Energy Medicine." *Journal of Rehabilitation* 67 (1): 26–32.

Tucker, Sherry Jill. 1980. "The Psychology of Spinal Cord Injury: Patient-Staff Interaction." *Rehabilitation Literature* 41(5–6): 114–21, 160.

Turk, R., M. Turk, and V. Assejev. 1983. "The Female Paraplegic and Mother-Child Relations." *Paraplegia* 21 (3): 186–91.

Turner, Aaron P., Charles H. Bombardier, and Carl T. Rimmele. 2003. "A Typology of
Alcohol Use Patterns among Persons with Recent Traumatic Brain Injury or Spinal
Cord Injury: Implications for Treatment Matching." *Archives of Physical Medicine
and Rehabilitation* 84 (3): 358–64.

Underwood, J. William, and Susan M. Atwood. 1983. "Sexuality and Severe Disability."
Chapter 26 in *Vocational Evaluation, Work Adjustment, and Independent Living for
Severely Disabled People,* edited by Robert A. Lassiter, Martha Hughes Lassiter, Rich-
ard E. Hardy, J. William Underwood, and John G. Cull, pp. 320–30. Springfield,
IL: Charles C. Thomas.

Union of the Physically Impaired Against Segregation (UPIAS). 1976. *Fundamental Principles of Disability.* London: Union of the Physically Impaired Against Segregation.

United States Census Bureau. 2001. *Current Population Reports. P-60–213. Money Income
in the United States: 2000.* Washington, DC: U. S. Census Bureau.

United States Census Bureau. 2003. "Educational Attainment in the United States:
March 2002 Detailed Tables (PPL-169)." Retrieved June 17, 2003, at landview.
census.gov.

United States Social Security Administration. 2002. *Ticket to Work and Work Incentives
Improvement Act of 1999.* Retrieved August 9, 2003, at www.ssa.gov.

United States Social Security Administration. 2005. *Working while Disabled: How We Can
Help.* Retrieved June 23, 2005, at www.ssa.gov

Urey, Jon Russell. 1986. *Marital Adjustment Following Spinal Cord Injury: An Analysis of Recreational, Sexual and Conflict Resolution Behaviors.* Unpublished doctoral dissertation. Memphis State University.

Urey, Jon R., and Scott W. Henggeler. 1987. "Marital Adjustment Following Spinal Cord Injury." *Archives of Physical Medicine and Rehabilitation* 68 (2): 69–74.

Urey, Jon R., Vicki Viar, and Scott W. Henggeler. 1987. "Prediction of Marital Adjustment among Spinal Cord Injured Persons." *Rehabilitation Nursing* 12 (1): 26–30.

Van Den Bout, Jan, Nel Van Son-Schoones, Jacob Schipper and Conny Groffen. 1988. "Attributional Cognitions, Coping Behaviour, and Self-Esteem in Inpatients with Severe Spinal Cord Injuries." *Journal of Clinical Psychology* 44 (1): 17–22.

Vander Kolk, Charles J. 1976. "Physiological and Self-reported Reactions to the Disabled and Deviant." *Rehabilitation Psychology* 23 (3): 77–83.

Vargo, Frances. 1984. "Adaptation to Disability by the Wives of Spinal Cord Males—A Phenomenological Approach." *Journal of Applied Rehabilitation Counseling* 15 (1): 28–32.

Vash, Carolyn. 1981. *The Psychology of Disability.* New York: Springer.

Vaughan, C. Edwin. 1997. "People-First Language: An Unholy Crusade." The National Federation for the Blind. Retrieved January 13, 2005, at www.blind.net/bpg00006.htm.

Verduyn, Walter H. 1993. "Spinal Cord Injured Women, Pregnancy, and Delivery." Chapter 11 in *Reproductive Issues for Persons with Physical Disabilities,* edited by Florence P. Haseltine, Sandra S. Cole, and David B. Gray, pp. 239–45. Baltimore: Paul H. Brookes.

Vernon, Ayesha. 1998. "Multiple Oppression and the Disabled People's Movement." Chapter 13 in *The Disability Studies Reader,* edited by Tom Shakespeare, pp. 201–10. New York: Cassell.

Ville, I., J. F. Ravaud, and the Tetrafigap Group. 2001. "Subjective Well-Being and Severe Motor Impairments: The Tetrafigap Survey on the Long-Term Outcome of Tetraplegic Spinal Cord Injured Persons." *Social Science and Medicine* 52 (3): 369–84.

Wada, Michael A., and Martin G. Brodwin. 1975. "Attitudes of Society toward Sexual Fun[c]tioning of Male Individuals with Spinal Cord Injury." *Psychology* 12 (4): 18–22.

Waites, Ken B., Kay C. Canupp, and Michael J. DeVivo. 1993. "Epidemiology and Risk Factors for Urinary Tract Infection Following Spinal Cord Injury." *Archives of Physical Medicine and Rehabilitation* 74 (7): 691–95.

Waldinger, Heidi C. 1999. *A Social Model Analysis of Identity Transformation Following Spinal Cord Injury.* Unpublished master's thesis. University of Illinois at Chicago.

Wang, Caroline. 1993. "Culture, Meaning and Disability: Injury Prevention Campaigns and the Production of Stigma." In *Perspectives on Disability,* 2nd Edition, edited by Mark Nagler, pp. 77–90. Palo Alto, CA: Health Markets Research.

Wang, Michael Y., Brian O'Shaughnessy, Iftikharul Haq, and Barth A. Green. 2004. "Pain Following Spinal Cord Injury." *Seminars in Neurosurgery* 15 (1): 99–105.

Warfield, Robert D., and Marc. B. Goldstein. 1996. "Spirituality: The Key to Recovery from Alcoholism." *Counseling and Values* 40 (3): 196–205.

Waters, Robert L., Jeffrey Cressy, and Rodney H. Adkins. 1996. "Spinal Cord Injuries Due to Violence." *American Rehabilitation* 22 (3): 10–15.

Waxman, Barbara Faye. 1993. "The Politics of Eugenics." *Disability Rag* 14 (3): 6–7.

Waxman, Barbara Faye. 1996. "Commentary on Sexual and Reproductive Health." *Sexuality and Disability* 14 (3): 237–44.

Weaver, Carolyn L. 1986. "Social Security Disability Policy in the 1980s and Beyond." In *Disability and the Labor Market: Economic Problems, Policies, and Programs,* edited by Monroe Berkowitz and M. Anne Hill, pp. 29–63. Ithaca: ILR Press.

Webster, George D. 1983. "Sexual Dysfunction in the Paraplegic Patient." *Medical Aspects of Human Sexuality* 17 (1): 32M–32AA.

Webster, Guinevere, and Lynne M. Hindson. 2004. "The Adaptation of Children to Spinal Cord Injury of a Family Member: The Individual's Perspective." *SCI Nursing* 21 (2): 82–87.

Weinberg, Nancy. 1988. "Another Perspective: Attitudes of People with Disabilities." Chapter 11 in *Attitudes toward Persons with Disabilities*, edited by Harold E. Yuker, pp. 141–53. New York: Springer.

Weinberg, Nancy, and Judy Williams. 1978. "How the Physically Disabled Perceive their Disabilities." *Journal of Rehabilitation* 44 (3): 31–33.

Weingardt, Kenneth R., Jeanette Hsu, and Michael E. Dunn. 2001. "Brief Screening for Psychological and Substance Abuse Disorders in Veterans with Long-Term Spinal Cord Injury." *Rehabilitation Psychology* 46 (3): 271–78.

Weisner, Thomas S., Laura Beizer, and Lori Stolze. 1991. "Religion and Families of Children with Developmental Delays." *American Journal on Mental Retardation* 95 (6): 647–62.

Weiss, Andor A. 1968. "Early Management of Spinal Cord Injured Patient." *New York State Journal of Medicine* 68 (15): 2029–31.

Weitzenkamp, D. A., K. A. Gerhart, S. W. Charlifue, G. G. Whiteneck, C. A. Glass, and P. Kennedy. 2000. "Ranking the Criteria for Assessing Quality of Life after Disability: Evidence for Priority Shifting among Long-Term Spinal Cord Injury Survivors." *British Journal of Health Psychology* 5 (1): 57–69.

Weller, Doris J., and Patricia M. Miller. 1977a. "Emotional Reactions of Patient, Family, and Staff in Acute-Care Period of Spinal Cord Injury: Part 1." *Social Work in Health Care* 2 (4): 369–77.

Weller, Doris J., and Patricia M. Miller. 1977b. "Emotional Reactions of Patient, Family, and Staff in Acute-Care Period of Spinal Cord Injury: Part 2." *Social Work in Health Care* 3 (1): 7–17.

Wendell, Susan. 1996. *The Rejected Body: Feminist Philosophical Reflections on Disability.* New York: Routledge.

Westbrook, Mary T., Varoe Legge, and Mark Pennay. 1993. "Attitudes towards Disabilities in a Multicultural Society." *Social Science and Medicine* 36 (5): 615–23.

Westgren, Ninni, Claes Hultling, Richard Levi, Ake Seiger, and Magnus Westgren. 1997. "Sexuality in Women with Traumatic Spinal Cord Injury." *Acta Obstetricia et Gynecologica Scandinavica* 76 (10): 977–83.

Westgren, Ninni, and Richard Levi. 1994. "Motherhood after Traumatic Spinal Cord Injury." *Paraplegia* 32 (8): 517–23.

Westgren, Ninni, and Richard Levi. 1999. "Sexuality after Injury: Interviews with Women after Traumatic Spinal Cord Injury." *Sexuality and Disability* 17 (4): 309–19.

Whipple, Beverly, Carolyn A. Gerdes, and Barry R. Komisaruk. 1996. "Sexual Response to Self-Stimulation in Women with Complete Spinal Cord Injury." *Journal of Sex Research* 33 (3): 231–40.

Whipple, Beverly, Eleanor Richards, Mitchell Tepper, and Barry R. Komisaruk. 1996. "Sexual Response in Women with Complete Spinal Cord Injury." *Sexuality and Disability* 14 (3): 191–201.

White, L. Jayne. 1983. *The Adjustment Process of the Spinal Cord Injured: Case Study Reports.* Unpublished doctoral dissertation. Oklahoma State University.

White, Mary Joe, Diana H. Rintala, Karen A. Hart, and Marcus J. Fuhrer. 1993. "Sexual Activities, Concerns and Interests of Women with Spinal Cord Injury Living in the Community." *American Journal of Physical Medicine and Rehabilitation* 72 (6): 372–78.

White House. 2001. "Fact Sheet: Embryonic Stem Cell Research." Retrieved June 1, 2005, at www.whitehouse.gov.

Whiteneck, Gale G. 1993. "Changing Attitudes toward Life." Chapter 16 in *Aging with Spinal Cord Injury,* edited by Gale G. Whiteneck, Susan W. Charlifue, Kenneth A. Gerhart, Daniel P. Lammertse, Scott Manley, Robert R. Menter, and Kathie R. Seedroff, pp. 211–18. New York: Demos.

Whiteneck, G. G., S. W. Charlifue, H. L. Frankel, M. H. Fraser, B. P. Gardner, K. A. Gerhart, K. R. Krishnan, R. R. Menter, I. Nuseibeh, D. J. Short, and J. R. Silver. 1992. "Mortality, Morbidity, and Psychosocial Outcomes of Persons Spinal Cord Injured More Than 20 Years Ago." *Paraplegia* 30 (9): 617–30.

Whiteneck, Gale G., Susan W. Charlifue, Kenneth A. Gerhart, Daniel P. Lammertse, Scott Manley, Robert R. Menter, and Kathie R. Seedroff, editors. 1993. *Aging with Spinal Cord Injury.* New York: Demos.

Whiteneck, Gale, Michelle A. Meade, Marcel Dijkers, Denise G. Tate, Tamara Bushnik, and Martin B. Forchheimer. 2004. "Environmental Factors and their Role in Participation and Life Satisfaction after Spinal Cord Injury." *Archives of Physical Medicine and Rehabilitation* 85 (11): 1793–1803.

Widerström-Noga, Eva G. 2002. "Evaluation of Clinical Characteristics of Pain and Psychosocial Factors after Spinal Cord Injury." Chapter 5 in *Spinal Cord Injury Pain: Assessment, Mechanisms, Management,* edited by Robert P. Yezierski and Kim J. Burchiel, pp. 53–71. Seattle: IASP Press.

Widerström-Noga, Eva G., Ernesto Felipe-Cuervo, and Robert P. Yezierski. 2001. "Chronic Pain after Spinal Cord Injury: Interference with Sleep and Daily Activities." *Archives of Physical Medicine and Rehabilitation* 82 (11): 1571–77.

Widerström-Noga, E. G., and D. C. Turk. 2003. "Types and Effectiveness of Treatments Used by People with Chronic Pain Associated with Spinal Cord Injuries: Influence of Pain and Psychosocial Characteristics." *Spinal Cord* 41 (11): 600–609.

Wilder, Esther Isabelle, and William H. Walters. 2005. *Voices from the Heartland: The Needs and Rights of Individuals with Disabilities.* Brookline, MA: Brookline Books.

Willborn, Steven L. 2000. "The Nonevolution of Enforcement Under the ADA: Discharge Cases and the Hiring Problem." Chapter 4 in *Employment, Disability, and the Americans with Disabilities Act,* edited by Peter David Blanck, pp. 103–17. Evanston: Northwestern University Press.

Williams, Gareth. 1998. "The Sociology of Disability: Towards a Materialist Phenomenology." Chapter 16 in *The Disability Studies Reader,* edited by Tom Shakespeare, pp. 234–44. New York: Cassell.

Williams, Margie. 1997. *Journey to Well: Learning to Live after Spinal Cord Injury.* Newcastle, CA: Altarfire.

Willmuth, Mary E. 1987. "Sexuality after Spinal Cord Injury: A Critical Review." *Clinical Psychology Review* 7 (4): 389–412.

Wilson, Walter C., and Donald D. Thompson. 1983. "The Virginia Community Cadre Network: Community Reintegration of Persons with Spinal Cord Injury." *Rehabilitation Literature* 44 (1–2): 19–23.

Wineman, N. Margaret, Ellen J. Durand, and Richard P. Steiner. 1994. "A Comparative Analysis of Coping Behaviors in Persons with Multiple Sclerosis or a Spinal Cord Injury." *Research in Nursing and Health* 17 (3): 185–94.

Withers, Sallie. 1996. "The Experience of Counselling." Chapter 9 in *Beyond Disability: Towards an Enabling Society,* edited by Gerald Hales, pp. 96–104. Thousand Oaks, CA: Sage.

Woodbury, Byron. 1978. "Psychological Adjustment to Spinal Cord Injury: A Literature Review, 1950–1977." *Rehabilitation Psychology* 25 (3): 119–34.

Woodrich, Frank. 1982. *Demographic and Disability Related Variables which Influence Acceptance of Disability in Spinal Cord Injured Men and Women.* Unpublished doctoral dissertation. Florida State University.

World Health Organization (WHO). 1980. *International Classification of Impairments, Disabilities, and Handicaps.* Geneva: World Health Organization.

World Health Organization (WHO). 2001. *International Classification of Functioning, Disability and Health.* Geneva: World Health Organization.

Wortman, Camille B., and Roxane Cohen Silver. 1992. "Reconsidering Assumptions about Coping with Loss: An Overview of Current Research." Chapter 18 in *Life Crises and Experiences of Loss in Adulthood,* edited by Leo Montada, Sigrun-Heide Filipp, and Melvin J. Lerner, pp. 341–65. Hillsdale, NJ: Lawrence Erlbaum Associates.

Wortman, Camille B., Roxane Cohen Silver, and Ronald C. Kessler. 1993. "The Meaning of Loss and Adjustment to Bereavement." Chapter 23 in *Handbook of Bereavement: Theory, Research, and Intervention,* edited by Margaret S. Stroebe, Wolfgang Stroebe, and Robert O. Hansson, pp. 349–66. New York: Cambridge University Press.

Wright, Beatrice A. 1960. *Physical Disability—A Psychological Approach.* New York: Harper & Brothers.

Wright, Keith C., and E. Davis Martin, Jr. 1987. "Ethical Considerations in Rehabilitation." In *Rehabilitation Counseling and Services,* edited by Gerald L. Gandy, E. Davis Martin, Jr., Richard E. Hardy, and John G. Cull, pp. 331–45. Springfield, IL: Charles C. Thomas.

Wrigley, Michael, and Mark LaGory. 1994. "The Role of Religion and Spirituality in Rehabilitation: A Sociological Perspective." *Journal of Religion in Disability & Rehabilitation* 1 (3): 27–40.

Wu, Sheng K., and Trevor Williams. 2001. "Factors Influencing Sport Participation among Athletes with Spinal Cord Injury." *Medicine and Science in Sports & Exercise* 33 (2): 177–82.

Yarkony, Gary M. 1993. "Aging Skin, Pressure Ulcerations, and Spinal Cord Injury." Chapter 4 in *Aging with Spinal Cord Injury,* edited by Gale G. Whiteneck, Susan W. Charlifue, Kenneth A. Gerhart, Daniel P. Lammertse, Scott Manley, Robert R. Menter, and Kathie R. Seedroff, pp. 39–52. New York: Demos.

Yarkony, Gary M., and Allen W. Heinemann. 1995. "Pressure Ulcers." Chapter 6 in *Spinal Cord Injury: Clinical Outcomes from the Model Systems,* edited by Samuel L. Stover, Joel A. DeLisa, and Gale G. Whiteneck, pp. 100–119. Gaithersburg, MD: Aspen.

Yasuda, Satoko, Paul Wehman, Pamela Targett, David X. Cifu, and Michael West. 2002. "Return to Work after Spinal Cord Injury: A Review of Recent Research." *NeuroRehabilitation* 17 (3): 177–86.

Yezierski, Robert P., and Kim J. Burchiel, editors. 2002. *Spinal Cord Injury Pain: Assessment, Mechanisms, Management.* Seattle: IASP Press.

Yoshida, Karen Kume. 1991. *Life Reconstruction among Individuals with Spinal Cord Injuries: A Sociological Analysis.* Unpublished doctoral dissertation. University of Toronto.

Yoshida, Karen Kume. 1994a. "Employment among Persons with Spinal Cord Injury: Work Trajectories, Resources and Barriers." *Research in Sociology of Health Care* 11: 151–71.

Yoshida, Karen K. 1994b. "Intimate and Marital Relationships: An Insider's Perspective." *Sexuality and Disability* 12 (3): 179–89.

Young, Mary Ellen, Wayne G. Alfred, Diana H. Rintala, Karen A. Hart, and Marcus J. Fuhrer. 1994. "Vocational Status of Persons with Spinal Cord Injury Living in the Community." *Rehabilitation Counseling Bulletin* 37 (3): 229–43.

Yuker, Harold E., editor. 1988. *Attitudes towards Persons with Disabilities.* New York: Springer.

Zasler, Nathan D. 1991. "Sexuality and Neurologic Disability: An Overview." *Sexuality and Disability* 9 (1): 11–27.

Ziolko, Mary Ellen. 1993. "Counseling Parents of Children with Disabilities: A Review of the Literature and Implications for Practice." In *Perspectives on Disability,* 2nd Edition, edited by Mark Nagler, pp. 185–93. Palo Alto, CA: Health Markets Research.

Zirpolo, Nicholas John. 1986. *Coping with Catastrophe: Dynamics of Adjustment to Spinal Cord Injury.* Unpublished doctoral dissertation. Stanford University.

Zola, Irving Kenneth. 1982a. *Missing Pieces: A Chronicle of Living with a Disability.* Philadelphia: Temple University Press.

Zola, Irving Kenneth. 1982b. "Denial of Emotional Needs to People with Handicaps." *Archives of Physical Medicine and Rehabilitation* 63 (2): 63–67.

Zola, Irving Kenneth. 1987. "Neither Defiant nor Cheering." *Disability Rag* (September/October): 16–18.

Zola, Irving Kenneth. 1993. "Self, Identity and the Naming Question: Reflections on the Language of Disability." In *Perspectives on Disability,* 2nd Edition, edited by Mark Nagler, pp. 15–23. Palo Alto, CA: Health Markets Research.

Zwerling, Craig, Nancy L. Sprince, Charles S. Davis, Robert B. Wallace, Paul S. Whitten, and Steven G. Heeringa. 2000. "Occupational Injuries among Workers with Disabilities." Chapter 12 in *Employment, Disability, and the Americans with Disabilities Act,* edited by Peter David Blanck, pp. 315–28. Evanston: Northwestern University Press.

Zwerner, Janna. 1982. "Yes We Have Troubles but Nobody's Listening: Sexual Issues of Women with Spinal Cord Injury." *Sexuality and Disability* 5 (3): 158–71.

# Appendix

## Study Participants

| Name | Sex | Age | Race/ethnicity | Religion | Marital status | Education |
|------|-----|-----|----------------|----------|----------------|-----------|
| Adam | m | 26 | white | None | single | some college |
| Al | m | 28 | white | Baptist | single | some college |
| Andrew | m | 36 | Latino | Baptist | divorced | associate's degree |
| Ben | m | 46 | white | Catholic | divorced | some college |
| Brad | m | 32 | white | Christian (nondenom.) | single | bachelor's degree |
| Chris | m | 48 | white | Baptist | married | high school |
| Cody | m | 42 | African American | Baptist | divorced | some college |
| Derrick | m | 39 | white | Baptist | divorced | high school |
| Doug | m | 38 | white | Christian/unspecified | married | associate's degree |
| Edward | m | 37 | white | None | single | some college |
| Fred | m | 39 | Native American | Christian (nondenom.) | single | less than high school |
| Harry | m | 33 | white | Christian (nondenom.) | divorced | some college |
| Jay | m | 37 | white | Catholic | single | some post-graduate |
| Jennifer | f | 21 | white | Baptist | engaged | some college |
| Jeremy | m | 46 | African American | Church of God & Christ | divorced | bachelor's degree |
| Jonathan | m | 49 | white | Methodist | married | some post-graduate |
| Kevin | m | 33 | white | Baptist | single | bachelor's degree |
| Leonard | m | 39 | white | Christian (nondenom.) | married | some college |
| Meghan | f | 42 | African American | None | divorced | graduate degree |
| Nathan | m | 49 | white | Assembly of God | single | bachelor's degree |
| Paul | m | 23 | white | None | single | some college |
| Roger | m | 43 | white | Catholic | married | some college |
| Rosa | f | 52 | white | Baptist | divorced | some college |
| Ryan | m | 20 | white | Baptist | single | some college |
| Shannon | f | 43 | white | Baptist | married | high school |
| Stacy | f | 20 | white | Baptist | single | some college |
| Stan | m | 50 | white | Methodist | single | graduate degree |
| Todd | m | 34 | white | Presbyterian | single | bachelor's degree |
| Tonya | f | 38 | white | Baptist | divorced | some college |
| Travis | m | 29 | Native American | Christian (nondenom.) | single | some college |
| Vibha | f | 33 | Asian | Catholic | single | bachelor's degree |
| Walter | m | 31 | white | Baptist | single | high school |

| Occupation[1] | Living arrangements | Age at injury | Level of injury | Complete/ incomplete[2] |
|---|---|---|---|---|
| student | brother | 20 | C-5 | complete |
| student | alone | 20 | C-4, C-5 | complete |
| computer analyst | alone | 20 | C-5, C-6 | incomplete |
| student | alone | 38 | C-5, T-10 | incomplete |
| PC technician | parents | 18 | C-5, C-6 | incomplete |
| not working | wife | 33 | C-6, C-7 | complete |
| programmer | children | 28 | T-2 | complete |
| unemployed | mother and stepfather | 35 | C-5, C-6 | incomplete |
| draftsman | wife | 23 | T-1, T-2 | complete |
| programmer | alone | 28 | C-7 | incomplete |
| not working | aunt and cousin | 34 | C-7, C-8 | incomplete |
| student | alone | 15 | C-5, C-6 | incomplete |
| programmer | alone | 1 | Unknown[3] | incomplete |
| student | fiancé and caregiver | 14 | C-6, C-7 | incomplete |
| math tutor | child | 27 | C-6 | incomplete |
| stock broker | wife and child | 7 | C-6, C-7, T-1, T-2 | complete |
| not working | parents | 18 | C-4, C-5 | complete |
| business owner | wife and children | 23 | C-5, C-6 | incomplete |
| unemployed | alone | 21 | C-5, C-6 | incomplete |
| prod. mgmt. specialist | brother | 27 | T-8 | complete |
| student | alone | 15 | C-5, C-6 | incomplete |
| construction estimator | wife and children | 40 | T-10 | complete |
| unemployed | single | 36 | T-12 | complete |
| student | alone | 7 | T-12 | incomplete |
| staff specialist | husband | 29 | T-10 | incomplete |
| student | alone | 15 | L-1 | complete |
| director, social services | alone | 17 | C-3, C-4, C-5, C-6 | incomplete |
| business services | alone | 22 | C-5, C-6 | complete |
| not working | children | 30 | L-1 | incomplete |
| student | girlfriend | 14 | T-4 | complete |
| student | alone | 0 | L-4 | incomplete |
| not working | girlfriend and child | 24 | T-6, T-7 | incomplete |

[1] "Unemployed" designates those who were actively seeking employment, as opposed to those "not working" and not seeking employment.

[2] Complete injury denotes no motor function and no sensation below the level of the injury. With incomplete injury, there is at least partial preservation of motor or sensory functioning below the level of the injury (Stover 1996).

[3] Respondent has paraplegia.

# Index

Page numbers in italic indicate figures, those in bold indicate tables.
Endnotes are indicated by a note number after the page, such as 282n5.